AT HOME
WITH AUTISM

DESIGNING HOUSING FOR THE SPECTRUM

KIM STEELE   SHERRY AHRENTZEN

First published in Great Britain in 2016 by

Policy Press
University of Bristol
1-9 Old Park Hill
Bristol
BS2 8BB
UK
t: +44 (0)117 954 5940
pp-info@bristol.ac.uk
www.policypress.co.uk

North America office:
Policy Press
c/o The University of Chicago Press
1427 East 60th Street
Chicago, IL 60637, USA
t: +1 773 702 7700
f: +1 773 702 9756
sales@press.uchicago.edu
www.press.uchicago.edu

British Library Cataloguing in Publication Data
A catalogue record for this book is available from the British Library

Library of Congress Cataloging-in-Publication Data
A catalog record for this book has been requested

ISBN 978 1 44730 797 6 hardcover

Cover design by Policy Press
Front cover image: Getty
Printed and bound in Great Britain by CPI Group (UK) Ltd, Croydon, CR0 4YY
Policy Press uses environmentally responsible print partners

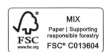

For my wonderful daughters,

Cecily and Zora

KS

To my ever-supportive siblings,

Shelly and Bill

SA

CONTENTS

Figures and tables   v
Abbreviations   x
Terminology   xi
About the authors   xiii
Acknowledgments   xiv

one   **Introduction**   **1**
     Why this book now?   1
     Numbers and names   5
     Adults on the spectrum and in the community   9
     Residential alternatives – or lack of   12
     Costs and competition of care and support services   22
     Advocacy and choice   25

two   **A research-informed approach for housing design**   **29**
     EBP in autism intervention   30
     EBP in environmental design: evidence-based design   31
     Our approach in this book   34
     Search protocol   37
     Assessing source information   38
     Documenting source information   39

three   **Quality of life design goals**   **41**
     Ensure safety and security   43
     Maximize familiarity, stability, predictability and clarity   47
     Enhance sensory balance   50

Offer multiple opportunities for controlling social interaction and privacy 54
Provide adequate choice and independence 61
Foster health and wellness 63
Enhance one's dignity 68
Ensure durability 71
Achieve affordability 72
Ensure accessibility and support in the surrounding neighborhood 76

four   Design guidelines   81
Neighborhood design guidelines 83
Overall home 91
Outdoor space 96
Floorplan strategies 102
Entry 109
Living room 111
Dining areas 114
Kitchen 115
Hallways, stairs, ramps & doorways 121
Bedrooms 124
Bathrooms 128
Multi-sensory environments 134
Laundry rooms 136
Storage 140
Support provider office 142
Ventilation 144
Heating and cooling 146
Lighting 148
Appliances 152
Acoustics 155
Technology 158
Materials 164

five   On the horizon   171
Introduction 171
New visions of housing types and models 172
Smart technologies for independent living 189
New directions in self-advocacy for housing choice 193

References 199
Appendix: Research and information sources used in developing goals and guidelines 247
Chapter Four image sources 257
Index 261

FIGURES AND TABLES

Figures

1.1	Health and medical conditions often associated with autism	8
1.2	Preferred residential type and arrangements: Response comparison between individuals with autism and caregivers	20
1.3	Example of en-suites in two-bedroom apartment at The Continuum, University of Florida	23
2.1	Three components shaping evidence-based practice (EBP) in medical/health practice	30
4.1	Neighborhood shops accessible by bike or walking	84
4.2	Local public transportation	84
4.3	Established neighborhood with welcoming entry areas: Milagros Independent Living, San Jose, CA	85
4.4	Example of new construction blending in with older homes	85
4.5	Pedestrian friendly neighborhood that minimizes vehicular interaction	86
4.6	Park supporting a variety of activities	87
4.7	Neighborhood street with central green space	87
4.8	District map providing visual cues to aid wayfinding	88
4.9	Dedicated two-way bike lane	88
4.10	Neighbors socializing	89
4.11	Layering of public to private spaces	89
4.12	Backyard deck areas separated by partial walls allow residents to interact or maintain privacy	90
4.13	Social gathering at neighborhood community garden	90
4.14	Involve residents in choosing their home	91
4.15	Create space for pets	91
4.16	Allow residents to choose whether or not to have roommates	92
4.17	Activity area within residential community; Sweetwater Spectrum, Sonoma, CA	92

4.18   Natural light filled living space with seating options   93
4.19   Low-rise townhomes and apartments within established neighborhood   94
4.20   Large window overlooking plant filled courtyard   95
4.21   Large windows and doors allowing views to landscape   95
4.22   Outdoor space with a variety of features allow for exploration; Sweetwater Spectrum, Sonoma, CA   96
4.23   Opportunity for gardening   97
4.24   Raised planters create interest and spaces for residents to garden   97
4.25   Water features provide soothing sounds   98
4.26   A mix of materials provides visual and tactile interest in an outdoor space   98
4.27   Protected courtyard viewed from inside home   99
4.28   Grouped swings offer opportunities to socialize and enjoy vestibular input   99
4.29   Front porch with rocking chairs allows residents to greet neighbors   100
4.30   Outdoor seating, paths and varied plantings provide opportunities for different experiences   100
4.31   Artistic fence that allows views out to surrounding neighborhood   101
4.32   Large living area with multiple seating areas and visual access to adjoining rooms   102
4.33   Computer nook clearly delineated from eating area by sliding glass doors   102
4.34   A window seat creates a spot for reading within the larger living area   103
4.35   Open, clutter-free living area with natural light   103
4.36   Barrier-free entry   104
4.37   Wide hallways to accommodate resident motor activity   104
4.38   Floorplan demonstrating multiple circulation options   105
4.39   Interior glass doors provide visual access to adjacent rooms   105
4.40   Activity rooms provide opportunities for socializing with friends at home   106
4.41   Wall decals add visual interest and are easily changed   107
4.42   Swing with fiber optic light strings in a sensory room   108
4.43   Clearly defined entry area with seating and storage   109
4.44   A covered entryway and a place to sit provides a calm transition space   110
4.45   Sightlines from the front entry through the apartment   110
4.46   Window seats create opportunities for people to participate from the periphery   112
4.47   Periphery seating allows individuals to feel secure and part of the action   112
4.48   Outdoor space is visually integrated into adjacent rooms   113
4.49   Variety of eating areas: breakfast nook, kitchen bar and dining room   114
4.50   Kitchen with multiple work areas to accommodate several people   115
4.51   Solid wood cabinets with non-toxic finishes are a healthy and durable choice   116
4.52   A pantry provides extra storage and good visual access   116
4.53   Different height work areas allow residents to sit or stand   117
4.54   Pull-out cabinets and drawers with inserts provided are accessible and easy to organize   117
4.55   Corner cabinets with rotating shelves increase accessibility   118
4.56   Wall-mounted oven is separate from stovetop   118
4.57   Utilize natural and mechanical ventilation   119
4.58   A visually interesting and durable backsplash adds texture without being too busy   119
4.59   Engineered quartz (such as Caesarstone) countertops are a durable choice   120
4.60   Although concrete requires some maintenance, it also is a good countertop choice   120

4.61	Wide hallways provide good visibility and accommodate resident activity	121
4.62	Seating in hallway provides a transition space and opportunity for socializing	122
4.63	Seating area at top of stairs	122
4.64	Wide hallways allow for jumping and pacing	123
4.65	Design should be flexible to accommodate couples	124
4.66	Personalized bedroom with desk space	124
4.67	Closet with built in organization system	125
4.68	Open shelving with organizing bins	125
4.69	Large bedroom window with views to landscape	126
4.70	Unobtrusive, quiet ceiling fan for the bedroom	126
4.71	Wall of built-in shelves	127
4.72	Inviting, non-institutional style bathroom	128
4.73	Accessible bathroom with roll-in shower and wall-hung sink	128
4.74	Communal bathroom or powder room for visitors	129
4.75	Hand-held showerhead	130
4.76	Spacious shower with built-in seat	130
4.77	Spacious bathroom with room for support provider if needed	131
4.78	Handrail in the shower	131
4.79	Concealed cistern toilet with push panel flush	132
4.80	Sink with concealed pipework	133
4.81	Sensory room with lighting, cushions and wall projections	134
4.82	Reclining chair and fiber optic lighting in sensory room	134
4.83	Snoezelen Room	135
4.84	Spacious laundry room able to accommodate resident and support provider if needed	136
4.85	Spacious laundry room with door to exterior	137
4.86	Laundry sink	137
4.87	Laundry room with folding area and ample storage	138
4.88	Textured, vitreous porcelain tile is a durable, non-slip flooring option	139
4.89	Laundry room with a fold-down ironing board	139
4.90	Bench seat with integrated storage	140
4.91	Visually accessible storage	141
4.92	Mudroom with storage doubles as transition space	141
4.93	Dedicated office with adequate workspace	142
4.94	A comfortable space for support providers to take breaks and do paperwork is essential	142
4.95	Operable windows for good ventilation	144
4.96	Adjustable, integrated window blinds	145
4.97	Mobile sun shades provide passive heating and cooling	146
4.98	Programmable thermostat	147
4.99	Solar panels	147
4.100	Clerestory windows provide indirect, natural light	148
4.101	LED bulb	148
4.102	Reduced glare under cabinet lighting	149
4.103	Adjustable task lighting	150

4.104   Durable pendant lamps   150
4.105   Accessible height light switches   151
4.106   Induction cooktop with cookware   152
4.107   On-demand hot water circulation system   153
4.108   Side-swing door oven   153
4.109   Wall-hung sink for accessibility   154
4.110   Rockwool cubes   155
4.111   Thicker walls are incorporated into sensitive areas such as bedrooms and laundry area   156
4.112   Wood flooring and other natural materials help absorb noise   157
4.113   Smoke and carbon monoxide alarm with visual and spoken notification   158
4.114   Keyless smart lock with lever-style handle for accessibility   159
4.115   Entry system with telephone and camera for previewing   160
4.116   Video doorbell with speaker and microphone   160
4.117   Telecare telephone prompt service   161
4.118   RFID sensor tag   161
4.119   Home monitoring system   162
4.120   Simon, the humanoid robot   163
4.121   Comfortable, personalized furnishings   164
4.122   Laminated glass stays in place when broken   165
4.123   Zero VOC paint   165
4.124   Low toxicity material samples   166
4.125   Non-toxic, water-based sealant available in different grades and applications   166
4.126   Marmoleum wainscoting   167
4.127   Untreated European Ash on left and thermally modified European Ash on right   168
4.128   Honeycomb blinds control light and are energy efficient   168
4.129   Hardwood flooring   169
4.130   Interface floor tiles   169
4.131   Homey, non-toxic environment in which to entertain friends   170
4.132   External shutters   170
5.1   First floor of TCFD Model Duplex for residents with ASC   176
5.2   Willakenzie Crossing in Eugene, OR, with community center at left   178
5.3   Entry vestibules and common courtyard area of 29 Palms, Phoenix, AZ   179
5.4   Hammock in quiet courtyard area, Sweetwater Spectrum, Sonoma, CA   181
5.5   Site plan of Sweetwater Spectrum, Sonoma, CA   182
5.6   Street front of Airmount Woods, Ramsey, NJ   183
5.7   Accessible kitchen, Airmount Woods   183
5.8   Cambridge Cohousing, Cambridge, MA   186
5.9   Gathering space in common housing with entry to dining room at right, Cambridge Cohousing 187
5.10   Visually-oriented cards for eliciting participation in housing preference, developed and used by   195
        Helen Hamlyn Centre for Design

Tables

1.1	Various residential building types and living arrangements	13
1.2	Post-1999 surveys of types of residences and living arrangements of adults with ASC	14
3.1	Sensory sensitivities often occurring with autism	52
5.1	Seven housing settings and affiliated models	173

ABBREVIATIONS

ASAN   Autistic Self Advocacy Network
ASC   autism spectrum condition
ASD   autism spectrum disorder
CMS   Centers for Medicare and Medicaid Services (a US federal agency)
DSM   Diagnostic and Statistical Manual of Mental Disorders
EB   evidence-based
EBD   evidence-based design
EBP   evidence-based practice
HCBS   Home-Based and Community Services (of CMS)
HVAC   heating, ventilation and air-conditioning
LEED   Leadership in Energy and Environmental Design (of USGBC)
MIT   Massachusetts Institute of Technology
NT   neurotypical
SSI   Social Security Income
USGBC   United States Green Building Council
WHO   World Health Organization

TERMINOLOGY

AUTISM

In this book, we use both identity-first and person-first terminology. This includes, for example:

Identity-first terms   Autistic individuals
Spectrum adults
Self-advocate

Person-first terms   Individuals with autism
Individuals on the spectrum
Adults with ASC (Autism Spectrum Condition)
Adults with ASD (Autism Spectrum Disorder)
We use the term *ASD* when particular organizations or researchers use this term in referring to specific diagnostic classifications, such as the American Psychiatric Association in DSM-5. Otherwise, we use *ASC*.

INTELLECTUAL DISABILITY   We use the term "intellectual disability" (ID) instead of the now-disbanded term "mental retardation." This condition encompasses significant limitations both in intellectual functioning (e.g. reasoning, problem solving) and in adaptive behavior, of a range of everyday social and practical skills. This condition originates before the age of eighteen (aaidd.org/intellectual-disability/definition). Also see Schalock and colleagues (2007) for history of this shift in terminology.

DEVELOPMENTAL DISABILITIES   "Developmental disabilities" is an umbrella term that includes intellectual disability (see above) and other disabilities apparent during childhood. They are chronic disabilities that can be cognitive or physical or both, and that appear before the age of 22 and are likely to be lifelong. Cerebral palsy or epilepsy are examples of developmental disabilities that are largely physical conditions (see aaidd.org).

NEURO—

Neurological   Pertaining to the body nervous system

Neurodevelopmental   Pertaining to impairments of the growth and development of the brain or central nervous system, disorders including those disorders of brain function that affect emotion, learning ability and memory and that unfold as the individual grows. Examples include: autism or ASC; fetal alcohol spectrum disorders; Down syndrome; attention deficit hyperactivity disorder

Neurocognitive disorders   Those affecting cognitive functioning such as dementia, delirium, amnestic disorders

Neurotypical (or NT)   A term initially coined in the autism community to refer to people not on the autism spectrum. It is sometimes used for anyone who does not have any atypical neurodevelopmental condition (Sinclair, 1998). In the United Kingdom, the National Autistic Society recommends the use of this term in its advice to journalists.

ABOUT THE AUTHORS

Kim Steele is Director of Urban and Health Initiatives at The Elemental Group where she works with individuals, communities and organizations to develop strategies and policies that advance equitable, healthy, accessible and livable communities. Her research has been widely disseminated at national and international conferences and in numerous published reports. As an associate professor at Auburn University and Arizona State University, she taught participatory design studios where students worked with community members, including those with autism and other disabilities, in crafting award winning design solutions. Currently, she is advancing this work in her doctoral research at UCLA. She is a mother of a daughter with autism.

Sherry Ahrentzen, PhD, is Shimberg Professor of Housing Studies at the University of Florida. She is a recognized leader in advancing social justice dimensions within the built environment and design education. Her research on housing and community design that fosters the physical, social and economic health of households has been published extensively, and presented at national and international conferences. In 2003 she received the Distinguished Professor Award from the Association of Collegiate Schools of Architecture; in 2009, the Career Award from the Environmental Design Research Association; and in 2014, the ARCC James Haecker Award for Distinguished Leadership in Architectural Research.

ACKNOWLEDGMENTS

At Home with Autism evolved out of research initially sponsored by the Urban Land Institute Arizona and Pivotal Foundation with support from Southwest Autism Research & Resource Center and Denise Resnik. Along the way there have been numerous people and organizations that have generously offered insight to help guide our endeavor. Thank you to the following individuals and organizations for their contributions and support: Tom Toronto of Bergen County's United Way; Jay Klein of Arizona State University; the people at the Center for Discovery in Harris, New York, especially Terry Hamlin and Peter Dollard; Marsha Maytum of Leddy Maytum Stacey Architects; Paul Harris and Teresa Brice of LISC Phoenix; Ricardo Lopez; Linda Messbauer; Jonathan Fogelson and Jason Bregman of Michael Singer Studio; Deirdre Sheerin of Sweetwater Spectrum; Julia Robinson of University of Minnesota. Angela Sinclair created the wonderful ten icons for our earlier report (Ahrentzen and Steele, 2009) which are reproduced here, courtesy of Arizona Board of Regents for and on behalf of Arizona State University. The assistance of Ryan Brotman, Lisa Dwyer, and James Erickson on that earlier report also helped lay the foundation for this book. We would also like to thank the owners, property managers, and housing developers, who allowed us to tour their developments, ask questions and speak with staff and residents. These include the following: Casa de Amma; Chapel Haven West; Community Housing for Adult Independence, Jewish Family and Children's Services; Community Living Options; Hello Housing; Housing Consortium of the East Bay; Imagine!; Laguna Senior Apartments; Marc Center of Mesa; Mid-Peninsula Housing; Mission Creek Senior Housing; Step Up on Second & Step Up on Fifth; Stoney Pine Villa.

ONE

INTRODUCTION

Why this book now?

Public attention on autism has soared in the last decade. In plays, movies and on television, characters with autism or autistic traits are expressively portrayed. For example, in 2009, three very popular movies – a romantic comedy, a biopic of an accomplished animal science professor, and an animated film of pen pals – all revolved around a character with Asperger's syndrome. Between 1997 and 2011 the number of books and articles annually published about autism increased more than sixfold (Solomon, 2012). For several years celebrity comedian Jon Stewart has headed a star-studded telethon – "Night of Too Many Stars" – to support the U.S.-based organization, Autism Speaks. Founded in 2005 by grandparents of a child with autism, Autism Speaks has become in less than ten years the leading private autism research advocacy organization in the world, with over $58 million from funding sources in 2012 alone (Autism Speaks, 2013). Not since the height of the AIDS crisis has there been such an aggressive campaign for funding and research, much of this spurred by parent-affiliated organizations (Solomon, 2012). One parent group, Cure Autism Now, pushed the U.S. Congress to pass the 2006 Combating Autism Act, providing a billion dollars of spending over five years for research on autism and related disorders over five years. In 2011, a three-year extension of over $600 million was ratified for further research. In 2012 the largest single grant for autism in the world ($37.8 million), and the largest for the study of any mental health condition in Europe, established European Autism Interventions – A Multicentre Study for Developing New Medications

(EU-AIMS), a multi-national, multi-industry initiative to discover and develop drugs for autism. In September 2013, the World Health Organization (WHO) convened its first conference on autism, the initial step in enacting the recently passed World Health Assembly resolution on autism.

Within this tempest of media attention and funding mechanisms are the lives, aspirations and frustrations of millions of individuals with autism, young and old, in homes, schools, and communities: an estimated 2 million Americans, over 3 million Europeans, and millions more worldwide. The numbers and increasing prevalence rates have spurred legislation, research and initiatives for not only discovering the cause of autism, but also how to treat, educate, and support individuals as they go about their daily lives.

Most of the research and interventions have focused on children and adolescents. Only recently has there been growing concern of how best to plan for individuals once they age out of the school system: working and earning money; meeting and socializing with friends; exercising and recreating; setting up a home and living in the community – and doing so with dignity and self-fulfillment.

With this growing attention on ways to support adults with autism spectrum disorder (ASD) – or autism spectrum condition (ASC) as it is increasingly referred to in Europe, see Terminology (p viii) – are questions concerning the types of places in which it is best to live. What is needed for those who wish to or must live outside their parents' homes? Is it best to live in urban neighborhoods with the mix of people, services, amenities, and intensity that cities bring – or on rural farmsteads and gated communities set up specifically for individuals on the spectrum? Are there advantages to living with roommates; and if so, how many, and with or not with others on the spectrum as well? What home layouts work best for these arrangements? Do individuals want to live in residential developments intentionally developed for people with disabilities; or do they want to live in housing that is marketed to everyone? Are there home technologies that can enhance security and independence without invading one's privacy? How appropriate is the present housing stock for those who may have sensory or chemical sensitivities, or who may have support providers come to the home on a daily – even a live-in – basis? When living in apartment or condominium complexes, what design features allow autistic residents to feel comfortable in public spaces, such as lobbies or corridors, when they come across neighbors or visitors? What are the best residential layouts, room sizes and configurations, lighting, colors, appliances, and other home features for those who may be sensitive to appliance noises, or who have never cooked and cleaned before, or who may need ample personal space to feel comfortable? How can individuals choose those places that are best for them when the options are so few and often unknown?

Questions like these led us in 2007 to begin researching what might work best and for whom. While there have been a few reports describing ways for advancing the design and development of housing for adults on the spectrum (including ours in 2009), this is the first published book on the topic. If autism has been around – or at least, medically identified – since the 1940s, why is it only now that we are writing about promising ways to create homes and communities that enhance residential living for adults on the spectrum?

The first of the reasons for "why this book now?" are the numbers. While the increase of many neurodevelopmental conditions among children has been mitigated in recent years, autism has been on the rise from a rate of 1 in 150 U.S. children reported in 2000 (the first year of systematic national surveillance by the Autism and Development Disabilities Monitoring network), to 1 in 68 in 2010 (Baio, 2014). Similar trends follow in other countries as well, as we will see later in this chapter.

Second, adults on the spectrum are more visible in communities today. This is partly the result of increasing numbers and public awareness, but also from legislation and advocacy efforts that mandate residential choice and de-emphasize institutionalized living. Yet this increased visibility does not mean that we know much about who they are, what they need, or how they want to live.

The movement towards community living, however, is impeded by what is available – or more likely, unavailable – in communities. The global recession and housing crisis of the last decade affected nearly all segments of the population in developed countries around the world. But it particularly compounded the challenges already existing for adults with disabilities to find affordable, accessible and appropriate housing – and homes that met one's aspirations as well. Understanding what type of housing would work best for individuals not typically addressed by conventional housing types is a third reason for this book appearing now: it remains a mystery for many potential residents as well as interested developers and architects who are contemplating designing, constructing, renovating or moving into residences in community settings.

The fourth reason for this book's timeliness is the escalating cost of care of individuals with health impairments – functional, physical, sensory, psychological, and neurological – and the limited means of governments and households to cover such care. In response, innovations are being pursued to support such care through housing designs and household technologies, with anticipated cost reductions in the long run.

The final reason is the parents, organizations, service providers, developers and individuals on the spectrum who recognize the impending demand for such housing. These individuals are asking, "What will happen to my child – and the millions of other adults like him or her – when I pass away or can no longer provide the care needed?" There are those spectrum individuals who plan to leave their parents' homes and move to residences and communities which, to date, have never been designed or constructed with their needs and aspirations in mind. For them, housing is not simply an accommodation but a springboard to enhance their quality of life.

This book, *At home with autism: Designing housing for the spectrum*, introduces housing providers, architects, developers, planners, service providers, public officials, and importantly, individuals with autism and their families and communities, to conditions and aspirations of adults on the spectrum who demand a new approach to how we provide, design and develop homes in which they live. There is no singular residential model, just as there is no singular prototype of autism. Based on research, interviews and site visits throughout North America and Europe, this book identifies resident-based quality of life goals, and profiles design guidelines directed to those goals, with examples from a range of residential settings. Our intent is to provide a robust platform that architects, housing providers, families and residents can use to identify, design, retrofit or construct homes that best respond to specific needs and aspirations of the residents. The content and organizational structure of the book also lends itself to those housing providers developing residences for adults with other neurodevelopmental conditions.

This initial chapter introduces the reader to the five key issues that drive this impetus for housing for individuals on the spectrum; as well as different approaches of how to understand and create homes and places in which to live a fulfilling life. Chapter Two describes our research-informed approach that underlies the shaping of the design goals and design guidelines in the rest of the book.

Ten quality of life goals that can direct design efforts are described in detail in Chapter Three, with an explanation of the icon system we developed for enabling readers to consider and select their own combination of goals and guidelines that work best for them. The most extensive section of this book is the design guidelines that form the heart of Chapter Four. A look at what is on the horizon is profiled in Chapter Five. Detailed matrices in the Appendix identify and profile the sources of our quality of life goals and design guidelines.

The well-worn adage, "if you know one person with autism, you know one person with autism," affirms that there is no single prototype of housing that works best for the vast spectrum of autistic adults. The optimal approach would be to have a range of residential options available within communities and to work with individuals to discover which best suits them. But while today there are more residential options than there were 20 years ago, and while there are fledgling efforts to evaluate their effectiveness and appropriateness, progress towards increasing the number, diversity and availability of residential options is glacial. This book, we hope, contributes to an avalanche of interest, research, design and development of residential settings for adults with ASC and other neurodevelopmental conditions. Given the growing numbers of adults on the spectrum – and the aging of their parents in whose homes most of them presently reside – architects, housing providers, policymakers and developers are being called upon as never before to plan, design, retrofit and develop homes and residential developments that best fit the needs and aspirations of these individuals. We are still on the path to determining how best to characterize what is currently available; to evaluate the strengths, shortcomings and appropriateness of these models; and also – importantly – to imagine what can be aspired, designed and constructed. We envision this book as a useful and engaging guide along that journey.

Numbers and names

Numbers associated with autism prevalence regularly make news headlines. The latest surveillance monitoring undertaken by the U.S.'s Centers for Disease Control and Prevention (Baio, 2014) claims prevalence of autism at an estimated 1 in 68 children aged 8, translating into over 2 million Americans. Age-specific prevalence rates for "classical autism" in the European Union (EU) vary between 3.3 and 16.0 per 10,000, with indications that these rates could reach between 30 and 63 per 10,000 once the full range of autism spectrum (that is, autism, Asperger's syndrome, childhood disintegrative disorder, and pervasive development disorder – not otherwise specified) are included (European Commission, 2013). The global prevalence ratio is estimated to be 1:160 (Elasbbagh et al, 2012).

Autism occurs in all racial, ethnic and socioeconomic groups, and is five times more common among boys than among girls. Historically thought to be rare, autism spectrum conditions are now second only to intellectual disabilities as the most common, severe developmental disability, as legally defined in the United States (Newshaffer et al, 2007). Over the last 12 years, the prevalence of all developmental disabilities has increased 17 percent in the U.S. with the prevalence of autism alone increasing 290 percent (National Center on Birth Defects and Developmental Disabilities, 2012).

Few prevalence studies exist outside the U.S. and Europe, but this is changing of late (Hughes, 2011). A prevalence study in Brazil found 27.2 cases of autism per 10,000 people; a study in Oman found 1.4. In the first comprehensive study of autism prevalence using a total population sample, an international team of investigators from the U.S., South Korea, and Canada estimated the prevalence of ASD in South Korea to be 2.64 percent, or approximately 1 in 38 children, suggesting that autism prevalence estimates worldwide could actually be higher if this particular surveillance methodology is used (Kim et al, 2011).

The World Health Organization estimates a global median prevalence of 62/10,000, which translates to one child in 160 with ASD, recognizing variability across countries. The differences in surveillance approaches among the various countries (and across years in a single country) further confuse the issue of how prevalent autism is in the global population. Even in those countries with well-established surveillance methodologies, counts of prevalence are confusing. In the U.S., for example, some of the highest autism prevalence are in states with the best autism health and support services such as Arizona (15.7 cases per 1,000 children aged 8) and New Jersey (21.9); compared with states with fewer services, such as Alabama (5.7) (Baio, 2014). Do the higher numbers in New Jersey reflect better informed, more extensive surveillance practices among healthcare professionals, and not necessarily more children on the spectrum? Or do parents avoid living in states such as Alabama when they discover services there may be sorely inadequate for the decades of support services their children will need?

Disentangling the many potential reasons for prevalence increases has been challenging: some of it is likely the result of a change in study methods and reporting standards; some can be attributed to changes in diagnostic and classification criteria;

some a result of increased awareness of ASC; and some a reflection of increasing risk factors (Rice et al, 2010).

Yet, ironically, even with this remarkable rise in prevalence we really do not know what autism is. There is no standard biological marker. We do know that autism is a syndrome rather than an illness because it is a collection of behaviors rather than a known and established biological entity. The syndrome, however, encompasses a highly variable group of symptoms and behaviors rooted in a disruption of social function. But to date researchers do not know why it occurs, what exactly triggers it, or what areas of the brain are affected. With such ambiguity, it is no wonder that we see so many different ways that people and professionals define, diagnose, socially construct, legislate, value and even label autism and individuals on the spectrum. Naming itself not only influences how and what we count (and how we value or treat those whom we count), but also establishes how behavioral symptoms – and those individuals manifesting them – are researched and treated. Research in neuroscience, gastroenterology, environmental science, immunology, epigenetics, systems biology, gut microbiology, nutrigenomics, metabolomics, psychiatry, developmental psychology, and education capitalize on funding streams for numerous neurobiological and neurodevelopmental disorders – as well as special streams for autism. In the U.K., Autism Act 2009 committed the government to developing an adult autism strategy to transform services for adults with autism, including for those living independently in the community. Naming and labeling "autism" has both regulatory and financial consequences.

The *diagnostic* definition of autism is repeatedly changing – frustrating some, encouraging others, mystifying many. The two major international classifications that provide criteria for diagnosis are the *Diagnostic and Statistical Manual of Mental Disorders* of the American Psychiatric Association (2013) and the World Health Organization's *International Classification of Diseases* (www.who.int/classifications/icd/en/), with the former being used most often for clinical diagnoses (Posada et al, 2007). Prior to the most current version of the *Diagnostic and Statistical Manual of Mental Disorders* (referred to as DSM-5) issued in May 2013, autism spectrum disorder (ASD) encompassed four separate disorders: autistic disorder, Asperger's disorder, childhood disintegrative disorder, pervasive developmental disorder not otherwise specified. The most current diagnosis in DSM-5 now uses a single umbrella to define ASD with symptoms falling along a continuum, some manifestations of symptoms being rather mild, others severe. To be classified with ASD, symptoms must appear in early childhood and the symptoms must impair the individual's ability to function in daily life. Usually diagnosis occurs when a child is under five years of age, with some diagnoses occurring much earlier – at six or eighteen months, for example. Diagnosis is based on careful observation, extensive interviews with parents, and medical and personal histories.

The two core criteria for diagnosis in DSM-5 are (1) communication and social deficits, and (2) fixed or repetitive behaviors. All individuals diagnosed with ASD have difficulties in reciprocating social or emotional interaction; severe problems in maintaining relationships; and non-verbal communication problems. Repetitive and restrictive behaviors are expressed in at least two of the following: extreme attachment to routines and patterns and resistance to changes in routines; repetitive speech or movements; intense and restricted interests; and difficulty integrating sensory information, or strong seeking or avoidance of sensory stimuli.

These clinical definitions are expressed when a person is unable to talk or talk much; flaps arms or engages in other self-stimulating behaviors; makes no or minimal eye contact; shows little interest in friendships; does not engage in spontaneous or imaginative play; demonstrates no or little empathy or emotional reciprocity; can be fairly rigid and with highly focused interests; may talk to others at great length and with extensive details about objects of a particular fascination, such as grasshoppers, fans or lampposts; or form attachments to seemingly random objects. A person may think in an extremely concrete manner and have difficulty understanding humor, irony or sarcasm. Some may engage in self-injurious behavior, including hand-biting and head-banging; some may have sensory-motor deficits. Food rituals and extremely limited diets are common. Many are acutely sensitive to sensory stimulation, whether that be from crowded rooms, human touch, flicking fluorescent lights, or the hum of a refrigerator motor. Some find minor tactile irritants such as clothing tags unbearable. Others find pleasure in having heavy objects – such as weighted blankets – laid on top of them. Extreme symptoms may include a tendency to spread feces on the walls, the ability to go many days without sleeping, being in a state of manic high energy, an inability to connect with or speak to another human being, or a propensity for seemingly random acts of violence, including self-injury (Solomon, 2012).

Characterized as a pervasive disorder, autism affects almost every aspect of behavior as well as sensory experiences, motor functioning, balance, the physical sense of where one's own body is, even inner consciousness. Intellectual disability is not part of autism *per se*, although there is a significant number of individuals having intellectual disability as well. Some authors and clinicians talk about "high functioning" autism spectrum disorder (HFASD), meaning someone with an IQ of 70 or higher who also is diagnosed with ASD (James et al, 2006; Matson and Wilkins, 2008; Roy et al, 2009; Geurts and Jansen, 2011). According to neuroscientist Martha Herbert (2010), behaviors in autism are a property of altered brain and body networks – differences in cellular function, gene expression or brain structure that manifest in behavior.

Many children on the spectrum have other physiological difficulties as well: seizures, sleep dysfunction, gastro-intestinal problems such as chronic constipation, diarrhea, colitis, abdominal pain and esophagitis. Sometimes pain from these physical problems manifest themselves behaviorally – such as head banging or biting oneself – because individuals may not be able to communicate about the pain or source of it, or because their sensory system may not localize the pain to convey what is happening (Herbert, 2010). From Autism Speaks, Figure 1.1 displays the myriad health and medical conditions associated with ASC.

As evidenced from the preceding descriptions, autism historically has been characterized in terms of disorders, deficits, impairments and deficiencies. Challenging this viewpoint is an increasing number of autistic activists who advocate an alternative perspective – *neurodiversity* – that considers autism as a variation of "brain wiring" or neurological development, and portrays autistic people as individuals who possess a blend of cognitive strengths and weaknesses in: language, communication and social interaction; sensory processing (or environmental input); motor skill execution; and goal-oriented and reflexive thinking, planning, and self-regulation (Biklen et al, 2005; Baker, 2006; Fenton and Krahn, 2007; Glannon, 2007; Clarke and Amerom, 2008; Robertson and Ne'eman, 2008; Pollack, 2009; Robertson, 2010).

While relative strengths and difficulties in these core domains remain specific to the individual, numerous commonalities exist among autistic people (Robertson, 2010). Key strengths include detailed thinking, expansive long-term memories, a comfort with rules and guidelines, and an affinity for analyzing complex patterns in the social and physical worlds. Key difficulties include managing simultaneous tasks, understanding social nuances and various forms of social communication, filtering competing sensory stimuli, and planning tasks of daily living.

While controversial within the autism community, the neurodiversity perspective demands re-examining premises of the status quo – not only of the construct and meaning of autism, but also the role and relevance of the context in which we live,

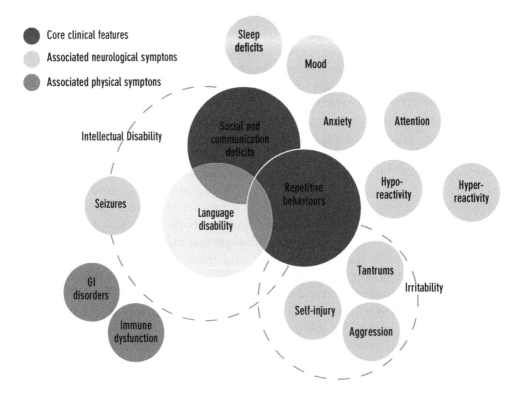

Figure 1.1: Health and medical conditions often associated with autism

(Adapted, courtesy of Autism Speaks)

and how successfully we live there, in defining and shaping autism. We return to this perspective at the end of this chapter.

A final note on how we use terms in this book is necessary. The American Psychological Association (2001, 63) has recommended that academic authors "respect people's preference; call people what they prefer to be called." Prominent autistic self-advocates James Sinclair (1999) and Scott Robertson (2010) call for using identity-first language (that is, "autistic individuals") rather than person-first language (that is, "people with autism"). However the vast majority of publications, directives, and media documents use the latter form. Given the vagaries of this ever-changing label and diagnoses, this book uses *both* identity-first and person-first terminology, recognizing the fluid and variable nature of "naming" at this time, as previously noted in Terminology (p viii).

Adults on the spectrum and in the community

To the general public, the face of autism is typically that of a child or teenager. But autism is not simply a childhood condition. Autism is considered nondegenerative and nonterminal. Children grow to be adults. Childhood and adolescence spans 18 years, whereas adulthood continues for 40, 50 and more. Clearly then, the adult population comprises the majority of those with autism.

Given recent medical advances and improved living conditions, the life expectancy for people with developmental disabilities is becoming similar to that of the general population although this may not be the case for certain individuals on the spectrum (Janicki et al, 1999; Bittles et al, 2002; Heller et al, 2010). Danish and California studies conducted in the 2000s concluded that mortality rates were nearly twice as high as expected (Shavelle, Strauss and Pickett, 2001; Mouridsen et al, 2008), with a study in Sweden reporting 5.6 times higher than expected (Gillberg et al, 2009). Shorter life expectancy seems to occur with those experiencing epilepsy and seizures, in accidents, and among those with severe learning disabilities (Shavelle and Strauss, 1998; Mouridsen et al, 2008; Pickett et al, 2011; Piven and Rabins, 2011). It is unclear, though, whether autism itself diminishes longevity, or whether the strong association with seizure disorders (affecting approximately 30 percent of those with ASC) and intellectual disability (25–50 percent) account for increased mortality (Happé and Charlton, 2012). Conversely, deaths due to smoking, alcohol, traffic and work accidents may be less common among autistic adults than among the general adult population (Shea and Mesibov, 2005).

Life expectancy estimates are not the only demographic forecast that are uncertain. Even the prevalence and numbers of adults on the spectrum are extremely difficult to gauge. Adults who as children were diagnosed with intellectual disability or a language disorder may today be diagnosed with ASC, given the changing nature and professional familiarity of neurodevelopmental diagnoses. Diagnosis of an adult is challenging since getting accurate developmental history of the first three or four years of a person's life can be difficult, particularly when parents are unavailable (Happé and Charlton, 2012). The only study that actually counted adults with autism was undertaken in the U.K., and estimated a prevalence of 1.1 percent among those between ages 16 and 44, 0.9 percent between ages of 45 and 75, and 0.8 percent over the age of 75 – a relatively stable figure across birth cohorts and similar to that in the population of children. Indeed, these figures may actually understate prevalence in adulthood since researchers did not sample those in institutional settings or those diagnosed with intellectual disabilities (Brugha et al, 2009; Brugha et al, 2011). Still, using the prevalence figures of the sample in this study means that approximately 700,000 American individuals age 65 and older in the next 15 years will be on the spectrum (Piven and Rabins, 2011).

While it is clear that there will be a much more visible presence and number of autistic adults residing in our communities in the coming decades, the overwhelming bulk of autism research remains focused on children and teens. Of the $408 million spent on nearly 1,500 autism research projects in the U.S. in 2010, only 2 percent went to researching needs of adults (IACC, 2011).

Of the research that does focus on adults, the bulk examines those transitioning out of the school system: that is, individuals under 30 years of age. There is only one published study of autistic adults aged 50 and older (Totsika et al, 2010). Will needs, experiences, service programs, and living situations of autistic adults in their 20s be relevant to those in their 40s, 50s and older? It is relatively safe to assume that there may be additional complications with older adults on the spectrum. Some symptom profiles common in people in their 60s and older – for example, late-life decline in sensory abilities – may differentially affect older individuals with ASC who already have existing sensory sensitivities. With much unknown, we need to be cautious when projecting the needs and conditions of young adulthood to those of older adults, particularly given neurocognitive and sensory changes that appear in typical aging years (Geurts and Vissers, 2012). Clearly more research and attention to the lifespan of autism is needed.

From the limited research we do have on adults, we know that for those diagnosed with ASC in childhood, a significant number will become adults with persisting social and communication difficulties, and, in many cases, with psychiatric and behavioral co-morbidity (Howlin, 2000; Howlin et al, 2004; Seltzer et al, 2004; Cederlund et al, 2008). The majority of adults on the spectrum will likely remain dependent on families or other support services to a greater or lesser extent, and face challenges in employment, housing, communicating and socializing, dating, and community participation (Howlin et al, 2004; Seltzer et al, 2004; Kuhlthau et al, 2010; Billstedt, Gillberg and Gillberg, 2011).

How such behaviors may manifest in adulthood, and to what degree, is a large unknown – whether that be improvement, deterioration, or stability (Seltzer et al, 2004; James et al, 2006; Geurts and Jansen, 2011; Gillespie-Lynch et al, 2011; Stuart-Hamilton and Morgan, 2011). One study of over 700 individuals with ASC aged

2 to 62 years (Esbensen et al, 2009) found that restrictive and repetitive behaviors were less frequent and less severe among older individuals than with the younger adult counterparts. Sensory sensitivities have shown to improve with age for some individuals (Seltzer et al, 2003; Kern et al, 2006); but whether that improvement continues when individuals experience age-related declines in hearing and vision is unknown (Happe and Charlton, 2012). Some individuals on the spectrum may attain educational, independent living, and relationship goals in adulthood, but do so a decade or more later than those of the general population (for example, Stuart-Hamilton and Morgan, 2011). Some researchers have noted functional and symptom improvements over time (Seltzer et al, 2003; Howlin et al, 2004; Seltzer et al, 2004). Some even suggest that between 15 and 30 percent of adults with autism will show more positive outcomes as they grow older (Seltzer et al, 2004; Cederlund et al, 2008). We do not know if the many concomitant health, psychiatric and medical conditions often associated with children on the spectrum – sleep disorders and gastrointestinal problems, for example – also prevail into later adulthood years (Pivin and Rabins, 2011). And whether symptom improvements and declines are the result of an aging process, or of childhood years of specialized educational training, medical attention and support opportunities, is still a mystery. With so much unknown, projections of the future must be cautious of relying on present-day moving targets.

While many believe the efficacy of childhood interventions and support programs will translate into later years, actual research on sustaining effectiveness is still unclear (Hendrick and Wehman, 2009). One study, for example, found that adult day activities are often not as intellectually stimulating as similar activities in high school, and as a consequence may result in a decline in an individual's improvement witnessed during school years (Taylor and Seltzer, 2010). The transition from the public school system with its supports and routine, to much more ambiguous educational, occupational, residential and relational arenas, can be particularly stressful for young people in general but may be even more so for autistic individuals who have difficulty coping with change (Smith, Greenberg and Mailick, 2012v). Families, too, may be under increased stress as their children lose insurance coverage and access to therapies as they transition to adulthood. One thing that almost all research studies show is a significant gap in the support services beyond the school years, witnessed internationally (Gerhardt and Lanier, 2011; Interagency Autism Coordinating Committee, 2011; Rydzewska, 2012; Ling-Yi, Shu-Hing and Ya-Tsu, 2012)

Most of the research examining adult outcomes has defined and measured outcomes goals in conventional ways. These may not be desired or appropriate for many on the spectrum (see Henninger and Taylor, 2012, for review). An emerging person-environment perspective – or person-centered planning – within the support and care service system moves away from established normative milestones to consider an individual's ideas and aspirations of adulthood and support systems to achieve those (Arnett, 2000; Henninger and Taylor, 2012). In person-centered planning, an individual determines what it means to be responsible for oneself, to establish a personal value system, to relate to parents as adults, and to become financially independent, as marks of becoming an adult. An autistic adult who enjoys living in a group home, does volunteer work he finds meaningful, and goes bowling twice a week with his roommates may feel a level of independence and maturity that cannot be matched if he were to struggle holding two part-time menial jobs to pay the rent on an apartment where he lives by himself and has to take two bus lines to a recreational center where he meets friends on the weekend. Person-centered planning considers whether the outcome is congruent with the desires and abilities of the individual, not a broad-sweep diagnostic (Taylor, 2009). Successful planning for adulthood, then, depends in part on having a diversity of residential types and living arrangements for a broad spectrum of adult individuals.

Residential alternatives – or lack of

Since autism is defined as a spectrum condition, it would seem that the population of individuals with ASC might best be served by having a spectrum or range of housing types and of residential arrangements from which to choose. This diversity, however, is rarely the case in a single community or even in a single metropolitan area. Table 1.1 lists a range of housing types and residential arrangements, although most of these are absent in a single community. (Chapter Five provides more detailed profiles of housing types.) If we combined the residential arrangements with housing types, we would see endless possibilities.

Even if, however, there was a spectrum of housing types and residential arrangements in all our communities, there still remains the issue of figuring out which would be a good match for an individual's personal aspirations, living situation, and needs. How can someone decide if an accessory dwelling unit or a cohousing community would be suitable if one has never seen or heard of such? Will living by oneself or with housemates be more suitable? To get a better grasp of the difficulty of envisioning what might be the best place to live, we can start by looking at places where autistic adults currently reside.

Once again we are left with no single comprehensive survey that identifies the residences and places where adults with autism live. From a research review of nine surveys conducted between 1960 and 1999 in various countries (Canada, Japan, U.K., U.S.) that identified place of residence of adults with ASC, Howlin and Moss (2012) found that the percentage of adults who were living independently or semi-independently ranged in these surveys from 1 to 44 percent, with a mean of 18 percent. Those living with their parents ranged from 22 to 93 percent, with a mean of 57 percent. Those living in hospital care ranged from 0 to 48 percent, with a range of 13 percent.

Table 1.1: Various residential building types and living arrangements

RESIDENTIAL BUILDING TYPE

Independent detached home (a.k.a. SFH)

Independent attached home (e.g. townhouse)

Cluster of detached homes, no shared/common spaces (e.g. planned residential development)

Cluster of detached homes, shared/common spaces in separate buildings on property

Attached home, 2–5 units (e.g. duplex, triplex, four-plex)

Attached home, 6 or more units (e.g. apartment, condominium), no shared or common spaces

Attached home, 6 or more units, with shared or common

Attached efficiency units or guest rooms (e.g. single-room occupancy housing)

RESIDENTIAL LIVING ARRANGEMENT WITHIN HOME

Solo or alone

With family

With self-selected friends or housemates, no live-in care providers (referred to as "shared housing")

With agency/provider-selected housemates, no live-in care providers

With roommates and live-in care providers (often referred to as "group home")

With spouse or domestic partner (with or without children)

TYPES OF CARE AND SUPPORT IN HOME

None

Supported: with personal support providers living off-site

Supervised: with support providers living on-site or with working office on-site

Long-term institutional care: extensive services spaces on site, staff present during sleeping hours, some
    staff may be live-in

Transitional training: supported or supervised, but intended only as temporary

Subsequent surveys of living arrangements and residences undertaken in different communities and countries after 1999 show similar substantial ranges, as evidenced in Table 1.2. Many of these surveys have small sample sizes, limiting their generalizability. In addition, young adults in their 20s dominate these surveys; again leaving unanswered questions about where those in their 30s and older live. Across all surveys, though, one trend holds true: few autistic adults live alone. Many live with their families, particularly with parents (Howlin, 2000; Krauss, Seltzer and Jacobson, 2005; Orsmond, Krauss and Seltzer, 2004), ranging from 37 percent to 87 percent in these various studies. Unfortunately these surveys rarely tell us the housing type or situation of these parents.

Table 1.2: Post-1999 surveys of types of residences and living arrangements of adults with ASC

UNITED KINGDOM: HOWLIN ET AL, 2004

Sample characteristics: 1985 and 1991 follow-up studies of children who were diagnosed with ASD between 1950 and 1959. Sample included 68 adults, ages between 21 and 49 with average age of 29.

	%
Living in family home*	38
Residential accommodations of:	
specialist autism provision with little independence	21
specialist autism provision with some independence	18
long-stay hospital provision	12
Semi-sheltered hostel-type accommodation, some support	6
Lived alone with limited parental support	4
Missing data	1

Note: *included one resident with separate dwelling unit on parent's property.

GOTHENBURG, SWEDEN: BILLSTEDT ET AL, 2005

Sample characteristics: 120 individuals diagnosed with autism in childhood, followed for 13–22 years. Residential survey at ages 17–40 years age, with mean age 25.

	%
Community based group homes	49
Parents' home*	38
Apartments with community-based support	8
Own apartment with occasional help from relatives	4
Apartment with girlfriend	2

Note: *61% of those living with parents were 23 years or younger.

WISCONSIN AND MASSACHUSETTS IN U.S.: KRAUSS ET AL, 2005

Sample characteristics: 133 mothers of families with adult (22 years plus) child with autism responding to questionnaire

	% of adults with autism	Average age of autistic adult (years)	Average age of mother (years)
Living in non-family setting	63	32.9	62.1
Living in parents' home	37	30.2	59.2

BRITISH COLUMBIA, CANADA: EAVES AND HO, 2008

Sample characteristics: 48 adults with autism born between 1974 and 1984, ages between 19 and 31 years old (mean = 24)

	%
Living with parents	56
Supported arrangements, such as group homes, foster care, home managed by microboard	35
Living "more or less" independently	9

UNITED STATES: EASTER SEALS, HARRIS INTERACTIVE, 2004

Sample characteristics: 1,652 young adults (ages 19–30) with ASD

	All adults with ASD (%)	With Asperger's (%)	With PDD-NOS (%)	With autism (%)
With parent or guardian	79	71	84	81
Supported residence for individuals with special needs	12	7	10	14
Independently, either with or without spouse or partner	4	9	3	3
With other family members/ spouse/partner	2	5	3	0
Other	3	7	0	2

ANDALUSIA, SPAIN: SALDAÑA ET AL, 2009

Sample characteristics: 74 adults with ASD, ages between 18 and 40 with mean age of 24. From interviews.

	%
Living with parents	87

UNITED STATES: AUTISM SPEAKS, 2013

Sample characteristics: 379 adults with autism responding to online survey; 55% male; median age 25 years, with 52% being 25 years or younger, 8% between 50 and 69 years. Approximate numbers below:

	%
At home with family	61
In own home	18
Other	12
Group home	3
Own home with roommates	3
With family other than one's own	1
At residential school	1

Living in a parent's home (also called "family co-residence") is even more pronounced among adults with ASC than those with other neurodevelopmental conditions. In comparing living arrangements of over 1,800 high school graduates (ages 21–25 years) who were diagnosed with either ASC, intellectual disability, learning disability, or emotional disturbance, researchers found that young adults with autism were more likely to live with their parents and least likely to live independently after leaving high school compared to those with other types of disabilities. Only about 17 percent of the young adults on the spectrum had ever lived independently, compared to 34 percent of their peers with intellectual disability, 65 percent with learning disabilities and 63 percent with emotional disturbance. They also stayed with their parents for a longer period of time than the other peer groups (Anderson et al, 2013). Young autistic adults had the highest rate of supervised living arrangements and the lowest rate of independent living following departure from high school, confirming trends identified in studies in Sweden (Billstedt et al, 2005), the U.K. (Howlin et al, 2004) and the U.S. (Newman et al 2011). Even after controlling for demographic characteristics and impairment severity, those with ASC were significantly less likely than young adults with other neurodevelopmental conditions to have ever lived independently since leaving high school.

Granted, family co-residence is not an unusual stage for adults in their 20s. Stretching out the road to independence from that of previous generations, 36 percent of the Millennial generation (that is, born between early 1980s and early 2000s) in the U.S. live in their parents' homes (Fry, 2013). Milestones and aspirations of young adults are continually in flux across generations, across decades. Leaving home to set up one's own household, finish college, find a job, get married, start a family – these achievements may no longer be the norm for the general population of young adults in their 20s, particularly in light of changing economic, environmental and social conditions (Furstenberg et al, 2005). So then, why consider these as milestones for similar-aged young adults on the spectrum?

Eventual desires to live more independently will depend in part on daily living skills – such as cleaning, cooking, grooming, healthy eating, managing money, shopping, and taking public transportation – perhaps more so than other types of adaptive behaviors (Kapp, Gantman and Laugeson, 2011). While many youth and adults with ASC have difficulties achieving such skills (Balfe and Tantam, 2010; Geller and Greenberg, 2010), from these surveys we witness a modest proportion of autistic adults having a moderate degree of independence in their residential settings.

Another prominent pattern revealed in these surveys of Table 1.2 is declining residency in institutional settings, such as developmental centers, nursing homes, and psychiatric hospitals. Whether this is or will be the case for adults in their later years remains an unanswered question. Few of these surveys included older adults with autism (that is, individuals in their 60s and older), where we may see larger numbers of individuals living in assisted living facilities, nursing homes, or other institutional care placements as we do in the general aging population.

The majority of comparative research of residential settings focuses on differences between institutions and group homes (Mahan and Kozlowski, 2011). The latter tend to have higher staff to resident ratios, thus increasing the availability of personal attention for residents (Hundert et al, 2003). There is also some evidence that group home residents have greater adaptive behavior functioning and increased family contact (Spreat, 1998; Spreat and Conroy, 2002).

For those living outside family co-residence or institutional facilities, we have very little information about the types of homes in which they live: A single-family home in a gated community? A one-bedroom apartment in a public housing complex? A shared room on a farmstead? A studio apartment of one's own in downtown Philadelphia or a condo in a retirement community in Florida? While the surveys give us a sense of how many roommates there may be in the home, we do not know if these are in homes where bathrooms are shared between two or three residents; or in homes where each individual has his or her own en-suite (that is, large bedroom with adjoining bath) and where family spaces – living room, kitchen, eating space – are shared among roommates, much like we see in contemporary residential complexes designed for university students. As architectural and housing researchers, we believe this lack of detailed description of the residential arrangements and housing types is problematic in determining not only the suitability of present residential living situations but also in envisioning how best to go forward. How one lives is in these spatial and social details.

So when we ask the question, "Where do spectrum adults *want* to live?" we first need to acknowledge that we do not have a solid, comprehensive map of the types of homes, residential arrangements and neighborhoods where individuals on the spectrum currently live.

The challenges of having spectrum adults communicate and express their preferences are often raised as a deterrent to getting an idea of predilections and needs. (As we see later in this chapter and in Chapter Five, we do not hold to this position since there are non-conventional survey techniques for eliciting and obtaining this information.) In cases where the spectrum individual does not express his or her opinions or predilections, family members or support providers are used as proxies, describing what they believe would be best or most suitable. Another challenge to gauging residential aspirations is that many individuals – parents, self-advocates and other individuals on the spectrum – have limited exposure to residential options beyond what they have immediately experienced or seen in their communities. There is then the challenge of making choices within severe financial constraints.

Since few adults with ASC are employed, and when they are employed they work few hours or for minimum wage, financing a home and the support services needed to live there is a major hurdle. In many North American and European countries, government assistance is provided to those with disabling conditions, and in most countries this financial assistance is meager. For example through the Social Security Income (SSI) program, the U.S. government pays benefits to people with disabilities who have limited income and assets. The typical monthly SSI payment in 2014 was $721 for an individual ($1082 for a couple), from which a person is expected to pay for rent, utilities, food, transportation, health services, and other necessities. (And if the recipient works to try to make ends meet, the SSI amount can be even less or absent.) But this public assistance is not only needed by the individual. When the recipient of that income – the autistic adult – moves out of the parents' home, so does that income which for many families has become essential in making ends meet.

Another difficulty is that some public entitlements restrict or define where one can live. In the U.S., low-income adults with disabilities (including those with autism) may be eligible to receive financial assistance under the Home and Community-Based Services program (known as HCBS, part of the federal Medicaid program). While only personal care and support services are financially supported, the HCBS program requires those services be provided in a Medicaid-approved setting. In 2014, the Centers for Medicare and Medicaid Services (CMS) that administers these funds changed the regulations to more specifically define what constitutes a qualified "home and community-based" approved setting, frustrating many self-advocates and housing providers (Centers for Medicare and Medicaid Services, 2014; The Arc, 2014). Some proponents claim that a substantial number of existing residential settings for those receiving HCBS funds may no longer meet the revised CMS criteria – particularly those living in settings where a predominant number of other residents receive HCBS waivers as well – potentially leaving them with a choice of either moving to a qualified residential setting or staying in place but relinquishing the public subsidy (http://ltoventures.org/news/articlesop-ed/choice-v-olmstead/).

Efforts to gauge where adults with ASC would like to live, and how, are rare. The most extensive study is a 2013 on-line survey sponsored by Autism Speaks. Not only does it capture a relatively large number of respondents – over 8,500 caregivers and nearly 400 youth and adults on the spectrum (average age of 25) – it also queried respondents about preferred living arrangements, housing styles, home locations and other residential conditions. While the survey entails some ambiguous terms – for example, the term "suburban environment" likely conjures different types of places and meanings given the diversity of suburban settings – the survey findings do affirm that there is no one type overwhelmingly desired by all (see Figure 1.2). Notably, the responses from caregivers – 89 percent whom were parents – differed in many ways from responses of individuals on the spectrum.

Having systematic research results of residential preferences and needs could provide housing providers and developers with valuable information of what and where to build and provide. It could also help inform policy initiatives and regulations, such as the HCBS definition of a qualified home and community setting described previously. But an underlying premise of constructing valid research surveys is having an array of true housing options from which to make informed choices.

Determining that choice is not easy. Conventional surveys do a poor job in ferreting out and providing to respondents detailed information of housing options. For example, the term "group home" conjures a dismal image for many, given that the public media has often broadcast crowded, miserable examples, usually in exposés of places being investigated by public health officials. But many upscale university campus residences (once called "dormitories") are essentially variants of the group or shared home model, but specifically designed so that each roommate has his or her own en-suite unit, sometimes in separate corners or in opposite ends of the apartment, so that personal privacy is maximized and can be maintained (see Figure 1.3). Shared areas can be spacious, amenity-rich and accommodating.

Even nursing homes are moving towards more individualized living space in a group or congregate setting. With support from the Robert Woods Johnson Foundation, the Green House Project intends to revolutionize long term care by providing a residential model that is healthier, more personalized, and more cost effective than the conventional nursing homes that prevail today. These residences are designed for ten to twelve residents. Each resident has a well-lit, private en-suite unit, in proximity to a common hearth area with a living room, open kitchen and dining area. Smart technology is used throughout the residence to provide comfort and safety for the residents and staff. Direct support providers, known as *Shahbazim*, function within self-managed work teams to provide the day-to-day care for the residents and act as managers of the home (http://thegreenhouseproject.org).

These housing options – and many more innovative settings – are not on housing preference surveys. And, unfortunately, not available or visible in many communities. Having real housing choice means having an array of different alternatives from which to choose. We believe that the currently narrow spectrum of housing choices for adults with ASC and other neurodevelopmental conditions does not have to remain so limited – simply witness the evolution of housing for older adults in the last few decades. Before the 1970s, older adults who found it difficult to live in their homes as they aged basically had four options. They could stay in their home and seek help of a family member to care for them; or they could move in with a son or daughter. If they had sufficient assets, they could hire staff for personal and healthcare needs, allowing them to stay in their own home. Or they could enter a nursing home. Options beyond these were rare.

Starting in the 1970s, residential opportunities expanded. Today, there is a wide array of housing choices for older adults: "active seniors" apartment complexes and condominiums; modular home communities; "granny flats," or accessory dwelling units; naturally occurring retirement communities (NORCs); shared housing; elder villages; assisted living and continuing care retirement communities; senior day care services; senior cohousing; Alzheimer's accommodations within a retirement community (sometimes referred to as the "memory wing"); Green House Project nursing homes; and others. One need only log onto the website of the American Association of Retired Persons (www.AARP.org) to see profiles and video-clips of these numerous options.

While, however, these options have expanded considerably over the last few decades for older adults, concern now rests with the support systems needed for making some of these residential arrangements feasible and affordable. It is also a concern for adults with autism and those with other neurodevelopmental conditions. That is the cost and competition of care and support services for living at home.

Figure 1.2: Preferred residential type and arrangements: Response comparison between individuals with autism and caregivers

(Source: Autism Speaks 2013 National Housing Survey[a])

Most appropriate living arrangements in next five years

Individuals with autism	Caregivers

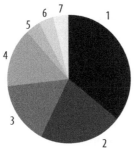
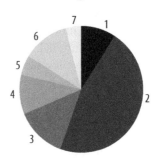

Individuals with autism:
- 1. Own home (36%)
- 2. At home with family (22%)
- 3. Other responses (16%)
- 4. Own home with roommate (15%)
- 5. Assisted living facility (4%)
- 6. In group home (4%)
- 7. Own home with multiple roommates (4%)

Caregivers:
- 1. Own home (9%)
- 2. At home with family (46%)
- 3. Other responses (13%)
- 4. Own home with roommate (10%)
- 5. Assisted living facility (5%)
- 6. In group home (12%)
- 7. Own home with multiple roommates (4%)

Levels of support in ideal situation

Individuals with autism	Caregivers

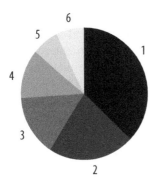
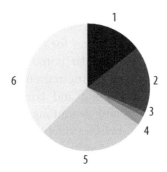

Individuals with autism:
- 1. Support only as needed (37%)
- 2. Minimal – few hours per week (22%)
- 3. No support (15%)
- 4. Ongoing support (12%)
- 5. Support throughout the day (7%)
- 6. 24 hour support (7%)

Caregivers:
- 1. Support only as needed (12%)
- 2. Minimal – few hours per week (14%)
- 3. No support (1%)
- 4. Ongoing support (2%)
- 5. Support throughout the day (23%)
- 6. 24 hour support (31%)

#1 choice for housing type

Individuals with autism

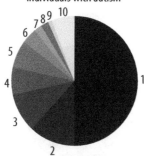

Caregivers

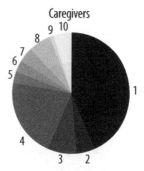

- 1. Single family home (51%)
- 2. Apartment/condominium without common/shared spaces (12%)
- 3. Apartment/condominium with common/shared living areas (10%)
- 4. Planned/intentional community (homes built in specific neighbourhoods with a common purpose) 7%
- 5. Townhouse (7%)
- 6. Duplex/triplex/fourplex (small apartment building) (4%)
- 7. Multi-family (attached) home (2%)
- 8. Assisted living facility (2%)
- 9. Room rental in home (1%)
- 10. Other (6%)

- 1. Single family home (43%)
- 2. Apartment/condominium without common/shared spaces (5%)
- 3. Apartment/condominium with common/shared living areas (8%)
- 4. Planned/intentional community (homes built in specific neighbourhoods with a common purpose) (21%)
- 5. Townhouse (3%)
- 6. Duplex/triplex/fourplex (small apartment building) (3%)
- 7. Multi-family (attached) home (4%)
- 8. Assisted living facility (6%)
- 9. Room rental in home (1%)
- 10. Other (5%)

Most appropriate community type[b]

Individuals with autism

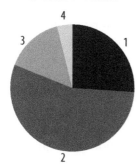

Caregivers

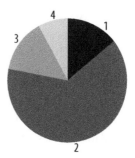

- 1. Urban: City with many people and buildings (26%)
- 2. Suburban: neighbourhood outside a city (55%)
- 3. Rural: Community with lots of open land and few businesses, people (15%)
- 4. Farmstead: A farm where people live and work together (4%)

- 1. Urban: City with many people and buildings (14%)
- 2. Suburban: neighbourhood outside a city (64%)
- 3. Rural: Community with lots of open land and few businesses, people (14%)
- 4. Farmstead: A farm where people live and work together (8%)

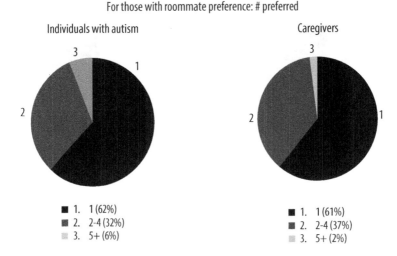

For those with roommate preference: # preferred

Individuals with autism

3

1

2

■ 1. 1 (62%)
■ 2. 2-4 (32%)
▨ 3. 5+ (6%)

Caregivers

3

2

1

■ 1. 1 (61%)
■ 2. 2-4 (37%)
▨ 3. 5+ (2%)

[a] Sample size for individuals with autism is 397; for caregivers, 8,164. Note 89% of caregivers are parents. Also note only 42% of caregivers provided care and support to individuals 18 years and older.

[b] Question wording differs between groups. Caregivers were asked "most appropriate community"; individuals were asked in what type of community they would like to live.

Costs and competition of care and support services

The soaring costs of long-term services and supports for persons with disabilities, chronic health conditions or functional limitations feed public concern around the globe. In the U.S., $210.9 billion is spent on long-term services and supports of individuals with disabilities and older adults with functional impairments and chronic conditions (O'Shaunghnessy, 2013). Unpaid support and care from families and friends – not typically included in these cost projections – are estimated to reflect hundreds of billions of dollars annually (IOM and NRC, 2013). With the projected aging of the global population, costs of long-term care and support are expected to increase substantially.

Changing family demographics likewise have affected the long-term care system (Parish and Lutwick, 2005). Smaller family sizes and increased mobility that characterize today's households mean extended families are less likely to live in the same community, reducing the availability of unpaid, informal supports for a family member needing assistance. Employed women and men have less time to care for family members with disabilities, or do so in ways that strain their lives and pocketbooks.

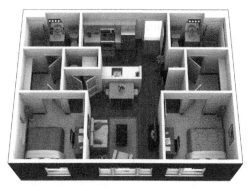

Figure 1.3: Example of en-suites in two-bedroom apartment at The Continuum, University of Florida
(Courtesy of The Continuum)

Another contributing factor to rising costs is the increased life expectancy of individuals with developmental disabilities (Roizen and Patterson, 2003). For the first time in history, large numbers of individuals with such conditions are outliving their parents who in many cases have provided home and informal support. With more individuals living longer, their assistance needs are in direct competition with those of the elderly population who is also living longer, growing in number, and placing increased demand on formal and informal long-term support services (Hooyman and Gonyea, 1995). The aging of the general population is one of the most pressing forces shaping domestic policy in many countries. A recent report of the Institute of Medicine (2008b) concluded that the U.S. workforce will not be prepared to care for the anticipated increase in the number of elderly individuals in the population. It is not only a deficit of available nurses and physicians, but a much larger demand for direct support providers who provide 70 to 80 percent of the daily hands-on care and assistance for disabled and chronically-ill older adults (Piven and Rabins, 2011).

This competition for support services is compounded by the fact that the long-term care workforce is seriously underpaid and lacks sufficient training (Braddock and Mitchell, 1992; Minnesota Technical College Task Force, 1993). The average wage of direct service staff in a group home is $8.50–$9.50/hour in the U.S., not much different from that of a Starbucks barista with a high school degree (ltoventures.org/our-model). The U.S. Department of Health and Human Services (2004) reports the annual average staff turnover rate for programs serving adults with developmental disabilities is 50 percent. Even if the turnover rate was lower – say, half at 25 percent – this would be considered debilitating and unacceptable in most other industries. Reasons for the high turnover and vacancy rates are low pay, inadequate benefits, excessive client-to-staff ratios, physical or behavioral challenges presented by clients, inadequate training, and limited professional status. Governments and agencies may eventually have to contend with not only complaints but even lawsuits as this situation continues to degenerate (Parish and Lutwick, 2005).

Indeed, starting in the 1970s, families of people with developmental disabilities used federal class action litigation to improve conditions in residential and institutional living settings, and to expand community-based long-term care, eventually moving people from a bureaucratic system of large public institutions to a network of community-based residential programs and supports such as group homes (Braddock, 2002; Prouty, Smith and Lakin, 2003; Parish and Lutwick, 2005).

The greatest responsibility for this assistance and care is, however, borne by families who constitute the largest group of support providers (Fujiura, 1998). Support services for these family members are often a lifeline: services such as respite, environmental adaptations, assistive devices, personal assistance, mental healthcare, crisis intervention and behavior management. Family members who use these support services suffer significantly less stress and feel less overwhelmed by their caregiving responsibilities. But when those children become adults, and their parents themselves may need care and support, public funds for such assistance drops precipitously (Floyd and Gallagher, 1997; Haverman et al, 1997; Freedman et al, 1999; Freedman and Boyer, 2000; Seltzer and Krauss, 2001; Parish and Lutwick, 2005).

Recent efforts to quantify costs of autism have been estimated for the United States and United Kingdom (Buescher et al, 2014). Given the spectrum of healthcare, education, social services, and medical care related to autism, figuring out costs can be painstaking, particularly in countries with multi-payer healthcare systems such as the U.S. (Sharpe and Baker, 2011). With estimates of the number of individuals with autism at 3.5 million in the U.S. and 605,000 in the U.K. and assuming a prevalence of intellectual disability among 40 percent of individuals with ASDs, researchers estimated the annual national cost of supporting children with autism at $61 billion in the U.S. and £3.1 billion in the U.K. Annual national costs for adults are $175 billion in the U.S. and £29 billion in the U.K. For adults, the largest contributor to total costs in both countries was accommodations (including costs of staff services), followed by direct medical costs and individual productivity loss. Medical costs were much higher for adults than for children.

Given these soaring costs and scenarios, governments as well as care and residential support industries are looking for alternative solutions. One venue is smart or assistive technology. A smart device may be situated in the home itself, or – such as an app on a smartphone, iPad or tablet – may be pervasive and ubiquitous, hence mobile with the individual. While public media often spotlights high-end technologies such as robotics, relatively simple technologies can solve common but extremely complex problems such as getting out of bed and dressing in the morning (IOM, 2013). The convergence of aging and disability is creating an economic and political opportunity to advance these technologies in the home at reasonable cost. More about advances in smart technology that assist autistic adults living more independently at home is described in the last chapter of this book.

Another venue being explored for reducing costs of care are innovative residential settings and programs that support not only residents but also support providers, resulting in reduced services for less essential care and in mitigating turnover. The

Green House Project mentioned earlier, a project initiated by the Robert Wood Johnson Foundation, is such an example. Nursing homes have been the most expensive residential care setting for older adults, costing upwards of $240 a day for a private room, $207 a day for a shared room (Genworth, 2013). With nearly 260 Green Houses open or in development in the U.S., preliminary cost analyses indicate improved health and reduced healthcare costs in Green Houses compared to traditional nursing homes, while staff and housing costs remain relatively the same (Jenkens et al, 2011; Horn et al, 2012). Residents also are happier with this model, and have demonstrated their preference by their willingness to relocate longer distances if such housing choices are available (http://thegreenhouseproject.org/doc/28/consumer-research.pdf).

Another model particularly tied to those with autism and other developmental disabilities is the Family-Teaching home model, pioneered by the University of Kansas and Community Living Options (Strouse et al, 2003). Each Family-Teaching home serves two or three adults with developmental disabilities. Since these homes are duplexes with an adjoining door connecting the two units, a married couple – with or without children – live in the separate but adjoining living quarters. This couple who has gone through extensive service training and receive competitive salary with benefits such as respite care, paid vacations, use of SUV, and the like, provide ongoing support and assistance to residents. In a quasi-experimental study comparing nine Family-Teaching homes, five conventional group homes, and eleven individualized living residences, the Family-Teaching homes had 43 percent lower staff turnover, 57 percent fewer vacancies, 8 percent higher wages, and 13 percent fewer direct-support employees involved in the support of the residents. It is an exemplary model associated with significantly better direct-support staff stability and lower costs.

Advocacy and choice

The disability rights movement views disability not as a physiological or psychological deficit needing to be "fixed," but rather as a social construction shaped in large part by the social and physical environments in which people live and work (Bagatell, 2010). That is, "disabilities" are embedded within the community or environmental setting, not the person – a perspective similar to that of the World Health Organization's International Classification of Functioning, Disability and Health (www.who.int/classifications/icf/en/).

This perspective resonated with many individuals with ASC, spawning the neurodiversity movement mentioned earlier in this chapter. Neurodiversity foregrounds assets and strengths of autism that are often ignored or devalued in biomedical or conventional perspectives. For instance, neurodiversity proponents challenge studies that identify societal costs of autism (for example, Ganz, 2007) because the underlying premise does not ask, or even consider, the benefits of autism, only costs. The neurodiversity viewpoint has begun to penetrate segments of the autism research community. One example is Simon Baron-Cohen, a leading autism researcher at Cambridge University, who stresses systematizing behavior as an important cognitive strength of autism, and calls for the term "disorders" to be replaced by the term "conditions." Changing terminology to conditions – as in autism spectrum conditions, for example – may also encourage others to understand and accept the differences that individuals on the spectrum exhibit (Wright et al, 2013).

What is important is that the neurodiversity movement has also questioned who "speaks" for autism (Bagatell, 2010). The self-advocacy movement began in Sweden in the 1960s when people with intellectual disabilities fought for the right to make their own decisions, speak for themselves, and take control over their lives (Ward and Meyer, 1999). By the 1970s, the movement spread to other parts of Europe and the United States. In the early 1990s, adults with ASC began attending autism conferences that were previously the domain of parents and professionals. When some of those self-advocates felt their needs and viewpoints were being ignored at these forums, small groups sprung up, run for and by individuals with autism (Sinclair, 2005). One of the most active and visible groups is the Autistic Self Advocacy Network (ASAN) whose members have testified in state and federal legislatures, and has been quoted and profiled in public media. Others include: Autism Network International (ANI), Association for Autistic Community, Autism Women's Network, Ollibean, The Art of Autism, TASH, The Thinking Person's Guide to Autism.

Among other issues, self-advocates have raised questions about the purpose, ethics, and focus of interventions. For many members of the autism community, interventions should be targeted to alleviate problematic and disruptive symptoms, such as allergies, unwanted movements, gastro-intestinal problems, and sensory sensitivities. They resent exorbitant costs spent on research that seek "cures," or behavioral interventions that target "normalizing" behavior (Robertson, 2010). Rather, they advocate interventions that help in coping with health conditions, assisting everyday life challenges, and enhancing quality of life (Bagatell, 2010) – which includes having a home and community in which to live and thrive.

What such a place may be is a premise of this book – not by providing a prescription or directive, but rather by offering a platform that can inform a resident's choice and that can broaden the landscape of residential alternatives from which one could truly choose.

In North America and many European countries, "choice" has replaced the previous emphasis on "normalization" (Wolfensberg, 1972). Retreating from the old ways of thinking of "normalization" as meaning having the same type of home and living environment that the typical population has or aspires to, today's advocacy efforts stress making one's own choices about what works best for oneself (Murray, 1996). That means, in part, having alternatives or options to choose from, and information about those options to make informed choices. ASAN suggests that U.S. federal guidelines governing the residential settings in which an individual can receive HCBS financial support (described earlier) should stipulate a setting must have been "selected by the individual following a meaningful opportunity to choose from among alternatives including the setting that is the most integrated setting appropriate for the individual," rather than a fixed type or definition. Among individuals with disabilities, the most common interpretation of the terminology "the most integrated setting" – that is promoted in these U.S. federal guidelines – was "a place where the person exercises choice and control." The second most common interpretation was "a home of one's own shared with persons with whom one has chosen to live, or where one lives alone" (National Council on Disability, 2010).

Yet because they are refused or lack self-advocacy skills, people with ASC often are denied the opportunity to express meaningful choices. Decisions about where they live, with whom to live, and how they live, are usually made by others, such as service providers, guardians, and family members. Whether these decisions that others make are consistent with the aspirations of autistic adults is an open question. But recent surveys suggest important differences particularly as it pertains to housing type and location, as seen in the Autism Speaks survey described previously (in Figure 1.2).

Whether online surveys are appropriate mechanisms for eliciting one's preference or gauging choice is debatable. The illusion of choice pervades most surveys. Even if there is a long list of possible alternatives, if a respondent is not knowledgeable or aware of the realm of possibilities, then the opportunity for gauging true choice vanishes. Choice implies the freedom to choose from a set of alternatives. It also suggests awareness and understanding of information in making a choice, being cognizant of the range of alternatives, and knowing what each means. That informative quality is absent in most conventional surveys (Ahrentzen, 1997).

As noted by Murray (1996), although involvement of consumers is encouraged in helping to make choices about their lives, there are few methods available or promoted to assist people with disabilities in making those choices. Given verbal and communicative aspects of autism, other means than conventional language-dominant surveys or interviews need to be developed to inform and gauge choice; and innovative techniques, technologies and strategies for developing such self-determination and self-advocacy tools are described in the last chapter of this book.

We believe that this book can also assist in these efforts. The visually oriented nature of the design professions can help inform autistic adults and those who support them in learning about a wider array of residential housing types and arrangements; what features of a home or neighborhood may work best for their particular living situation, health conditions, life goals and ideals; and enable them to reflect upon and express their residential aspirations.

This book also can help with the other dimension of choice, by advancing the development of a wider array of residential alternatives from which to choose. This book implores those involved in housing design, production and policy to expand their exposure to what is possible, what is desirable, and to direct their efforts towards expanding the horizon of residential choice to those on the spectrum.

TWO

A RESEARCH-INFORMED APPROACH FOR HOUSING DESIGN

The modern evidence-based (EB) movement in medicine began in the 1990s to advance "the conscientious, explicit and judicious use of current best evidence in making decisions about the care of the individual patient. The practice...means integrating individual clinical expertise with the best available external clinical evidence from systematic research" (Sackett et al, 1996). In other words, doctors and healthcare professionals would make decisions about treatments – if, which, and how they should be applied – based on the best available research, one's clinical or professional experience, and how it suited a patient's clinical state, predicament, preference, and choice (Sackett et al, 2000) (see Figure 2.1). Formalizing this movement was the formation of the Cochrane Collaboration in 1993, which today is an international network of over 31,000 people whose mission is to systematically identify, evaluate and summarize scientific evidence for specific healthcare treatments or practices.

The EB approach in medicine eventually morphed into other fields: public health, nursing, social work, criminal justice, management, education, among others. In addition to the Cochrane Collaboration, other professional organizations established assessment criteria and procedures for identifying evidence and effective interventions in respective fields and professions. With a legacy of empirical research and funding over the past several decades, researchers and practitioners in these fields have been able to assemble extensive portfolios of research studies that shape evidence-based practices (EBP).

What appeared as clear-cut definitions and thresholds for EB medicine, however, often becomes a quagmire in other fields. What constitutes "evidence," for example,

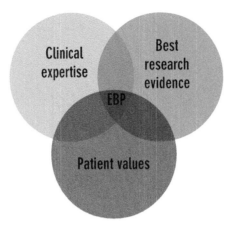

Figure 2.1: Three components shaping evidence-based practice (EBP) in medical/health practice

and are there different types? How does one evaluate "best" when alternatives are few? What criteria are used to judge whether one technique is "better" than another? Does "evidence" constitute only empirical investigations? Is evidence allowed only when the outcomes are measurable and observable? How do we base decisions when non-measurable outcomes – such as the homelike "feel" of a place compared to an institutional one – are issues at hand? How does one proceed when there is insufficient research or evidence?

We wrestled with these fundamental questions when trying to lay an evidence-based foundation for the design guidance in this book. The research roots of that foundation are the knowledge fields and the professional/clinical practices of autism and of environmental design.[1] Neither of these fields has a long history of EBP, and each draws upon different ways of knowing, or what encapsulates "evidence." In developing our approach for a research-informed process to craft and empirically ground design goals and guidelines, we combined qualities and perspectives from each.

EBP in autism interventions

Given a history when doctors pointed to parental pathology – the "refrigerator moms" – as the source of autism, evidence-based approaches to diagnoses, causes, treatments, and interventions have for the most part been soundly welcomed in the autism community. Empirical research has allowed the field to move beyond testimonials and anecdotes based on fairly egregious information. National professional organizations, such as the American Academy of Pediatrics, have established guidelines for practices of early screening and diagnosis for ASD. Efforts to identify EBP for effective therapeutic and educational interventions have taken root in the last decade (for example, Mesibov and Shea, 2011; Giarelli and Gardner, 2012; McHugh and Barlow, 2012).

For example, in 2007 the Office of Special Education Programs in the U.S. Department of Education funded the National Professional Development Center on Autism Spectrum Disorders (NPDC) to cultivate the use of EBP in programs for infants, children, and youth with ASC and their families. To be considered an EB practice for individuals with ASD, the NPDC stipulates that one of the following needs to be met through peer-review research in scientific journals (Odom et al, 2010):

- two high quality experimental (randomized) or quasi-experimental group studies
- three different investigators or research groups must have conducted five high quality single subject design studies
- a combination of evidence, that includes one high quality randomized or quasi-experimental group design study *and* three high quality single subject design studies conducted by at least three different investigators or research groups

In addition to the NPDC project, five other systematic reviews of ASD interventions have been undertaken that are considered exemplars in the field (see Missouri Autism Guidelines Initiative, 2012, for list and description). By and large, all stipulate methodologies must employ either experimental or quasi-experimental research designs, whether group or single subject. For some, this methodological restriction is a rather frustrating threshold given that there is fairly limited scientific research on interventions and treatments, and what there is has almost exclusively focused on children and, to some extent, youth.

The EBP approach in autism intervention research is not without its critics. The population of people with autism is too heterogeneous and autism intervention programs too complex, they say, for an overall singular solution to be practical or informative. Some criticize the premise that randomized controlled trials are the only or best research methodology for autism intervention studies. In examining systematic reviews on EB interventions for autism, Mesibov and Shea (2011) note that the various reviewers examined different literature, used different definitions of 'evidence-based,' lumped or split interventions at different levels of specificity, and reached different conclusions. As they claim, "As a result, although there is *some* (although not universal) consensus about *some* aspects of interventions for *some* sub-groups of individuals with autism, particularly young children…there really is no agreement within the field about what constitutes effective, evidence-based treatment for the entire range of people with autism" (p. 119).

EBP in environmental design: evidence-based design

EBP in environmental design is relatively new. There is no established agenda for organizing, disseminating and advancing the state of knowledge of how good design is best employed to create long-term economic, social and human value in buildings. Empirical research does not have a long or pervasive history within environmental design practice except for structural, material and mechanical performances of buildings. And while there is a 50-year history of empirical research examining the effects of building characteristics on human perceptions, social interactions, health and human performance (that is, the field of environment-behavior studies or environmental design research), very little of this research actually directs the bulk of design and building decisions unless specifically embedded in building codes and regulations.

So, it is not simply a lack of empirical evidence that is a hurdle. By and large, environmental design – architecture in particular -- has not been an evidence-*seeking* culture. Many designers believe "evidence" is foreign to the design process (Brandt, Chong and Martin, 2010). While the field is replete with design awards and "best practices," most best practice profiles provide little evidence of what makes them "best" or even establishes the criteria for why they are judged so (Ahrentzen, 2006). Most design professionals are not educated as researchers, nor do they have familiarity with research methodologies. They may be unable to distinguish good, solid evidence from misinformation. They typically rely upon intuition and past project experience to make design choices. While experiential knowledge does have value within certain contexts and situations, it is limited and shaped by the individual practitioner.

This attitude within the profession is changing, slowly. Where this is most apparent is in the healthcare facility design field. There designers and researchers are promoting evidence-based design (EBD) and are convincing healthcare administrators to invest the time and money in EBD to build better buildings (Ulrich et al, 2008; Viets, 2009; Brandt, Chong and Martin, 2011). Based on EBP, for example, the American Institute of Architects required new acute care hospitals to include only single rooms in their 2006 *Guidelines for the Design and Construction of Health Care Facilities* which are used as a code or reference standard in most U.S. states and by the U.S. federal government. The U.S. Department of Defense requests that all design teams apply patient-centered and EBD principles across all military construction projects, affecting 77 hospitals, 500 clinics and 9.6 million people globally (Ulrich et al, 2008). With serious fiscal, liability, safety and health issues at stake, many architects and interior designers of healthcare facilities welcome the emerging research foundation on which to base design decisions (Hamilton, 2003).

Outside of healthcare facility design, however, EBD is in its infancy and there are endless debates of how to do rigorous research that is useful to practitioners and clients, the relative value of qualitative and quantitative methods, what criteria should be used to evaluate and define evidence, and other contentious issues (Ulrich et al, 2008). Although quantitative methods are used in much of the environmental design research and there is a growing body of rigorous studies related to healthcare design (Ulrich et al., 2008; Viets, 2009), research methods and approaches vary widely and there are very few with randomized controlled trials, systematic reviews, or meta-analyses.

In building and strengthening an evidence-based foundation for EBD, the healthcare design research community – organizationally represented by the Center for Health Design – has started to establish certain criteria for identifying "evidence." For example, a recent review of evidence-based research literature used the following selection criteria (Ulrich et al., 2008):

- The study should be empirically based and examine the influence of environmental characteristics on patient, family, or staff outcomes.
- The quality of the study is to be evaluated in terms of its research design and methods and whether the journal was peer-reviewed.

Another researcher commenting on EBD, Viets (2009) suggests three general sources for EBD:

- peer-reviewed quantitative studies
- peer-reviewed, triangulated qualitative studies
- traditional authority, which is less emphasized and should be approached and used with caution

Both of these approaches mandate peer-review publications. The peer-review process has its merits, as a check against researcher bias and conflict of interest, and an independent assessment of research integrity (Kassirer and Campion, 1994; Weller, 2001; Benos, 2007). But the peer-review criterion is a hurdle in environmental design research which has very few academic or scientific journals, only a fraction being peer-reviewed research ones (most serial publications are trade-oriented magazines). In addition, since practicing architects and designers rarely read academic journals, those researchers who want to disseminate their findings to practitioners are more likely to seek media venues that are more accessible to design professionals such as trade magazines, webinars and presentations at professional, non-academic conferences. A growing effort to disseminate peer-reviewed research findings to practitioners in an accessible version is *Research Design Connections* (researchdesignconnections.com), yet its readership is still only a small segment of the environmental design field.

Viets's (2009) inclusion of a cautious and judicious use of "traditional authority" in EBD places the "clinical expertise" component of the tripartite scheme of EBP (in Figure 2.1) not on an equal footing but a more transparent one. EBP in environmental design may be more open than other fields to explicitly recognizing and including the value of experience, in part because of the lack of peer-reviewed empirical research and research training in the field. Critics like Henry (2012) deride the non-scientific claims of architectural interventions assumedly beneficial to those with autism. Most of these derive from post-occupancy evaluations of a single case study, which because of their nature are fraught with potential selection bias and confounding factors. We believe that Viet's (2009) "traditional authority," single case studies, and non-experimental studies have to be examined and interpreted with a degree of vigilance and circumspection (as would experimental studies carried out in contrived settings and contexts). But under such scrutiny and with cautious interpretation and extrapolation, it may be that "untested" sources of information such as one's own personal experience (when extensive and reflective) and non peer-reviewed case studies can suggest solutions when empirical evidence is absent or scant, particularly when the issue does not present major health risks or personal harm. Further, such sources can be launching points for future scientific testing to determine whether such practices or "rules of thumb" have empirical merit. Importantly, these non-scientific findings – as well as those derived from solid empirical research – can be used as springboards for engaged discussion between design professionals, housing providers, and intended clients about the viability of design choices in light of the context of the place and the aspirations and needs of the occupants.

Our approach in this book

In developing the design goals and guidelines in this book, our intent was to ground them in research demonstrating how and what environmental features support or undermine adults on the spectrum. We faced a dilemma, however: a deficit of empirical research on residential environments for such individuals. There are only a handful of empirical studies that examine how the design or physical features of homes – or most settings for that matter – are responsive to the needs and aspirations of residents with ASC. And of this handful, only a small fraction has been published in peer-reviewed journals.

Yet architects, designers, housing providers, developers, counselors, parents and individuals themselves want to know what works best, and how to proceed in producing such housing before all the "evidence" comes in. Our hope is that more empirical studies are conducted and peer reviewed. But given the current track record, it will not be anytime soon at the scale needed to address the growing demand for such housing. An example of this quest is Daniel Silverstein, now an engineering student at Ohio State University, whose brother is on the spectrum. Daniel contacted us a few years ago. Working on his capstone project when a high school senior, Daniel had chosen to design a residential complex for adults. Even though he had lived with his brother his entire life, he wanted concrete, evidential information on which to base his design decisions. While he used our 2009 guidelines in the *Advancing full spectrum housing* report (Ahrentzen and Steele, 2009) and contacted us several times during his project with questions about issues not covered there, he came to realize that sometimes he simply had to make reasonable guesses of what would work effectively given the lack of research information. At those times he considered his brother's experiences, although Daniel realized that those singular experiences certainly did not represent the gamut of experiences of the intended residents. But designers, like physicians, do not have the luxury *not* to take action simply because there is not sufficient empirical evidence for the situation at hand. We hope that by the time Daniel finishes college and starts his career, there is more solid research and evaluation on which to make design decisions for him and for many others.

Until then and at this pioneering stage of EBD of autism-responsive settings, however, we crafted what we call a *research-informed approach* (RIA) that assessed and documented reliable sources of information and research at this point in time. We needed to balance three goals: (1) being comprehensive and inclusive, without prematurely eliminating resources that might provide valuable insights and directions (Wright et al, 2013); (2) creating a transparent process of search and selection that honed in on research and insight that demonstrated either research integrity or what educator Donald Schön (1983) calls "reflective practice" (explained further below); and (3) relevancy to a spectrum population of adults. We recognized early on that science's "gold standard" of double-blind, randomized experiments published in peer-reviewed journals was simply not available in environmental design research. Yet we also knew that other indicators of research integrity and relevance could be identified and used as guides.

Research integrity encompasses empirical research that follows a sound research methodology appropriate and relevant to the research domain (for example, ethnography, survey, quasi-experimental). In this sense, it follows the criterion of "credible research" in the EBD definition in healthcare facilities design described in an earlier section of this chapter. Instead of ruling out non-experimental research, we deemed non-experimental research approaches that followed a disciplined, well-crafted and documented methodology, such as ethnography, as important to understanding *in situ* everyday practices of those with autism. Such data and information is particularly key to understanding the environmental context of living in homes and communities (Solomon, 2010). It also is important in gaining the emic perspective, the worldview of those on the spectrum.

Relevancy was achieved when the research (1) identified and specified physical features of the residential built environment (interiors, housing structure, residential outdoor space, neighborhood components, for example); and (2) targeted or included adults with autism.

Honing in on just these two criteria, however, would still have left us with very little empirical research, particularly of relevancy. So we also considered empirical research of residential environments for *children* with autism, or for non-autistic adults *with other neurocognitive or neurodevelopmental conditions* that reflected, in part, similar symptoms or behavioral characteristics associated with ASC. Also included were building or equipment performance studies that were applicable (for example, decibel ratings of HVAC equipment when considering guidelines for sensory sensitivities). On a rare occasion we included studies pertaining to general populations when the issue was vital but we could not locate any research targeting individuals with ASC or other neurodevelopmental conditions.

We also made a decision, one that might be controversial within EBP fields, to consider statements and accounts of lived experiences and reflective practice. While empirical research is a guidepost, we believe that so is experts' reflective experience (see Hamilton, 2004, and Brandt, Chong and Martin 2010, for using a blend of experts' assessments and empirical research evidence in environmental design and architectural practices). Reflective practice involves paying critical attention to and reflecting on one's actions in a process of iterative learning. Recognizing the value of one's lived experience in a home and in a community, we wanted to incorporate the reflective thinking and practice of this lived experience by "experts" – not simply family members or professionals who have worked or lived with an adult with ASC for a period of time, but also autistic adults themselves. Since communication can be a challenge that many individuals on the spectrum face, this was not a simple matter of conducting a survey. Rather we considered reflections of how they experienced their physical world and built environment when written, profiled or translated in memoirs or videos. We discovered auto-ethnographic and biographical profiles of adults with autism that revealed insightful statements of the built environment context of their lives and activities. *Disability Studies Quarterly* (dsq-sds.org), for example, is an excellent source for such material. While the term "reflective practice" is typically applied to service professionals, such as architects and educators, we use this term to also refer to reflection of one's own lived experience in the built environment.

Our decision to seek and include such material reflects Duffy and Dorner's position (2011, 214) of recognizing and integrating more "first-person" accounts of autistic individuals who are "active agents of their own definition." Such accounts can greatly expand the conceptual thinking of much empirical research, and in so doing proffer an enriched sensibility of living in the residential environment with autism. Often holding a strengths-based viewpoint, these authors on the spectrum offer not just additional information but also an alternative and discerning perspective that goes beyond the disorder/deficit models underlying some of the more traditional bio-medical oriented and clinical research. As Wright and colleagues (2013, 58) note, individuals with autism are changing the perspective of the autistic condition, transforming it from "the autism landscape of 'cure' to 'community.'" Including this material allowed us not only to fill in knowledge gaps when empirical research was lacking, but also to provide a fresh perspective of this landscape of possibilities.

We had no elaborate rating system for ranking or weighing the relative contribution of different pieces of evidence, as is being done in EBP of autism interventions. The strength of the evidence – how much one can rely on the data to predict design impacts – is critical for application. But there is simply a lack of research standards and protocols necessary for widespread development, application and dissemination; and – as mentioned earlier – a deficit of empirical research to even consider "adding" and "weighing" one or more studies. Lacking metrics to establish the strength of evidence, we knew it was necessary to provide credible, straightforward and clear documentation of how and what we gathered and used to craft our design goals and guidelines (described in the next section of this chapter).

This book, and its quality of life design goals and guidelines, is not a mandate. The guidelines are not intended for rote application. Rather, following the tripartite scheme presented earlier in the chapter, these recommendations and guideposts should be used by housing and design professionals in conjunction with intended residents. We thus tried to advance a collaborative approach, advocated by many in the neurodiversity movement, of basing these design goals and guidelines on the work of professional researchers, reflective practitioners, and autistic adults themselves in order to achieve meaningful solutions to challenges of autism in adulthood (Robertson, 2010; Wright et al, 2013). We see the book as an insightful, seasoned and reflexive partner in making decisions about designing, constructing, remodeling, and planning residential settings that work best for various individuals on the spectrum. It is itself at the adolescent stage of its lifespan of design research, one that will grow and flourish as it continues to experiment, expand and be examined in the years ahead.

Since we include both empirical research and reflective practice as source material, we call this a "research informed" approach instead of an evidence-based one. Doing so implies that research is also needed to systematically analyze and understand the clients' needs, aspirations, and situations. How this self- or client-analysis research can be used to better understand the appropriateness of the various design guidelines in this book is further explained in Chapter Three.

The remaining sections of this chapter describe our process of identifying and selecting informational resources that form the foundation of the design goals and guidelines of the book. A list categorizing these resources is available in the Appendix. Full bibliographic sources are included in the references.

Search protocol

A broad search was undertaken to identify relevant research, studies, and accounts in databases pertinent to autism interventions and to environmental design research. We began by searching through several electronic databases, including ProQuest, EBSCOhost, Google Scholar, Avery Index to Architectural Periodicals, Social Sciences Abstracts and Full Text, and PubMed. Search terms we used are listed in the Sidebar. As Wright and colleagues (2013, 23) similarly discovered, "the beauty of the serendipity of the search process is that it renders further connections." We not only examined relevant articles derived from these searches of databases, we also pursued studies that cited these. We were only able to select English-language studies.

In our cascading search process, we also discovered essays and non-empirical articles that referenced empirical studies; we examined these sources as well. Websites of over 100 organizations, agencies, and research institutions involved in autism or developmental disabilities were checked for relevant source materials. A few of these organizations compiled bibliographies and reference lists on housing for those with ASC; these also were consulted and references followed. Index searching of relevant journals in the autism field – notably *Autism, Autism Insights, Autism Research, Journal of Autism and Developmental Disorders, Research in Autism Spectrum Disorder* – was also

Search terms included:

Asperger's,
autism, autism
spectrum disorders,
cognitive disability,
developmental disability

AND

architecture, design,
environment, home,
housing, interior design,
residence, residential

conducted. We looked at various online communities operated and used by bloggers on the spectrum, such as Autistic Self Advocacy Network, for source material. There are also a number of books and videos authored, co-authored or produced by adults with ASC. Those with insightful statements about their engagement with and feelings about the built and landscaped environment were considered and included in our listing.

In addition, we identified several housing developments or homes that targeted adults with ASC, either exclusively or with other populations. Our method of identifying and selecting these "case studies" is described in our earlier report *Advancing full spectrum housing* (Ahrentzen and Steele, 2009). However there have been several developed since that 2009 report that we were able to identify. Of these places, we visited and toured the development, and spoke to the director, staff and, when available, with residents and/or family members. We took photographs of physical features that came up in conversations, or that we felt were important to the design goals that were emerging. In some cases we were not physically able to visit the site, and we held phone conversations with staff and received photo-documentation from them (as well as other print or electronic material of relevance). These were not rigidly structured interviews, but we did develop an interview guide to make sure various topics/issues were brought up consistently.

Even with this intensive literature and source search, we recognize that we did not exhaust and exhume every published or public document pertaining to residential environments for adults on the spectrum. We are encouraged by the growth of publications addressing adults with ASC in the last couple years alone – indeed, even in the last few months before this book went to press. Nonetheless, we are confident that our process and diligence surfaced some of the most exemplary findings and insights of adults living at home with autism.

Assessing source information

We divided the source material into two groups: empirically-based and reflective practice. For the empirical source materials, we considered and incorporated material when a study met the characteristics listed in the Sidebar. Research of poor methodological integrity was discarded; however, a small sample size was not considered a deficiency of sound methodology.

In selecting reflective practice material, the documents were much less numerous than one might expect since the document had to address, in part, reactions to residential settings or the built environment. Some of the information was from written sources, such as manuals or blogs; and some was from personal or verbal communication with the authors, including those observations and interviews during our case study visits.

In drawing upon this material for our design goals and guidelines, we selected those insights and experiences when it was expressed by more than one expert or by a committee or commission. Further, we acknowledged two types of experts. *Practitioners* included professionals or support providers in autism-related services, education, or care with years of experience, particularly in residential living. But experts were also those individuals on the spectrum who were able to express their experiences about their living environments; these we call *self-advocates.*

Documenting source information

Once source material was selected and assessed, we needed to document its particular relevance and contribution to the development of the quality of life design goals and guidelines. Each source document was marked for its application to each of these ten goals, and whether it pertained to identifying appropriate design guidelines, substantiating the design goal, or both. Each source was also characterized by the relevancy of the population: adults with autism; children or teens with autism; those with non–autism but having similar behaviors/symptoms; general population. These are documented in the Appendix.

In addition, the process of developing the design guidelines included a comprehensive review, analysis, and integration of research material as it corresponded not only to quality of life design goals but also to: the particular spaces or areas of the dwelling (and immediate surroundings); the particular design feature at issue; supporting reason for its applicability; and, when relevant, its sustaining nature. These references are also included in the Appendix.

Selection criteria for source information

1. empirically derived and with at least partial focus and measure of the residential environment, with sound methodology appropriate to the research domain (e.g. survey, ethnographic) and including a sample of adults with ASC

2. same as #1 but instead of residential environment, another environment (e.g. school) was examined

3. same as #1 but instead of adults with ASC, adults with other relevant neurobiological or neurocognitive conditions, or youth with ASC

4. same as #1 but instead of adults with ASC, sample is typical or general population; used only for salient design issues when no research reflecting #1, 2, or 3 above was available

5. building systems, materials or landscape performance research in which occupant information is unnecessary

Note

[1] In this book, the term "environmental design" encompasses architectural, interior, urban, and landscape design.

THREE
QUALITY OF LIFE DESIGN GOALS

The homes and neighborhoods where adults with autism live may significantly affect the quality of their lives. Yet most housing providers, developers, architects and sometimes even family members are unaware of how specific residential features and neighborhood amenities can affect the comfort, pleasure and well-being of those on the spectrum. Designers and housing providers need to know how best to foster and create autism-friendly environments and how residents can be supported to not only live but thrive in their homes and communities. Optimal design and neighborhood selection at the outset can help avoid later problems that may require a subsequent move, which could prove difficult for residents who need stability and consistency in their lives.

As previously mentioned, there is no single "type" of autism. Likewise, there is no single type of housing solution. In order to let potential residents as well as housing providers and architects decide which housing features may work best for whom, we developed ten quality of life design goals, crafted from a synthesis of available research. Residences and neighborhoods should be designed and selected to facilitate opportunities for residents to realize those goals. Most of these goals – foster health and wellness, ensure safety and security, for example – pertain to any individual, with autism or not. However, *how* these goals are achieved and *what they mean* to those on the spectrum may be quite different or unexpected from what an architect or housing provider has encountered in prior experiences with neurotypical clients. The pleasure of "being social" by sitting quietly in the same room with someone else, not communicating or interacting but engrossed in one's own pursuit or activity, may not appear to be very enriching social behavior to an architect familiar with designing college student residence halls. In fact, it may remind the architect more of children who engage in "parallel play" than of adults "being social." But having a quiet place for such "parallel play" may be much more desirable for a spectrum adult than being in a lounge with many others who are bellowing at a missed touchdown pass as they watch a football game on a large-screen monitor.

The challenges facing those on the spectrum do not simply reside in human neurology. Challenges exist in legislation, within policy arenas, among cultural beliefs and practices, in educational and employment settings, within our communities at large, and in the physical environments where we live, work and play (Dicker and Bennett, 2011; Lin et al, 2011; Rydzewska, 2012; Yudell et al, 2012). Housing providers and architects need to know how best to create autism-friendly environments and how residents can be supported to manage in their homes and their wider communities with dignity, productivity, purpose and pleasure.

Good design and community access is also critical for support providers since the quality of care, and their desire to continue their service, can be facilitated in part by the environment in which they work and the resources available to them. Not only does turnover of support providers result in considerable financial costs, it can trigger behavioral and emotional upheavals among residents as well (United States Department of Health and Human Services, 2004). The more that support providers feel the environment strengthens them in their work and allows them opportunity for respite and restoration, the more likely they will be to stay in their positions (Strouse et al, 2003).

In identifying and developing these quality of life design goals, we moved away from a singular focus on rectifying "impairments" often associated with autism. Granted, there is a need to recognize how health problems can be ameliorated, and at the very least not exacerbated, by the environmental qualities of the spaces we inhabit. But we did not want to frame these quality of life goals within a dominant medical perspective, as mentioned in the first chapter. The goals emanate from a broader perspective and scholarship that embraces "positive biology," "positive psychology," and "positive or humanistic neurology" which recognizes autism not as a disease or developmental disorder, but as a spectrum of behavioral and health patterns deserving of rich and supportive environmental conditions that can facilitate self-fulfillment for those on the spectrum (Seligman, 2011; Farrelly, 2012; Wright et al, 2013).

This approach is relatively new terrain within autism research and interventions. A person-in-environment (PIE) approach offers a dynamic and broad framework for identifying "successful" or desirable outcomes that encompass both subjective and objective characterizations of independence and functional abilities (Henninger and Taylor, 2012); and seeks to discover how individuals interact with conditions of the social environment to effect or provide opportunities for those outcomes to be realized (Pelphrey et al, 2011; Wright et al, 2013). We expand this PIE orientation by emphasizing the physical environment as well.

Most of the research on ASC focuses on impairments, treatment modalities, psychopathology, developmental disabilities and individual limitations (Sigman, Spence and Wang, 2006; Brugha et al, 2011). Few lines of research – and most of this is relatively recent – focus on positive attributes and potentials, or quality of life (Renty and Roeyers, 2006; Jordan and Caldwell-Harris, 2012; Kamio, Inada and Koyama, 2012; Wright et al, 2013). The latter is slowly emerging in academic and professional research, but it is much more pronounced in books, blogs and videos produced and authored by individuals on the spectrum. To the extent possible, the quality of life design goals reflect *general* ways in which the designed environment can enhance and optimize residents' needs and predilections. In some instances the design goals may overlap; and sometimes even conflict with one another. Nevertheless, an understanding of such goals can sensitize those who wish to create meaningful and suitable homes to the ways in which our physical surroundings can play a role. They should also be key considerations when quality control or cutbacks in construction, design or materials are being debated, to better recognize behavioral and health consequences for residents of such trade-off decisions.

The ten quality of life design goals described in this chapter establish a basis for the design guidelines of Chapter Four. Each goal is associated with its own icon, which facilitates identifying those design guidelines in Chapter Four that are particularly responsive to specific goals.

What follows will not apply to everyone. Particular design features can be experienced differently among individuals. Clearly, there is no one perfect model. We advocate a range of options so that individual circumstances, needs and inclinations can be accommodated. The aim of these design goals and subsequent guidelines is to provide a robust platform that architects, housing providers, families, support providers and residents can use to identify and select design features that best respond to needs and aspirations of various individuals on the spectrum.

 ## Ensure safety and security

Ensuring that residents sustain no harm is the first priority of any home. Safety and security risks in residential structures are typically covered in building codes (for example, handrails and bannisters on stairways), with no specific attention on persons with unique conditions or needs. Minimizing opportunities for criminal behavior in our homes and communities is the thrust of Crime Prevention Through Environmental Design (CPTED) a strategy promoted in many law enforcement jurisdictions throughout the U.S. and Europe (for example, Armitage, 2013; Fennelly and Crowe, 2013). CPTED is intended to reduce crime opportunities and to promote witnesses reporting criminal activities by incorporating design features that promote *natural surveillance* (placement of physical features that maximize visibility, such as strategic use of windows that look out to a building entrance); *access management* (guiding people by using signs and well-marked entrances and exits, as well as limiting access to certain areas by using real or symbolic barriers); *territoriality* (a clear delineation of space, expressions of pride or ownership, and the creation of a welcoming environment); *physical maintenance* that demonstrates general upkeep and sense of ownership and protection of a place; *order maintenance* (attending to minor unacceptable acts and providing measures that clearly state acceptable behavior); and *target-hardening mechanisms* such as locks and electronic surveillance systems. While CPTED has been supported strongly by law enforcement agencies, whether individuals with autism will similarly "read" environmental cues that convey a person's territory, or other CPTED factors, is still an unknown. (The role the environment plays in becoming familiar with and supported by one's neighbors is also relevant to enhancing security and safety, and is described in a later quality of life goal, Ensuring Accessibility and Support in the Surrounding Neighborhood).

In addition to basic life safety factors and criminal threats, there are, however, other safety and security issues of concern to those in the autism community, particularly the potential of self-injury and injury to others, and elopement and wandering. Also, how physical spaces may enhance a sense of security to those intimidated or threatened by social situations is of relevance to many of those on the spectrum.

The potential for self-injury is of particular concern because high rates of seizures are documented among children and adolescents with autism, with estimates varying between 22 percent to 30 percent (Olsson Steffenburg and Gillberg, 1988; Kawasaki et al, 1997; Tuchman and Rapin, 2002; Kogan et al, 2008; Tuchman, Moshe and Rapin, 2009). These rates of seizures in ASC are about ten times higher than rates in the general population, and much higher than those found among individuals with other neurologic conditions such as schizophrenia (Hyde and Weinberger, 1997; Theoharides and Zhang, 2011). Seizures can result in unintentional self-injury, from falls and from crashes into walls, counters, furniture, and fixtures.

While almost all of these studies focus on children and teens, a recent long-term study in Britain of young adults aged 21 years and older found that 22 percent had epilepsy, with the majority of them having their first seizures after ten years of age. For some, seizures did not appear until adulthood (Bolton et al, 2011). In over half of these individuals, seizures occurred weekly or less frequently; and for the majority, seizures were controlled with anticonvulsant medications.

Individuals on the spectrum who have difficulties with balance, postural stability, gait, joint flexibility and movement are also at risk for self-injury. A higher percentage of children with ASC have such motor conditions than is found in the population at large (Manjoiviona and Prior, 1995; Ghaziuddin and Butler, 1998; Page and Boucher, 1998; Minshew et al, 2004; Jansiewics et al, 2006; Green et al, 2008). While no similar prevalence assessments of motor and balance difficulties have been made for adults on the spectrum, it is likely that some difficulties continue into adulthood for many. Among those with epilepsy or motor/balance control difficulties, accidents and movement in the home becomes particularly problematic. Selecting furniture and materials that are resilient to "soft landings and bumps" may help reduce bruises, cuts, scrapes and the like. There is extensive environmental design research and recommendations for deterrence of falls among older adults, as well as for reducing the extent of injury should a fall occur (see Pynoos et al, 2012). Many of the design guidelines in Chapter Four draw upon this research since there is an absence of fall prevention research on adults with ASC.

The potential for injury also resides among those individuals with what clinicians call "challenging behaviors": aggression/destruction, disruptive behavior, self-injurious behavior and stereotypy (Matson and Rivet, 2008). Longitudinal research indicates that challenging behaviors tended to decline with age although it still persisted (Murphy et al, 2005). In studies of adults with autism and intellectual disability living in large residential facilities, the frequency of challenging behaviors increased with severity of autistic symptoms, suggesting that for many adults living in such places, self-injury or injury to their surroundings remains a potential occurrence. Still unknown is whether this pattern exists among those living in smaller and community-oriented settings or whether early intensive behavioral interventions have diminished the risk of challenging behaviors carrying over into adulthood. There is some indication that challenging behaviors may be unlikely to disappear without treatment (Matson and Rivet, 2008).

Self-injury also may result among those who need assistance with basic self-care, such as taking a shower or brushing their teeth. Since accidents in the home – especially those involving motor and balance conditions – often occur in bathrooms, kitchens and stairs (Lowry, 1990; Graham and Firth, 1992), selection and placement of appliances and fixtures need to be carefully considered to prevent injury among those with balance problems or a tendency to fall. Determining the amount of bathroom space needs to take into account that a support provider may be accompanying the resident. Many effective design strategies, such as non-scalding water fixtures, come from recommendations for assisted care and senior living residences. Most of these are not based on systematic research studies but from hands-on experiences of support staff and administrators with home care and independent living training (National Research Council, 2011; Greenhouse, 2012).

Elopement and wandering present another facet of security and safety. Wandering or elopement is the tendency for an individual to try to leave the care of a responsible person or of a safe area, sometimes resulting in potential harm or injury. Reasons for elopement remain speculative. Do those who wander do so because they are escaping a social or environmentally stimulating situation that is unbearable? Are they seeking places that have greater appeal? Are they just wanting to move or engage in some form of unstructured exercise? (Anderson et al, 2012). While still speculative, it may be that elopement is pleasing, even purposeful. As Naoki Higashida (2013), the author of *The reason I jump: The inner voice of a thirteen-year-old boy with autism*, claims: "Sometimes people say that I'm very good at running away, but really it's just that when someone's chasing me, I find it both funny and frightening when the chaser is catching up to me." Since many individuals on the spectrum have engrossing fascinations and interests, wanting to walk to places where they can pursue these interests may be an impetus – such as Lori McIlwain's son who had an irresistible attraction to highway exit signs, and one day walked from his house to a local highway to look at them (McIlwain, 2013).

Within autism research, studies of elopement primarily focus on young children. The extent to which it occurs among adults on the spectrum is entirely speculative. However, dementia research has a long history of studying wandering among older adults with Alzheimer's and other forms of dementia. This research and characterization of the nature and scope of wandering (for example, Zeisel et al, 2003; Algase et al, 2009) has helped identify environmental features that can facilitate and direct purposeful wandering in safe areas, such as visually engaging paths around the home dotted with points of interests and ending with identifiable destinations (Zeisel and Tyson, 1999; Fleming and Purandare, 2010; van Hoof et al, 2010; Edwards et al, 2012; Zeisel, 2013). Controlling access to the home or yard may be necessary for those who tend to wander and are unaware of potentially dangerous situations on public streets. Environmental design research focusing on wandering behavior of those with dementia suggests ways to do this without "imprisoning" residents or making them feel that way. While there are many characteristics of dementia that do not correspond to autism, design guidance for enhancing security among those who wander does have particular relevance.

Finally, while it is important for the home to "do no harm," the residence should not be perceived as a minefield. Too many manuals on independent living make it seem that threats are lurking around every corner of the house. Indeed, how we feel about our home surroundings should reflect a sense of security that is akin to comfort. The popular phrase "home-sweet-home" suggests that a sense of security derives from being surrounded by family and friends. But for some of those on the spectrum, these feelings or experiences may likewise derive from the more stable physical attributes of the residence itself.

From analyzing autobiographies and interviews of adults with autism, researchers Stijn Baumers and Ann Heylighen (2010; 2014) note that for some people on the spectrum the physical entity of space "offers a grip," as they call it. Physical features are visible, tangible, and understandable components of their immediate environment; and as such, they can provide a sense of certainty and confidence unlike entities that are not directly perceptible, such as feelings or expectations of people. Physical entities can become anchorages to the world. An example is a statement from Birger Sellin's 1993 autobiography: "Because of important reasons I can find safety only in things. People are incalculable and distinct monsters." Or this statement from Liane H Willey: "Whenever things became too fuzzy or too loud or too distracting; whenever I began to feel as though I would come unraveled, I knew I could crawl into my alcove and crunch up into it until I felt as square and symmetrical as the alcove itself" (Baumers and Heylighen, 2010). Much of this "grip," or sense of security, may derive from the clarity and predictability of elements of the physical world, to which we turn in the next quality of life goal.

◆

In sum, in addition to addressing basic life safety factors and criminal threats, residential design should also enhance security and safety by selecting materials, furnishings and design features that minimize falls, slips, and imbalance, and reduce the extent of injury should such occur. Controlling access to and from the residence and surrounding outdoor space needs to skillfully minimize features that result in feelings of "imprisonment" or unnecessarily restrict resident's choice and autonomy. Meaningful places to wander and explore under safe circumstances provide opportunities for productive exploration and exercise. Also, the design of the residence should be crafted to help anchor residents' sense of security through attachment to familiar physical objects and spaces.

 ## Maximize familiarity, stability, predictability and clarity

Many adults with autism seek a sense of order and familiarity in their surroundings, as evidenced by statements in the Sidebar. Autism researchers have interpreted expressions like these – of living in a visually or cognitively fragmented world, of seeking a sense of order and clarity in that world, of being comforted by familiar settings – as consequences of the way the brain is "wired" for perceptual functioning or executive functioning (EF). When this system is not working typically, adapting to changes in everyday life can be difficult (Frith, 2003). Some studies show that EF does not operate as effectively in individuals with autism above 16 years of age as it does with their developmentally typical peers (Pennington and Ozonoff, 1996; Hill, 2004; Geurts, Corbett and Solomon, 2009; Geurts and Vissers, 2012).

EF is usually couched in deficit terms in autism research. Other perspectives frame

Recollections of stability, fragmentation and clarity from those on the spectrum

"…I came to recognize and accept certain autistic traits in myself, chief among which was a strong attachment to familiar people, places, and things. I felt safe and secure living back in my hometown, even though my childhood friends had long since grown up and moved away. Walking down streets on which I had biked as a child and shopping at stores where I had shopped for years kept my inner chaos at bay. When people asked me why I did not go back to the city to look for a "real" job, I replied that I was needed here to care for an elderly aunt. In truth, it was the other way around. My elderly aunt was taking care of me."

(Charli Devnet, a New York tour guide and legal freelancer on the spectrum. In Grandin, 2012, 36)

"Small changes in routine can disrupt my entire day. Also, transitions are extremely difficult for me at times. Even today, I can have significant trouble with this. With regard to inflexibility, I have preconceived ideas of how things are going to work in any given situation, and when they don't meet my expectations, I can become quiet and snappish. In all honesty, I am very easygoing when I am comfortable with my environment. It's when I get anxious or tired that I become more rigid in my thinking."

(Sean Jackson, a Kentucky real-estate executive on the spectrum. In Grandin, 2012, 347)

> "Whatever object we spin, this is always true. Unchanging things are comforting, and there's something beautiful about that."
>
> (Thirteen-year old Naoki Higashida, 2013)

> "Our brains are wired differently… I take over a thousand pictures of a person's face when I look at them. That's why we have a hard time looking at people."
>
> (Carly Fleishmann, who began typing her thoughts and expressions as a teenager after years of being non-verbal. From: http://abcnews.go.com/2020/MindMoodNews/story?8258204&page=1)

such behaviors as *strong systemitizing*, a highly adaptive human ability (Baron-Cohen et al, 2009), or as *enhanced perceptual functioning* (EPF), a term coined by a group of researchers in Canada including Michelle Dawson who is herself autistic (Mottron et al, 2006). EPF suggests that autism may result from enhanced perception of low-level perceptual information and attention to detail (O'Connor and Kirk, 2008). And much research (Happé and Frith, 2006) and autobiographical accounts (for example, Birch, 2003; Grandin, 1995; Higashida, 2013) confirms that many individuals with autism are superior to their typically developing peers at processing details. For these individuals, enhanced attention to details can dominate or supersede the whole gestalt of a scene, its central coherence: in a sense, it means not being unable to see the forest for the trees (Armstrong, 2010).

Debilitating or enhancing, productive or counter-productive? The *situation* when this behavior or cognitive processing occurs, and what the individual is wishing to accomplish or experience within that situation, makes this enhanced or selective attention meaningful – whether that be frustrating, exhilarating, insightful, confusing, or inhibiting.

Recognizing that residents may be extremely attentive to the myriad details of a space rather than the gestalt of it, that they desire the comfort of continuity instead of stimulation of change, that they may gravitate to ritualistic behaviors involving a spatial object, that the transfer of skills and activities from one setting to another may not be smooth and simple – recognizing these and similar behaviors can help architects and housing providers enhance residential settings for these individuals.

Also, environmental stress research contributes to our understanding of how the physical environment can be manipulated to reduce or manage information or cognitive overload, particularly along the lines of perceptual or informational input (sensory inputs are addressed in a separate quality of life goal). The overload model of stress maintains that too much information or environmental input produces stress by taxing the information-processing system of the individual. In their evaluations of residential settings for adults with autism in Aberdeen, Scotland, researchers Sergeant and colleagues (2007) observed that changes in routines, structure and support staff could result in increased anxiety for individuals with ASC. They speculated that these individuals may be receiving an overload of information or stimulation when such changes occurred, resulting at times in increased anxiety, depression or outward displays of aggression or self-injurious behavior.

In addition, there are also accounts of adults on the spectrum favoring smaller spatial volumes (for example, Temple Grandin, Donna Williams), with large, unfamiliar and complex spaces producing anxiety. In his memoir *Born on a blue day,* writer and savant, Daniel Tammet (2007), speaks of his experiences in supermarkets: "I would regularly switch off and become anxious and uncommunicative because of the size of the store, the large numbers of people and amount of stimuli around me…The solution was to go instead to smaller, local shops, which are much more comfortable for me to use."

To cope with environmental stress, various adaptive strategies are employed: filtering or blocking inputs, increasing routinized habitual behavior, or attempting to redefine the source of information (such as Tammet going to smaller shops), to name a few (Evans, 1982). Environmental design researchers have identified a number of physical qualities of settings that can effectively reduce or manage such overload by providing coherence, affordance, control and restoration (Evans and Cohen, 1987; Evans and McCoy, 1998). Some of the design guidelines in Chapter Four draw upon this research when applicable.

Environmental stress researchers, such as Sheldon Cohen (1978), argue that information overload can be affected more by the *meaning* of the environmental stressor than by the intensity of the physical element itself. Cohen contends that predictability and controllability of the stressor and one's expectancies about its effects are important factors in interpreting a situation as stressful, and in designing environments that allow the occupant the opportunity to manage and have control. Take, for example, the situation described by Kinnaer and colleagues (2014) of an autistic child who does not enter a room through a closed door since he cannot see what is behind it. The child needs to know what is behind the door before considering whether to open it and enter the adjoining room. A closed door does not provide this needed information.

As a form of non-verbal communication, physical environments "tell" us something about the places we are in, about the people who live or work there (Rapoport, 1990). Messages we "read" might involve personal identity, social relationships, affect, or what we are expected to do there (Ahrentzen, 2002). Just as verbal or sign language can be the basis for communication as long as the grammar and linguistic structure is known and shared among individuals, so too with non-verbal communication such as that conveyed through environmental cues (Rapoport, 1990).

One meaning of a space we inhabit is its function. But, commonly, a single room in a home has multiple functions. A clear example is the kitchen in North American and Western European cultures. Kitchens are primarily built and used for making meals and cleaning up after meals. But they are also places for socializing during family and friend get-togethers or for children's play. For many persons, understanding these multiple functions of a space is learned through acculturation and socialization. But it may not be the case with those who process such environmental information in a more restricted or focused manner. An example is a situation encountered by Baumers and Heylighen (2010) in their participant observation research of a residential facility for people with developmental disabilities. When one woman on the spectrum discovered the researcher in the hallway writing down notes, she reprimanded him to go to the living room to sit and write. He was violating the primary function of the corridor. Writing notes, sitting and reading were acceptable behaviors in the living room. Hallways were for moving from one space to another.

The environment then is a form of non-verbal communication relaying "messages" – such as the function of a place – but only among those acculturated to read and interpret those messages similarly. Conversely, it may be the case that autistic people attend to information, including environmental messages or input, according to what *they* think important, regardless of whether it holds the same value or content of what neurotypical people think important in a setting (Bogdashina, 2003).

What is interesting is that environmental design researchers have found that compatibility between a room and its primary function is a prominent factor in reducing agitation among those with dementia. Design of dining rooms or other shared common spaces that reflect their intended, primary use encourages appropriate behavior in these settings (Zeisel, 2013). That design is reflected in the scale of the space, the type and style of furnishings, and features and fixtures that are compatible with its primary function. When physical settings and activities taking place there both "communicate" what is appropriate behavior, persons with neurological conditions such as dementia are more likely to behave appropriately. Zeisel and other environmental design researchers working with older adults with dementia have crafted design guidelines that address these considerations; and once again we have drawn upon these when they seem applicable to those on the spectrum in achieving a sense of clarity, familiarity, and predictability in their residential environments.

◆

In sum, potential for environmental overload and divergent interpretations of environmental cues can be addressed by design that fosters coherence, clarity, predictability, control and restoration. Functional clarity of rooms or residential spaces with their primary or functional purpose may help diminish confusion of what is appropriate behavior or use of those spaces. The scale of space, type and style of furnishings, fixtures and features play a role in clarifying environmental "messages."

 ### Enhance sensory balance

The new DSM-5 diagnostic criteria for autism spectrum disorders includes sensory disturbances in addition to the long-running symptoms of communication and social deficits that has defined the diagnosis for decades. Including these in the diagnosis reflects the overwhelming numbers of spectrum individuals who report being hypersensitive, hyposensitive, or a combination of both to sensory inputs (Marco et al, 2011; Stevenson et al, 2014). Indeed, an estimated 90 percent of those with autism have sensory conditions that can be characterized as oversensitivity, unresponsiveness, or sensory-seeking behaviors, with the most common sensitivities involving olfaction and touch (Woo and Leon, 2013). These range broadly, from being sensitive to labels on clothing, to the color orange or to phone rings, to name just a few of many examples (for example, Williams, 1991; Grandin, 1995; Wilson, 2008).

While there is some evidence that such sensory sensitivities occur across all ages and IQ levels (Watling, Deitz and White, 2001; Kern et al, 2007; Leekam et al, 2007; Tomcheck and Dunn, 2007; Ben-Sasson et al, 2009; Hilton et al, 2010; Woo and Leon, 2013), there is also evidence that hypo- and hypersensitivity to auditory process, visual processing and hypersensitivity to touch become more like those of neurotypical adults with increasing age; only hyposensitivity to touch seems to remain unchanged (O'Neill and Jones, 1997; Kern et al, 2006). Researchers do not know what will happen as individuals on the spectrum approach their senior years when a general decline in sensory processing, especially for hearing and vision, is common among aging adults (Happé and Charlton, 2010; Saxon, Etten and Perkins, 2010; Perkins and Berkman, 2012).

Many designers and housing providers assume those on the spectrum who will be living in their residences will be *hypersensitive*, that is with acute, heightened or excessive sensitivities to sound, textures, colors or other sensory stimuli. But individuals may also be *hyposensitive*, not getting sufficient sensory stimulation. Take, for example, John Robison (2007). In his memoir *Look me in the eye*, he recalls the many years he worked for and relished the concerts of the band KISS, designing their special-effects programs and instruments including the legendary fire-breathing guitars.

A video by Miguel Jiron (2013) provides an insightful glimpse into what these sensory experiences are like for those with autism, and how they may affect everyday life (http://anim.usc.edu/videos/sensory-overload-interacting-with-autism-project-by-miguel-jiron/). This video was created as part of Mark Jonathan Harris' and Marsha Kinder's "Interacting with Autism" series, a three-year transmedia project funded by the U.S.'s Agency for Health Research and Quality (AHRQ), with a team of filmmakers and artists developing an interactive, video-intensive website on understanding autism. Table 3.1, from this Project, provides a useful profile of hyper- and hypo-sensory conditions experienced by many on the spectrum.

The distress caused by particular sensory stimuli may be internalized until it overwhelms an individual – resulting sometimes in self-injurious and aggressive behavior, particularly among those unable to communicate their duress (Marco et al, 2011). Those who are hyposensitive may react by actions that create their necessary stimulation. Sensory researcher Bogdashina (2003) claims that autistic individuals often describe their stims as defensive mechanisms from hyper- or hyposensitivity.

Clinical interventions conventionally focus on sensory integration, sensory-based interventions (for example, massage, brushing) and auditory integration training (Case-Smith and Arbesman, 2008). Ethnographic research has turned a keen eye to the sensory-based environment of everyday settings. Such investigations generally reflect the perspective of the disability rights movement that it is not the individual

Table 3.1: Sensory sensitivities often occurring with autism

	Over-responsive	Under-responsive	Seeking out sensation
Tactile	Dislikes being touched or hugged, hair cut or washing, teeth brushing, nail clipping; avoids touching messy substances; complains about tags and/or seams in clothing	A hard fall causes no reaction; not always aware of touch	Bumps into people or furniture to get physical contact / sensation; seeks out messy substances such as finger paints
Auditory	Puts hands over ears to block out sound; shows extreme fear to sounds like vacuum, sirens, toilet flushing, coffee grinder and so on	Difficult to get child's attention; seems oblivious when spoken to; does not look around for the source of sounds	Craves loud noise or music; likes to talk, hum or make noise
Movement and motor planning	Afraid of heights; dislikes spinning, swinging or sliding; needs continuous physical support from an adult	Does not object to being moved, but does not initiate movement; once movement starts, can keep going for a long time; does not realize he is falling and makes no attempt to break fall	Needs to keep moving as much as possible; may repeatedly shake head, rock back and forth or jump up and down; craves intense movement experiences such as bouncing on furniture; likes active play (teeter-totter, swinging)
Visual	Overwhelmed by moving objects or people; avoids direct eye contact; complains of sunlight or that lights are too bright; may squint in ordinary light	Unaware of light/dark contrast; unaware of movement; bumps into moving objects; delayed response to visual information, such as an obstacle in his path	Seeks visual stimulation, such as finger flicking or spinning; seeks bright lights, including direct sunlight; stares at moving fans
Olfactory (smell)	Complains of strong odors or smells that may not be evident to others	Not responsive to typically offensive odors	Seeks strong smells; sniffs everything, including hair and clothing
Food taste or texture	Aversion to certain tastes/textures of foods; gags often	Easts most foods; no reaction to unusual textures or tastes	Licks nonfood objects; seeks items to put in mouth
Proprioception, vestibular (orientation in space, balance)	Prefers not to move; avoids weight-bearing activities such as running, jumping	Awkward motor movement abilities; fatigues easily; appears weak, floppy, loose-limbed; poor grip; has low tone	Bumps or crashes into objects or people; rubs hands on tables; craves active movement, such as pushing, pulling; likes being squeezed or swaddled
Interoception (internal body stimuli)	Tantrums easily when hungry or thirsty; prefers wearing as little clothing as possible	Unaware of hunger, thirst, toileting needs; no sense of satiation; will keep eating beyond hunger; oblivious to body temperature (will not remove jacket if too warm)	Craves strong taste, such as very spicy or sour; may prefer foods (or bathwater) to be either very hot or very cold

(Adapted with permission from Dr. Ricki Robinson, "Autism Solutions," Harris and Kinder (2013), "Interacting with Autism," Miguel Jiron, artist) who is disabled, but the environment that disables the individual. From this work and perspective, lessons can be drawn for designing the residential environment, such as from the ethnographic work of Kinnaer and colleagues (2014).

Given variation among individuals, architects and housing providers should strive for *balance* of sensory experiences when providing housing with multiple occupants. Having a myriad of different spaces – each with its own level of stimulating features – allows alternatives for residents to choose those spaces that work best for them. Another approach is to create a sensory-neutral residence where visual, acoustic, olfactory and tactile qualities of a setting can be easily modulated to suit a resident's particular preferences and to eliminate their sensory dislikes (Brand and Gaudion, 2012). It is easier to add a stimulating but moveable object like a painting or iPod, than to remove a feature that is relatively permanent or structurally embedded.

This approach is illustrated in a design research project in London, sponsored by the Helen Hamlyn Centre for Design at the Royal College of Art in London and the Kingwood Trust. As illuminated by the lead researchers and designers of this project (Brand and Gaudion, 2012), adults with very different sensory preferences may find themselves living together in the same residence. The team's research led to the development of a profiling tool that adults could use to express their sensory preferences in partnership with their support providers. It also generated a collection of sensory props and design guidelines demonstrating how lighting, fabrics and other materials could be used to create temporary, affordable and adaptable sensory spaces within home settings (more about their technique is described in Chapter Five).

From this work, Brand and Gaudion recommend that communal spaces in shared residences be designed and furnished to address the preferences of the most sensitive residents. Props then can be brought in when appropriate. Private spaces, such as bedrooms, can be personalized in ways most relevant to the particular resident. Another suggestion they make is having multiple common spaces in a shared residence or residential complex, ones that are sensory-neutral and others sensory-rich, allowing individuals to choose which best accommodates them. Many of the sensory-focused concepts, spaces and features developed in their project are reflected in the design guidelines of Chapter Four.

To date, research on sensory issues has focused on immediate stimuli and disruptions emanating from that. Accumulated effects and delayed responses are getting increased attention, however. As described by James C Wilson (2008, 46) of his autistic son, Sam: "Sometimes it's not any one particular event that 'causes' a meltdown. Rather, tension will build during a day or a week until one seemingly innocuous occurrence will trigger an explosion. This makes it more difficult to foresee or prevent a meltdown."

Research being undertaken at the Center for Discovery in New York suggests that simple one-to-one observations of what we may consider sensory triggers of such outbreaks may be limiting. Northeastern University professor, Matthew Goodwin, notes that some children sit and look calm in their classroom, but may actually be deeply anxious with a racing heart rate to match that anxiety (Singer, 2013). Since individuals on the more severe end of the autism spectrum can be nonverbal, they have difficulty communicating their feelings or identifying what is bothersome. Small wristband sensors that measure heart rate, movement, body temperature and skin conductance as indicators of stress, allow real-time monitoring of these physiological conditions while children are in the classroom or therapy room. Coupling and syncing the real-time monitoring of the sensory band with videotapes of what is happening in the therapy room – capturing the sounds, the movements, the visual displays, the touching, and all the rest – helps reveal the gradual build-up of physiological stress to disturbing triggers that eventually are displayed in outbursts, at times several minutes from the initiating annoyance that started the stress response. This work by Goodwin and others at the Center for Discovery demonstrates not only breakthroughs in research, but also suggests innovative ways to better understand and express the environments surrounding individuals on the spectrum.

◆

In sum, designing residential spaces requires a *balance* of sensory experiences – tactile, odors, visual and auditory – when providing housing with multiple occupants. This may be effected by having multiple spaces, each with its own level of stimulating features, so that residents can choose which spaces best suit them. Or an overall sensory-neutral residence can be provided in which stimulating furnishings, wall hangings, special lighting fixtures, and other features can be added to enhance the quality of the space for specific individuals.

 ## Offer multiple opportunities for controlling social interaction and privacy

A common perception of autism is that those on the spectrum are asocial, withdrawn, self-absorbed, even trapped inside oneself. But as the reflections in the Sidebar suggest, aspirations and experiences of "being social" or "being private" among those on the spectrum are not clear-cut. Research challenges conventional assumptions that spectrum individuals are not interested in pursuing intimate or social relationships, or that they are oblivious to the social workings of the world around them. A number of adults and teens feel isolated, have difficulties initiating social contact and interaction, and rarely participate in social and recreational activities (Orsmond et al, 2004; Liptak, Kennedy and Dosa, 2011). After leaving the public school system, nearly 40 percent report having no friends (Shattuck et al, 2012). Yet many long for greater intimacy, and some express a desire to contribute to one's community (Orsmund, Krauss and Seltzer, 2004; Muller, Schuler and Yates, 2008).

Some researchers suggest that friendships of autistic persons often lack a rich quality regarding intimacy, empathy and supportiveness (Baron-Cohen and Wheelwright, 2003). And there is some indication that many young adults with ASC limit their social opportunities by rarely initiating social connections or by withdrawing from social settings altogether (Shatyermann, 2007). But much of this research predates the proliferation of Internet websites and individuals' widespread access to them. It also typically profiles "social success" from the perspective of standardized tests or clinical definitions of therapists. As indicated by the remarks in the Sidebar, adults with ASC do not necessarily prefer to be alone and may spend as much time in social company as their neurotypical peers – but do so with people more familiar to them (Hintzen et al, 2010).

Although it is difficult for most autistic individuals to seamlessly engage in the socialized world, we live in cultures where socializing and social capital are important values; and when positive, these social connections can have enormous benefits (Armstrong, 2010). Health benefits of supportive social relationships are increasingly affirmed in the research literature (Wickelgren, 2012). The value of social capital – or social networks – derives from trust, reciprocity, information and cooperation (Putnam, 1993), and can be expressed in a number of ways, from simply watching a friend's pet when on vacation to coming together to advocate for zoning change in one's community.

Particularly in the last decade, educators, parents and therapists have spent enormous effort to assist those on the spectrum to interact, communicate with and relate to other people (Farmer-Dougan, 1994; Schreibman, 2005; Turner-Brown et al, 2008; Mahan and Kozlowski, 2011). Parents often play an active role in social coaching or facilitating friendships for their adolescent and young adult children (Orsmond et al, 2004; Howard, Cohen and Orsmond, 2006). What happens when parents are absent or less involved is not clear. Kapp and colleagues (2011) suggest that by adulthood, some individuals with ASC adopt diverse strategies of presenting

Thoughts on "being social"

"[M]any descriptions of autism and Asperger's describe people like me as 'not wanting contact with others' or 'preferring to play alone.' I can't speak for other kids, but I'd like to be very clear about my own feelings: *I did not ever want to be alone.* And all those child psychologists who said 'John prefers to play by himself' were dead wrong. I played by myself because I was a failure at playing with others. I was alone as a result of my own limitations, and being alone was one of the bitterest disappointments of my young life. The sting of those early failures followed me long into adulthood, even after I learned about Asperger's."

(Diagnosed with Asperger's in his thirties, John Robison recalling his childhood before diagnosis, in his book *Look Me in the Eye*, 2007, 211)

"The truth is, we'd love to be with other people. But because things never, ever go right, we end up getting used to being alone, without even noticing this is happening. Whenever I overhear someone remark how much I prefer being on my own, it makes me feel desperately lonely. It's as if they're deliberately giving me the cold-shoulder."

(Thirteen-year old Naoki Higashida in his book *The Reason I Jump*, 2013)

themselves in public, with some trying to "pass" and others openly self-disclosing their diagnoses for educational and advocacy purposes (Davidson and Henderson, 2010).

While a desire for social connection and friendships exists, what *being social* means to those on the spectrum may be profoundly different from conventional and clinical interpretation. Self-advocate, James Sinclair, co-founder of Autism Network International (ANI), writes about being social in what he calls autistic and NT (neurotypical) space. Sinclair (2010) claims that autistics' ways of interacting are different from general social norms – and also different from each other's. What is desired can range from not wanting any social contact at all at times (the common stereotype, although not often the reality) – to wanting some social contact but needing more "down time" than most neurotypicals need – to needing excessively constant contact, more so than even extroverts could tolerate. Close friendships may lack an affective quality that are found among neurotypicals, but instead may be valued simply for sharing activities and being in close proximity (Bauminger, Shulman and Agam, 2004).

Ethnographer, Nancy Bagatell (2010), reports how surprised she was to discover the highly social nature of autistic adult group meetings – those established and run *by* those on the spectrum, not *for* them. Socializing there involved practices she did not originally perceive as social, instead

> **More thoughts on "being social"**
>
> "Personally, I would much rather have someone walk up to me and tell me some interesting fact I hadn't known before about grasshoppers, or helicopters, or forensic dentistry, than have someone approach me uninvited to tell me something I'm perfectly aware of, such as the fact that it's a sunny or rainy day. If you're going to interrupt my train of thought and place demands on my cognitive processing to focus on you and comprehend what you're saying, at least say something that's intellectually engaging!"
>
> (Self-advocate James Sinclair, 2010)
>
> "Striking up conversations with strangers is an autistic person's version of extreme sports."
>
> (British journalist Kamran Nazeer, who is autistic, in his book *Send in the Idiots: Stories from the Other Side of Autism*, 2007)

reflecting Sinclair's characterization of "autistic socializing." There was no eye contact, small talk or back-and-forth dialogue. As one person mentioned, "What is the point of asking 'How are you?' if you don't really care and the person is just going to say 'I'm fine'?" Conversations sometimes appeared to be monologues, while at other times they were animated, sometimes even heated, dialogues. Individuals used humor and enjoyed jokes, riddles and puns, many of which she did not understand. Autistic socializing in these group meetings did not necessarily require conversation, but rather what Sinclair (2005) describes as "interactive stimming" – a kind of spontaneous sharing of pleasure in fixations and stimming (that is, self-stimulation or a form of stereotypy such as hand flapping and body spinning or rocking). From a biomedical perspective, stimming is undesirable. But Bagatell mentions a scene where she watched as two men sat next to each other, each stimming. After a while she noticed how synchronized their motions were. Socializing also meant being in proximity to others, or as one participant explained: "We don't have to talk. We can just share energy to be social" (Bagatell, 2010, 40).

Her observations of these gatherings resonant with James Sinclair's (2010) personal recollections. "My own words to describe the 1992 visit with Xenia [Grant] and Donna [Williams, both autistic women] during which ANI was founded were feeling that, after a life spent among aliens, I had met someone who came from the same planet as me." This "same planet" metaphor, along with metaphors about "speaking the same language" or "belonging to the same tribe," are descriptions commonly used by autistic individuals who have had this experience of autistic space. At the first Autreat in 1996 – ANI's annual three-day retreat-style conference run by autistic people and focusing on positive living with autism – one participant summed up her experiences by saying "I feel as if I'm home, among my own people, for the first time. I never knew what this was until now."

During the past 20 years, facilitated in large part by the Internet, more and more individuals on the spectrum have been reaching out and forming social connections, creating community and discovering their own styles of autistic togetherness (Sinclair, 2010). Virtual space means not having to go into noisy, crowded public spaces and risk uncontrollable sensory assaults. In the virtual world, individuals can absorb and respond to communications at their own pace. At the same time the upsurge in Internet autism forums appeared, the number of local live-meeting social or support groups for autistic people increased around the world, such as Autscape in the U.K., Empower-Paivat in Finland, and Aspeies e.V. Sommercamp in Germany (Sinclair, 2010). Each one has different rules and forums, but provides multiple opportunities for social connection that individuals can pursue according to their own predilections.

As Sinclair notes, many autistic individuals need undisturbed time to observe people and activities in a setting before deciding whether or not to join in. "Sometimes we'll decide to start participating after we've watched for a while. Sometimes we decide we don't want to participate, but we're still interested in watching what other people are doing. It's a great relief to be able to be among people, participating in whatever aspects of the situation we're interested in, without pressure to do more socializing" (Sinclair, 2010). Having a common point of interest may facilitate mutual interaction. But a lot of spontaneous initiation of social contact is unlikely, particularly between people who do not already have established social relationships (Sinclair, 2010).

To some extent, Sinclair's comments reflect the nature of social behavior in general – many people of all types prefer socializing with other people who hold common interests. Indeed, Sinclair's and Bagatell's trenchant observations resonant with concepts of privacy and social interaction framed by environmental psychologists and anthropologists (Altman and Chermers, 1980; Hall, 1990; Rapoport, 1990). The foundation of privacy and socializing is the *control* individuals have in regulating boundaries, whether those boundaries are interpersonal or physical ones. Privacy is a cultural universal. But how privacy is expressed experientially, socially and spatially varies across cultures – and within cultures along the lines of ethnicity, age and other personal and social conditions. What is seen as a boundary in one culture – whether that is one's body posture or a physical structure – may not be similarly perceived as a boundary in another culture.

The ability to choose solitude or the company of others endows us with a sense of self-determination; not having that choice makes us feel helpless (Westin, 1967). The essence of privacy, then, is controlling the management of information about one's self and the management of social interaction. The environment in which desired social and private encounters occur makes a difference – not simply the physical characteristics of the space but who controls and operates the setting is also important. We believe that this perspective of privacy as "selective control of access to the self or to one's group" (Altman, 1975) is a valuable way in understanding how *being social* and *being private* happens within the various facets and individuals of the autism community.

How the built environment is structured can facilitate or hinder individuals in regulating this distribution of information on which social interaction and privacy depends. Architect John Archea (1977) carefully identified how such physical arrangements could pace and convey social information. *Visual access* is the ability to monitor one's immediate spatial surroundings by sight – as a function of doors, walls, mirrors, and opaque and reflective surfaces relative to one's position. *Visual exposure* is the degree to which one's behavior can be monitored from the immediate surroundings. This depends on how barriers, spaces, lighting levels, and surveillance devices are placed relative to people's positions. A *gradient*, the dynamic dimension of a setting, is the amount of change of visual access and/or visual exposure available as a function of proximity to edges or openings, shifts in position, the movement of doors and other barriers, and the size of the space. *Terminals* are formal communication or information networks (for example, telecommunication systems, Internet).

These socio-spatial concepts of controlling privacy and social interaction are illustrated in various profiles of spectrum individuals in their homes. For example, from interviews with autistic adults, Kinnaer and colleagues (2014) found diverse reactions to having multiple small rooms or one big open space in a home. A sense of "overview" – or what Archea refers to as "visual access" – was often mentioned as desirable or comforting, such as being able to look into the kitchen from the living room (although some people noted that seeing too much, particularly too much mess, could be disturbing). The opportunity to close doors into these available spaces was a reccurring theme that cropped up in the interviews as well; that is, being able to control the visual clutter, noise or visitors. The need for privacy also seemed to influence how much space was needed and how it should be subdivided. Living with someone else is a daily negotiation until set patterns are established. Having space to concentrate on one's work as well as a space to withdraw to when visitors or roommates become too stimulating were also common themes.

In their observations of a group home of adults on the spectrum, Baumers and Heylighen (2014, 65) found that each occupant appropriated his or her own spaces in the house. These retreat spaces could be in the same room. "In the sitting corner, different worlds coexist simultaneously. The collective room seems to be subdivided into different spaces. The counselors confirmed this: Yes, even in a large room, you could tell these guys…define it: 'You only on that chair, you only from here till there; that's your space.' Even within one room, delineated places can function as separate spaces in the occupants' world." Apparently a sense of one's personal territory could be defined both spatially and temporally (the crafting and occupancy of these personal territories in the collective room happened only after sharing dinner together).

Sinclair (2010) likewise recognizes the creation of mutually agreed upon structure for people to maintain their own personal boundaries and recognize other people's boundaries. This need for providing a variety of different options and allowing people to make their own personal choice is illustrated in Sinclair's depiction of the dining room at an Autreat:

> The Autreat dining room may be the quintessential example of this phenomenon. It's a common stereotype that autistic people in a group dining situation sit alone, as far away from other people as possible. And indeed there are people who choose to sit alone in the Autreat dining room, or to take their meals out of the dining room to someplace more private…But there are also people at Autreat who not only choose to sit together, but who actually crowd *closer* together in order to fit more people around a table than the table was designed for…I've seen this happen again and again with person after person, until as many as ten people – most or all of them autistic – are happily crammed around a table that was meant to seat six."

Providing opportunities for controlling the desired gradient of privacy or sociality is particularly keen in residences where there are multiple residents.

Which then begs the question, "How many individuals should live together in one residence?"

Having one's own apartment is often viewed as a hallmark of independence by many young adults with autism and developmental disabilities (Jackson, 2008). For those who wish to live alone, loneliness can be an issue. In the general U.S. population, over one quarter of households is occupied by a single person and this number continues to grow. How their homes are accessible to other opportunities to social contacts, and how the homes themselves can be rich sources of pleasure rather than gloomy cells, are ways housing providers can minimize the potential for loneliness while maximizing the desire to live by oneself. (This issue is addressed more thoroughly in the last quality of life goal, Accessibility and Support in the Surrounding Neighborhood.)

In many instances, however, adults on the spectrum will be living with housemates, companions or spouses. In considering how many individuals should reside together, there are numerous parameters to consider, including that of location, cost and affordability. Program guidebooks of group homes and shared living arrangements for those on the spectrum suggest a range from two to three to no more than six (for example, Autism Society of Delaware, 2006). Even with these numbers of housemates, when you add the number of visitors who come on a regular basis – therapists, support providers, family, etc – typically-sized apartments or homes can become crowded fairly quickly. The desired number of housemates also rests on compatibility: whether or not residents share similar interests, or can accommodate or tolerate disparate activities by a housemate. Then there are also individuals who prefer not to have housemates.

Nonetheless, these rules of thumb are not backed by research documentation. Nor do they take into account the size (for example, square meters), numbers of bedrooms and bathrooms, configuration of the residence, availability of outdoor space, and other environmental qualities of the residence. It is not the number of residents itself that is the defining issue. Rather it is how the space is configured for that number which can best accommodate privacy and opportunities for desired socializing among residents and support providers.

What the adult with ASC perceives as crowded may not be what architects and designers typically perceive (Harker and King, 2004). Even two or three individuals in a residence may appear crowded, and residents may begin to be disturbed by competing stimuli and lack of space given the residential configuration. If a residence is designed to allow for both common areas where people can mix and separate places where individuals can withdraw – with boundaries appropriately controlled by residents – then residents have the opportunity to manage social discomfort more easily. Clearly defined boundaries between shared and private spaces reduce ambiguity in knowing which spaces are shared and where social interaction is expected to occur, and those that are private and belong to an individual.

Not only residents, but also support providers need spaces where they can effectively interact with residents as well as spaces for personal retreat and privacy. The ability to view residents without invading their personal space can help reduce stress among support providers as well (Whitehurst, 2006).

◆

In sum, desired levels of privacy and sociality lies in the *control* individuals have in regulating boundaries, whether those boundaries are interpersonal or physical ones. A number of spatial treatments can provide opportunities for allowing residents to control the level of privacy or openness they desire in their homes, through visual access, visual exposure, gradients and terminals. When a residence is shared, the number of housemates depends upon a number of individual and economic circumstances, as well as the size and configuration of the residence that does, or does not, allow for ample control of access and privacy. But the number of housemates should be relatively small since homes also are regularly visited by support providers and families, adding to the number of occupants and different levels of privacy needs.

Provide adequate choice and independence

Our sense of independence and self-worth, indeed the quality of our lives, is often shaped by our ability and opportunity to make choices, control events and environments, and have a level of independence. Yet as mentioned in Chapter One, choice can be a potential minefield for many adults with ASC who may view multiple options with uncertainty or find them possibly threatening.

Being able to make meaningful choices depends in part on having a field of viable options from which to choose. This has been a central tenet within the disability rights movement, particularly the right to choose one's home and living companions. Article 19a of the United Nations Convention on the Rights of Persons with Disabilities (United Nations, 2006) states: "Persons with disabilities have the opportunity to choose their place of residence and where and with whom they live on an equal basis with others and are not obliged to live in a particular living arrangement." Similar declarations are embedded in statues and administrative documents of countries across the globe (Stancliffe et al, 2011).

Yet constraints to residential choice are experienced by many people, oftentimes as a result of limited income, lack of affordable housing, proximity to work, or simply a lack of desirable or adequate homes in a location where one wishes to live. A U.S. survey showed that 64 percent of the general adult population felt they could maximize their choice of where to live, and 85 percent said they could choose with whom to live (Sheppard-Jones et al, 2005). But people with developmental or intellectual disabilities rarely have this level of choice, with constraints resulting from health conditions and healthcare availability, employment and/or financial resources, nature of support services, and the availability of the type of residence where an individual wants to live (Stancliffe et al, 2000; Lakin et al, 2008; Stancliffe et al, 2011).

There is also the matter of living independently within one's chosen home and neighborhood. The extent to which one needs assistance in daily household activities such as dressing, grooming, housekeeping, preparing meals and eating, managing finances, and getting around, affects an individual's ability to live independently at home. But it is not simply a matter of being able to "perform" these activities – or ADLs (activities of daily living) – with or without assistance. It is also a matter of choosing *how* they are performed that shapes one's sense of independence. A person may be able to prepare dinner, but if she is not able to choose what she wants to eat for dinner or when to eat, her sense of self-determination plummets. Self-determination extends beyond ADLs. It means not simply being able to answer the front door, but also being able to choose whom to invite in – or refuse – as company.

Having the opportunity to engage in meaningful activity gives a person a sense of purpose as well as self-satisfaction and confidence and autonomy, and environments can be designed to enhance these. Designers of senior living complexes are well aware of this, recognizing the declining physical abilities of many residents. Lean rails along corridor walls, toilets that are high enough to rise up from without help, chairs with arms to lift oneself up by, are all simple design solutions that increase the opportunity for older residents to maintain activity and a level of independence. When the physical environment is planned to enable the older adult to continue to use whatever capacity remains, the person stays independent from others and from intrusive technologies for longer periods of time (Zeisel, 2013).

Viable choice, though, means having options. Since too many options may present ambiguities which can be difficult to process for some persons on the spectrum, the challenge is to design environments with some but not overwhelming numbers of options, and allowing design and spatial features to be sufficiently flexible so that they can be altered according to the changing needs of residents (Brand, 2010).

Being able to maintain a home can be challenging for anyone, yet is also important in reinforcing one's sense of independence. Preparing meals can seem overwhelming for residents who have low tolerance for frustration or who may be regularly depressed. Maintaining one's home or personal hygiene can also be challenging for residents with intellectual and mental health difficulties. For these reasons, how bathrooms and kitchens are designed, what finishes are specified, and the amount of storage space available, can make such daily living tasks more manageable.

Independence does not mean going it alone – very few people truly go it alone. We are supported in varying ways and degrees by family, friends, co-workers, teachers, sometimes neighbors, and by public institutions such as libraries, schools, law enforcement services and the like. *Natural supports* are loosely defined as individuals who provide informal and unpaid support for persons with disabilities within their local communities – as distinguished from more formal supports such as paid case workers or independent living coaches. Unfortunately the scope and number of these natural supports are often rather restricted for those on the spectrum. Adults with disabilities can experience social exclusion because they do not have natural supports that enable them to participate as they wish in their homes and communities, instead relying more on formal supports or simply forgoing opportunities (Duggan and Linehan, 2013). An emerging option to the diminished availability of natural supports, and in lieu of more formal ones, is technological supports.

Within the last decade, home and mobile technology has allowed adults with autism and others to live more independently by providing a means to support, monitor, deliver therapy and comfort (Chan et al, 2008). But many devices available today can be overly protective, invasive, even demeaning, by accomplishing and performing everything for the individual, thereby not allowing for one's own engagement and sense of accomplishment. On the other hand are technology researchers and developers, such as those of MIT's Home of the Future Consortium, who believe that the most effective technology will not be that which automatically controls the residence – and consequently the resident – but instead helps residents learn how to control the environment on their own (Intille, 2002). Technology requiring a level of human effort helps keep lives as mentally and physically challenging as possible. Research has long shown that making even a slight effort or undertaking a slight challenge to accomplish an activity can enhance health and a sense of well-being (Rodin and Langer, 1977; Lawton, 1980). Devices that provide "just-in-time-teaching" unobtrusively inform the resident of actions that might be taken to make the home secure or comfortable or efficient. These devices leave residents in control of making decisions with preset options without confusing them. Such examples are prompting systems that provide timely reminders of upcoming tasks and completion of multiple step tasks (for example, Carmien et al, 2005; Wu et al, 2008). Increasingly, devices incorporate personalized information to tailor the current situation to specific information about the individual. These and other devices are described further in Chapter Five.

◆

In sum, design options should provide the opportunity to engage in meaningful activity. When the physical environment is planned to enable residents to use capacities and skills they have, residents achieve a level of independence and a sense of accomplishment. The most effective assistive technological devices are those that help residents learn how to control the environment on their own. Design features and technologies that require a level of human effort – but not an overwhelming or frustrating level – help keep lives as mentally and physically challenging as possible.

 ### Foster health and wellness

Maintaining a healthy living environment is important for everyone. This ranges from minimizing toxicological and bacterial harm in the home's environment – to eliminating hazardous features – to providing opportunities for more physical exertion and activity that can diminish harmful effects of sedentary behavior (such as obesity) and stimulate positive effects (such as alertness and muscle tone).

Since many individuals on the spectrum have other health complications, maintaining a healthy residence is even more critical. In addition, many adults will encounter health issues of the typical aging population such as cardiovascular disease, cancer, diabetes, dementia or memory loss, declining vision and hearing, hypothyroidism, and osteoarthritis (Smith, 2008; Perkins and Berkman, 2012; Schuhow and Zurakowski, 2012). In the general older adult population, for example, air pollution worsens the severity of asthma and COPD, and can trigger hospitalization for congestive heart failure and cardiac arrhythmias (Adler, 2003). Given the high frequency of comorbid conditions and frailer health, aging adults with autism may be even more susceptible to environmental stressors than the general senior population (Tyler et al, 2008).

While there is a well-established pediatric literature on medical comorbidity for children with autism, this extensive research does not incorporate middle-aged and older adults in their samples, so the chronicity or evolution of these conditions in adulthood is relatively unknown or has weak associations (Fombonne and Chakrahart, 2001; Erikson et al, 2005; Fernell et al, 2007; Piven et al, 2011; Howlin and Moss, 2012). We do know that several etiologies of intellectual disability are associated with autism, including Rett syndrome, Fragile X syndrome, tuberous sclerosis, Prader-Willi syndrome, Angelman syndrome, Velo-cardio-facial syndrome, and Down syndrome, and that these conditions typically persist into adulthood (see Perkins and Berkman, 2012). As mentioned previously, between 11 percent and 39 percent of people with autism have been reported to develop epilepsy, which is significantly higher than in the general population (Bolton et al, 2011). A recent survey of medical records of 2,100 adults with autism enrolled in a Kaiser health plan in northern California found them more likely than the similarly enrolled 21,000 non-autistic adults to suffer from depression (38 percent vs. 17 percent), high blood pressure (27 percent vs. 19 percent), high cholesterol (26 percent v. 18 percent), obesity (27 percent vs. 16 percent). They were also less likely to smoke (16 percent vs. 30 percent) and drink alcohol (23 percent vs. 53 percent) (see Diamond, 2014; Salemon, 2014).

For the most part, however, researchers do not know to what extent the status of chronic medical and psychiatric comorbidities can either stabilize, improve or deteriorate across the lifespan for those with autism. Drugs and medications administered in childhood may have effects that last into adulthood. As Perkins and Berkman (2012) point out, the likelihood of long-term medication use for epilepsy and mental health conditions can result in an acceleration of osteopenia, the aging-related reduction in bone mass leading to increased risk for developing osteoporosis. Long-term use of psychotropic drugs might result in development of tardive dyskinesia.

Estimates of mental health conditions in adults with ASC vary considerably, with general epidemiological or follow-up studies suggesting rates of around 25 to 30 percent. The most common diagnoses include anxiety, obsessive-compulsive disorder (OCD), and depression, often in combination (Happé and Charlton, 2012). Catatonia (that is, increased slowness, difficulty in initiating and completing actions, reliance on prompting, passivity) may occur disproportionately in adults with autism, with onset typically in the teens. But restricted and repetitive behaviors seem to be less severe in older than in younger individuals with ASC (Esbensen et al, 2009) and sensory sensitivities may become more similar to neurotypicals as age increases (Kern et al, 2006). Rates of schizophrenia and other psychoses are generally no higher than in the general population (Howlin and Moss, 2012).

An often overlooked health issue among those with autism is stress, a physiological reaction to life situations than can be either positive or negative (Groden et al, 2005; Goodwin et al, 2006). Stress occurs when a demand is placed on an individual who must respond by making an adjustment (Selye, 1974). A stressor is any stimulus or circumstance that compromises an individual's physical or psychological well-being and that requires an individual to make an adjustment (Selye, 1956). As one experiences stress, changes in the cardiovascular system, the immune system, the endocrine glands and the brain regions involved in emotion and memory are activated. Physiological actions are engaged that enable an organism to respond to a stressor by preparing the body to fight or flee – accelerations in heart rate, respiration and pupillary dilation. Coping with a stressor and these physiological reactions can involve responses where the individual tries to directly alter the stressful situation; for example, by leaving the environment where the stressful event is occurring. Palliative coping also may be engaged: the individual responds to the stressful situation by altering his or her "internal environment" – by taking drugs or alcohol, engaging in meditation or relaxation exercises, or creating arousing psychological defense mechanisms (Lazarus, 1966).

Goodwin and colleagues (2006) suggest that characteristics associated with autism – communication and socialization deficits, sensory problems, deficits in executive function – may make this population vulnerable to stressors and limit their ability to cope. Ineffective coping can lead to anxiety and even physiological harm, and research suggests that anxiety is more prevalent in persons with autism than in those who are typically developing (see Goodwin et al, 2006).

Groden and colleagues (2005) point out that many behaviors associated with the diagnosis of autism or developmental disability are related to stress. Maladaptive and stereotypic behaviors, such as self-injury, tantrums, hand flapping, or rocking, are frequently precipitated by stressful events. They suggest these behaviors may in fact be a functional strategy for responding to stressors and regaining equilibrium. They are currently testing ways to measure cardiovascular responses to stressors in individuals (teens to 30s) with autism and other developmental disabilities, in order to gauge an individual's specific environmental stressor.

Important to note is that stressors can be environmental ones (Evans, 1982), emanating from sounds, thermal conditions, lighting, air quality, density, congestion, even spatial layouts of buildings (Ahrentzen et al,1982; Evans, 1982; Zimring, 1982). They can also be "daily hassles" (Lazarus and Cohen, 1977), those stable and repetitive problems encountered in daily life that typically do not present great adaptive difficulty, such as a cataclysmic event like a hurricane, but still can induce a stress reaction – such as chronic dissatisfaction with one's job, neighborhood problems, or erratic and unpredictable bus schedules. Whether a stressor is acute or chronic, the physiological response and coping still requires adaptive energy. On the surface, low-level chronic stressors, such as these daily hassles, may not seem severe. But over time they may require far more adaptive responses than others stressors, gradually reducing an individual's ability to cope with subsequent acute stressors and resulting in exhaustion (Baum, Singer and Baum, 1982).

Research by Kloos and Shah (2009) on adults with serious mental illness characterizes poor quality and deleterious housing and neighborhoods as *active* stressors, increasing health risks. People who lived in better quality apartments and neighborhoods also were likely to report positive coping and lower perceived stress. Those who had more positive neighbor and landlord relations were more likely to report higher perceptions of their own recovery from mental illness.

In addition to the physiological and mental health conditions associated with many on the spectrum, there are also activities and behaviors that can be either health-promoting or deleterious. Some research shows that older individuals with developmental disabilities, including autism, who reside in community settings may be living dangerously sedentary lifestyles (Temple et al, 2000; Draheim et al, 2002). Health problems related to sedentary lifestyle include cardiovascular disease, insulin resistance syndrome, and obesity – conditions more common among individuals with intellectual and developmental disabilities than among those without (see Lang et al, 2010). When exercise is increased, improvements in physical health, intellectual functioning, perception, behavior, affect and personality have been reported (Gabbler-Halle, Halle and Chung, 1993; Lang et al, 2010). Sleep duration and quality also are linked to physical and mental health conditions.

While this litany of health concerns may seem daunting, the physical environment can play a role in diminishing opportunities for some of these debilitating health conditions and in fostering wellness. While a cadre of research endeavors are examining genetic mechanisms that might create vulnerabilities of autism and the environmental factors that might trigger the symptom onset (Institute of Medicine, 2008a), the impact of environmental conditions and substances on the health of individuals extends beyond the etiology of autism. Environmental exposures can foster or further exacerbate additional health problems including asthma, dermatologic conditions, headache, and certain cancers (Tyler et al, 2008). Neurotoxins in the environment have been steadily on the rise, from industrial waste polluting soil to synthetic chemicals in materials of everyday life including building materials and furnishings (Grandjean and Landrigan, 2006; Landrigan, 2010). There are over 80,000 commercially important chemicals in use today with 3,000 of these classed as high-production-volume (HPV) chemicals. Shockingly, in the U.S. nearly 80 percent lack adequate toxicity testing for risk assessment (Institute of Medicine, 2011). Environmental toxicology policy is more extensive and regulated in Europe. The EU's Registration, Evaluation, Authorization and Restriction of Chemical Substances (REACH) legislation, enacted in 2007, places the responsibility on industry to generate substantial amounts of data on potential risks of commercial chemicals and to register this information in a central database (European Commission on the Environment, 2011).

The indoor air and environmental quality of our homes is related to building materials, ventilation, temperature, humidity, furnishings and activities, such as household cleaning and cooking. Van Hoof and colleagues (2010) identify many building-related solutions responsive to populations with health and neurological conditions. The Institute of Medicine in the U.S. (2011) has compiled a monograph highlighting key human health concerns of various aspects of indoor environmental qualities, recognizing increased risks among more vulnerable populations especially in light of climate change. While many "green" building certificate programs – such as Building Research Establishment Environmental Assessment Methodology, or BREEM (www.breeam.org) and U.S. Green Building Council's LEED program (www.usgbc.org/home) – initially focused on building practices that enhanced energy and water efficiency, there have been substantial revisions over the years to incorporate building practices that address human health, particularly that involving indoor environmental quality. Perhaps the most extensive to date that addresses both green residential building practices and health is Enterprise Green Communities (http://www.enterprisecommunity.com/solutions-and-innovation/). Another certification program, Living Building Challenge, also incorporates design-based criteria associated with health (for civilized environment, healthy indoor environment, biophilic environment), requiring performance measures rather than prescriptive ones to qualify (www.living-future.org). A very recent building certification program focusing exclusively on health is WELL Building Standard, an evidence-based standard created through six years of research and development with researchers and physicians in health, medicine and the building industry. The WELL Building Standard sets performance requirements in seven categories: air, water, nourishment, light, fitness, comfort, and mind. It is administered by the International WELL Building Institute, which was founded by Scialla and Delos, and has been supported by the Clinton Global Initiative (http://www.wellcertified.com).

Outdoor spaces often are forgotten when considering designing for health. Researcher Ward Thompson and colleagues (2012) have found associations between reduced stress and green space close to home. Based on their research with adults with autism, the Hamlyn Centre for Design, in partnership with the Kingwood Trust and BEING, demonstrate how well-designed gardens can enhance focus and attention and reduce anxiety among those with autism. Many of their design recommendations also target opportunities for exercise as well as other benefits such as social activities, predictability, and sensation (Gaudion and McGinley, 2012). Similarly "green care" is increasing in Western European countries (Haugenhofer et al, 2010). Green care is an umbrella term for a broad spectrum of health-promoting interventions that use biotic and abiotic elements of nature in their treatments to promote a person's well-being. Most prominent examples include care farming, healing gardens, green exercise, wilderness therapy, horticultural therapy, and animal-assisted therapy. Research has not yet been conducted on a large scale to substantiate many of these claims, but anecdotal examples of the benefits of healing gardens, horticultural therapy and green exercise to the mental health of those with autism suggest the time is ripe for such research.

Light plays a significant role in regulating important biochemical processes, immunologic mechanisms and neuroendocrine control via the skin and eye. Light exposure is the most important stimulus for synchronizing the biological clock, suppressing pineal melatonin production, elevating core body temperature and enhancing alertness. Ambient qualities such as daylighting affect the health and well-being of individuals, although there has not been research yet that targets the effects of those with autism. Chronobiology studies show that the timing, intensity and duration of exposure to daylight and darkness can affect how well people sleep, how well they function while awake, and how well they feel (Terman and McMahan, 2012). Depression among adolescents seems linked to levels of sunlight experienced indoors (Sansal, Edes and Binatli, 2007). Low arousing (that is, cozy, relaxing) and high arousing (that is, activating, exciting) lighting created by lux levels and colors of the light source may affect people's mood. Lighting can also influence feelings of mental fatigue, with bright light (1000 lux and over) having an immediate positive effect on feelings of alertness and vitality (Smolders and de Kort, 2014). By manipulating the size, number and orientation of windows, interior window treatments, the color, location and levels of artificial lighting, and other lighting conditions, designers and residents can enhance healthier living conditions.

The location and nature of the residence itself might be associated with health-promoting qualities. Researchers have demonstrated that individuals in supported independent living (SIL) placements are presented with a larger variety of community activities and more frequent opportunities to participate in such activities compared to residential facilities such as institutions or group homes (Howe, Horner and Newton, 1998). With an emphasis on community participation, a wider social network is created, and opportunities for increased activity – formal and informal – may be available. However, other researchers have noted that severely developmentally disabled individuals in SIL may not receive sufficient opportunities to engage in preferred activities while at home; although with increased training of support staff, such activities actually increased (Wilson, Reid and Green, 2006).

◆

In sum, the physical environment of our homes and immediate outdoor settings can enhance and promote health. Many adults with autism have health issues associated with general aging. But autism is also more highly associated with other health conditions, such as epilepsy, mental health symptoms such as OCD and anxiety, stress, sedentary living, to name a few. Poor and even toxic indoor air quality is deleterious to many residents, but particularly those with chronic health conditions. A number of "green" certification standards now incorporate design and building features that can minimize health risks associated with poor indoor environmental quality and that also enhance wellness.

 ## Enhance one's dignity

Human dignity is the foundation of numerous human rights declarations. In everyday life, displays of how we respect and value others are evident in daily actions and negotiations between people – such as sharing toys among young children or knocking on a person's bedroom door before entering – and in laws and policies, such as providing equal access to education regardless of race, creed or health.

How spaces are designed and constructed also can enhance or diminish a sense of dignity of the occupants (Gibson et al, 2012). A home of a size, style, or quality that blends in with neighboring residences suggests that those residents living in the home "fit in" with neighbors. Or a particular house form may stigmatize residents when it is more "institutional-looking" than the domestic structures around it (Thompson, Robinson and Dietrich, 1996). Most housing design and siting recommendations advanced by organizations promoting autism-friendly housing – such as those of The Kingwood Trust (Osborn, 2009) and the National Autistic Society (Harker and King, 2004) in Britain, or the Autism Society of Delaware in the United States (n.d.) – recommend compatibility of the style, type and size of the designated residence with surrounding structures for this reason.

However, living in a distinctive residence – if it reflects increased value or worth in the community – may likewise convey a sense of dignified distinction among those residents. Residents with cognitive disabilities residing in a technologically-sophisticated, environmentally-sustainable group residence in Boulder, Colorado, appreciated the attention they received in the community by living in a place with amenities highly valued within the Boulder community (Muselman and Woodruff, 2010). While the Charles House residence was larger than neighboring ones (but skillfully designed not to look so) and the interior layout quite different, the curb view was appealing and appropriate to a style of living in this Rocky Mountain city.

A sense of self-determination and social dignity carries through to the interior of the residence as well. As noted previously, having one's own apartment may be viewed as a hallmark of independence and autonomy by many young adults. But in many instances – because of finances, preferences, or level of care needed – sharing one's home may be the only option available or appropriate. In such case, having a bedroom of one's own allows not only a sense of privacy and a place to escape undesired social interaction (discussed previously in quality of life goal for Privacy and Socializing). It also allows a place for personalization: furnishings, decorations and mementos that reflect one's personal interests, history, and tastes – that is, a sense of one's self. Not every roommate may agree that Kirsten's collection of *My Little Pony* memorabilia is something they want to be surrounded by in every room of the house. Allowing such displays in Kirsten's own room recognizes the dignity of her interests and passions. In many cultures, particularly Western ones, social dignity enhanced by a room of one's own is also extended to the bathroom where privacy is afforded to self-care, grooming, hygiene and ablutions.

Acknowledging the value and dignity of one's particular interests and abilities is increasingly respected among those living and working with individuals on the spectrum. Acknowledging the *dignity of intimacy* of those on the spectrum is less so. For much of history, recognizing individuals with any disability as sexual beings was inconceivable (Gerhardt and Lanier, 2012; Urbano et al, 2013), their sexual nature and longings for intimacy ignored and sometimes vehemently denied. Indeed, those with developmental disabilities were sometimes subjected to involuntary sterilization in the first half of the twentieth century in some countries. Parents, support providers, even housing providers may explicitly or implicitly dismiss a person's desire for romantic or sexual intimacy by suggesting that characteristics associated with autism –

sensory sensitivities to touch, lack of flexibility, social and communicative difficulties, emotional expressions – make intimate relationships and actions virtually impossible.

While, however, some individuals on the spectrum have publicly acknowledged celibacy or no desire for romantic or sexual intimacy (for example, Temple Grandin, in Goldman, 2013), others – while recognizing challenges they confront – seek and pursue these relationships (Ousley and Mesibov, 1991; Siebelink, 2006; Farley et al, 2009). Only recently has it been publicly acknowledged within the autism care and therapeutic communities that persons with ASC have the universal right to learn about relationships, marriage, parenthood and appropriate sexuality (Mesibov and Schopler, 1983; Travers and Tincani, 2010). One's realization of these needs and desires may develop later than same-age neurotypical peers; may take longer to establish because of poor social skills (Stokes, Newton and Kaur, 2007); and may be expressed differently depending upon the individual's sexual knowledge, beliefs and values (Urbano, 2013). Yet there is increasing evidence that the importance of romantic intimacy in their lives is no less significant than it is for neurotypical persons (Wedmore, 2011). Indeed, autism characteristics that are deemed as deterrents may actually be facilitators, as noted by reporter, Amy Harmon (2013), in her profile *Asperger love*, of a couple both with Asperger's syndrome: "But if the tendency to fixate on a narrow area of interest is sometimes considered a drawback for individuals with the condition, it may also explain one couple's single-minded determination to keep trying."

While challenges to achieving this intimacy may stem from autism characteristics such as sensory/processing or social/communication conditions, the environment too can exacerbate or enhance the dignity of intimacy. Some support providers and parents are not supportive of the desire of people with ASC to date or be sexual with others, resulting in rules set against intimacy, or avoiding situations where the likelihood of developing intimate relationships might occur (Stokes and Kaur, 2005; Wedmore, 2011; Kapp, Gantman and Laugeson, 2011). Wedmore (2011) found that in some group homes, roommate restrictions or house rules interfered with the resident's ability to have time alone or privacy, such as not allowing the door to a bedroom be shut when a boyfriend was over.

In accommodating those desires, the environment can play a role. As noted previously, many adults on the spectrum live with their parents, support providers, or with housemates. Having visual and auditory privacy in one's residence provides a more appropriate and comfortable setting for intimate relationships from the rest of the home's occupants. Often bedrooms are sized to accommodate a single individual. Such sizes may be constraining when occupied by a couple. Or each individual of a couple may have his or her own personal room, sharing one or the other when together.

A final facet of dignity is the *dignity of risk*. Like others, those with autism may choose to engage in behaviors that carry some degree of risk to their health, their confidence, even their livelihood. However, self-determination practices that are increasingly promoted among many of those on the spectrum subscribe to the philosophy that individuals must be provided the dignity to make their own choices that go beyond their "comfort zone," doing so with a clear understanding of the possible harmful consequences of their actions (National Gateway to Self Determination, n.d.).

Indeed, creating residential settings that cater to every single need and whim without allowing for some level of challenge to the individual can be disabling and unhealthy, as noted in the quality of life goal for Health and Wellness (Lawton and Nahemow, 1973). Slight or moderate levels of challenges engendered by one's environment can promote a sense of accomplishment and even pleasure. When the environmental situation is too intense or demanding, however, in relation to a person's physiological or mental competence, failure to achieve can result in loss of confidence, fear, and even physical harm. Using this "environmental press" perspective, environmental design researchers have amassed findings of a myriad of residential features that provide opportunities for individuals to engage in challenges that go slightly beyond their competence levels – which can be useful for housing providers and designers to consider for enhancing the dignity of risk for those on the spectrum (see Lawton, 1980; Wahl and Weisman, 2003; Geboy, Diaz Moore and Smith, 2012; Zeisel, 2013; Golant, 2015).

◆

In sum, how spaces are designed can enhance or diminish a sense of dignity of the occupants. Exterior design that blends in with neighboring residences – or incorporates features that are socially valued in the community – suggests that residents "fit in" with neighbors. In the interior, providing a room of one's own provides opportunities for personalization. The dignity of intimacy is too often overlooked; but having visual and auditory privacy in one's spaces provides appropriate and comfortable settings for intimate relationships from the rest of the home's occupants when the residence is shared. Finally, providing slight or moderate levels of challenges engendered by one's environment can promote a sense of accomplishment and even pleasure, allowing for opportunity of a dignity of risk.

 ### Ensure durability

Some individuals with autism are agile and well-coordinated, while many others have problems with gross motor skills and motor coordination. This includes poor upper-limb coordination during visuo-motor and manual dexterity tasks, and poor lower-limb coordination during tasks requiring balance, agility and speed (Fournier et al, 2010; Bhat, Landa and Galloway, 2011). These motor difficulties may in part be a result of neurological impairments associated with the cerebellum (Mostofsky et al, 2009), or a result of physiological conditions such as proprioception problems (that is, awareness of one's body in space), limited strength or muscle endurance, or poor muscle tone. Also, such motor difficulties may emanate from social conditions:

a lack of practice, confidence or motivation to participate in motor-related activities; avoidance of motor-related activities because of the social nature of many of these activities, such as team sports; or difficulty problem solving in order to develop such skills (Brereton and Broadbent, 2007).

Movement difficulties – or ease – may also rest in part on environmental conditions in which residents live, work and play, as described in the Safety and Security quality of life goal presented earlier in this chapter. In addition to falls, trips and bumps that may result from motor difficulties in the designed space, outbursts of repetitive or stereotyped movements – such as jumping, pacing, running and banging against surfaces – that some autistic individuals engage in can threaten not only the resident but also the durability of the home itself.

As part of a three-year study on built environmental factors responsive to people with ASC, Sergeant and colleagues (2007) interviewed a series of housing and service providers who identified damage in the residential settings they managed that resulted from resident behaviors: damage to walls and ceilings, including holes in plasterwork, due to excessive gross movement or aggressive outbursts; damage to paintwork from excessive touching and rubbing; doors damaged from holes punched or excessively slammed; radiators, toilet cisterns, shower fitments, washbasins, curtain rails, skirting boards and plasterwork pulled from the walls; toilet seats and bowls broken due to heavy wear and tear; even joists and kitchen units damaged by excessive and inappropriate use. A number of interviews of housing providers during our own visits to residential sites also mentioned similar damages on an occasional to frequent basis, as well as renovations and replacements to amend the damages and prevent occurrences in the future (see list of these sites in Appendix).

◆

In sum, specifying materials and equipment that are durable and easily maintained is essential not only for the resident's safety and wellbeing but also for minimizing long-term maintenance costs of the home. The challenge is finding hard-wearing materials and fixtures that do not have an institutional or commercial appearance but rather reflect a residential quality. The physical environment needs to be robust, ensuring that the risk of injury to the residents, support providers and damage to the property is all kept to a minimum.

 ## Achieve affordability

In many cities there are thousands of people who need affordable, safe living options in the community but are unable to find or pay for such homes. Most cities simply cannot provide sufficient numbers of decent, affordable and accessible homes in good neighborhoods at a cost that is affordable to many low-income and working households. This affordable housing deficit is acutely experienced by adults on the spectrum who wish to move from their parents' homes.

While there are no national statistics indicating the extent of available affordable homes to those with autism, national figures of housing costs relative to income of those with disabilities is a useful means to portray the degree of mismatch between available income and housing costs. In the U.S., federal standards consider a household "cost burdened" when rent or mortgage, utilities, and insurance and property taxes (for homeownership) exceeds 30% of monthly income.

Based on current income statistics and average housing costs in the U.S., an estimated 14.4 million households with at least one person with a disability are cost burdened, i.e. can not afford housing without paying more than 30 percent of their income – representing 41 percent of all households with disabilities (National Council on Disability, 2010).

Both household income and housing price play into this mismatch. Americans with disabilities experience higher unemployment rates than the general population and those who are employed tend to have low-paying jobs, work part-time and earn less than their counterparts, according to the U.S. Census Bureau (Bureau of Labor Statistics, 2015).

Take for example an adult on the spectrum who is unable to work or find employment. This is indeed the prevalent situation: 77 percent of U.S. adults with cognitive disabilities are unemployed. The full-time, full-year employment workforce for those with cognitive disabilities is only 11 percent, indicating underemployment is a major factor among many of those who do have a job (Erickson et al, 2014). In such case, this individual would qualify in the U.S. for Supplemental Security Income (SSI), the federal program that provides financial support for people with significant long-term disabilities, who have virtually no assets and minimal income, and who are unable to pay market rate for rental or for-sale housing. In 2014, the average annual income of a single individual receiving SSI was $8,995, well below the federal poverty level ($11,670 in 2014). With such a low monthly income, housing options – much less other necessities such as transportation, food, and clothing – are extremely restrictive. No state in the U.S. has an average-priced one-bedroom or studio apartment that would be affordable to someone whose income was exclusively SSI, as is the case for most adults with autism or neurodevelopmental disabilities. In fact, the average rental payment in the U.S. for a one-bedroom apartment would require spending every penny of the SSI payment with nothing remaining for other vital expenses such as food or transportation (National Council on Disability, 2010). In fifteen U.S. housing markets (e.g. Honolulu, New York City, Boston metro, Washington DC metro), such rents exceed 150% of SSI (Cooper et al, 2015)

Clearly, most of the 4.2 million people receiving SSI in the U.S. cannot afford housing in their communities unless they receive some form of housing subsidy, choose unhealthy and inadequate living units, live with their parents or other family members who will pay for much of their living expenses, or live in group or shared housing with several roommates, sometimes sharing a bedroom.

For those individuals who do work, the wages they receive are far from ideal, especially when considering the costs of housing. In the U.S., a single person or household with one worker would need to earn at least US$14.97/hour, for 40 hours a week, 50 weeks a year, to be able to afford the average rent for a one-bedroom rental unit. But housing costs vary from place to place. A wage needed to rent a one-bedroom apartment in Hawaii would be US$24.15 per hour, and in North Dakota, US$8.38. But for many of those with developmental disabilities who do work, it is at minimum wage which is currently set at US$7.25 per hour in most states (National Council on Disability, 2010).

Employment and income prospects remain dim for many of those on the spectrum. While many autistic adults wish to work, employment challenges arise from social skills that may not fit with workplace practices and expectations, noisy or stimulating environments that may be disturbing for many autistic adults, and a lack of training and on-the-job supports (Resnik, 2009). And should a person become employed, the SSI benefit system significantly limits the amount a qualified beneficiary can earn, making it even more difficult to support oneself from multiple meager sources.

There is no well-established national census or survey of unemployment rates of adults with autism; they are typically grouped with other adults who have various types of mental or cognitive abilities. But a recent longitudinal survey of over 11,000 young adults with disabilities graduating from high school found on average, young adults with autism earn an average $8.90/hour compared to $10.40/hour for all young adults with disabilities. When employed, nearly half of those with autism worked less than 20 hours a week, four times the rate for all employed young adults with disabilities (42 percent vs. 11 percent). Twenty-six percent of those with autism worked full time, compared to 71 percent of young adults with non-autistic disabilities. The proportion of those who worked in a sheltered workshop environment (that is, only working with other people with disabilities) was seven times greater than that for all employed young adults with disabilities: 34 percent vs. 5 percent (Standifer, 2011). To what extent these patterns also occur among the adult population beyond their early 20s is unclear.

We cannot take the factor of financial support lightly in supporting more independent living in the community. Two high-achieving older individuals on the spectrum who have been profiled in the public media as examples of successfully aging adults are Temple Grandin and Donald Triplett. While they were young, both of their families – in different parts of the country – refused institutionalization and insisted on them being included in public school and recreational activities. Their families encouraged participation in community events as well as attending college and becoming employed or having a vocation. But as Perkins and Berkman (2012) note in their review of older adults with autism, both Grandin and Triplett came from families who were financially advantaged, which allowed for continuing access to appropriate support and sources at later times in their lifespan.

The other side of the coin of the affordability issue is housing cost itself. Public financing options in many countries are generally insufficient in size and scope to support the creation or preservation of appropriate housing at the scale needed (Resnik, 2009). Some recent affordable housing construction is of rather high quality and standards, often with green amenities and in transit-efficient locations – but the numbers produced only meet a fraction of the demand for low-cost housing for all populations. Waiting periods for a housing subsidy or for an opening in a low-cost quality apartment can stretch to years for many of the eligible.

There are isolated cases of alternative residential financing sources that have had a modicum of success. In the U.S., shared equity homeownership and community land trusts have been successful in some markets to provide homeownership for low-income individuals. However, these models are unfamiliar to most people, including those with disabilities. In Great Britain, HOLD (Home Ownership for People with Long-Term Disabilities) helps individuals who qualify buy any home that is for sale on a shared ownership basis (Housing and Support Alliance, n.d.). Shared ownership plans are provided through housing associations where an individual or household buys a share of the home (usually between 25 percent and 75 percent of the home's value) and pays rent to the housing association on the remaining share.

In the U.S., community development financial institutions (CDFIs) are mission-driven organizations that serve low income people, often working in a market niche that is underserved by traditional financial institutions. The CDFI "Disability Opportunity Fund" was launched in 2007 in Albertson, New York, but operates nationally. It provides housing opportunities for and advances the needs of people with disabilities through pre-construction and construction loans, acquisition-rehab, and bridge loans. Many of the projects serve those on the spectrum (thedof.org/).

Architects and builders can do their part with careful attention to the physical design and layout of residences to help reduce construction, development and operation costs, thereby bringing down mortgage or rental prices. There are a number of excellent design guidelines for affordable housing (for example, Jones et al, 1995; Global Green USA, 2007). Key components that can help reduce both capital and long-term costs while still providing quality space include:

- green design features and systems for energy efficiency and water conservation;
- building shape, layout, appearance, and window treatments that when done skillfully can minimize square footage costs;
- durable materials that pay for themselves in the long run by lowering maintenance and repair costs;
- location efficiency, so that the location of the residence is in close and easy proximity to employment, retail, parks and transit opportunities, minimizing costs associated with long commutes or transit rides.

◆

In sum, the increasing difficulty of obtaining affordable housing is a factor of low income relative to high housing costs. Public funds for constructing and providing affordable homes are unable to keep up with the numbers needed. Building shape, appearance, layout, mechanical systems, and density – as well as that of parking and outdoor space – can be designed in such a manner to not only reduce construction and operational costs but also produce pleasing and well-designed homes. However, efforts to trim construction costs by cutting corners in design, specifications and construction can have long-range negative impacts on residents if what is cut is key to their health and well-being.

 ## Ensure accessibility and support in the surrounding neighborhood

Ask any real estate agent what are the three most important characteristics of a good home, and you will get the reply: location, location, location. While a somewhat glib response, the neighborhood qualities of where our homes are located are key not simply to property values but also to how easy, pleasing and secure it is to live the way we want. The locational and neighborhood characteristics are even more important to those who are transitioning out of institutional settings or parental homes to "community living."

Locating the residence in an area with good and easy access to services such as shopping, banking, entertainment, health clinics and places of employment – or what is termed "location efficiency" – is particularly important to many adults on the spectrum who do not drive or cannot afford personal automobiles. With the right location, individuals may be able to live more independently by accessing community services without having to be chaperoned by support providers. Yet too much intensity of the everyday world outside one's door also can seem threatening with its noise, traffic, people, and colors. Clear routes and target locations need to be identified, even mapped. In some cases, technology can assist residents in mapping and "testing" what could be a potentially difficult excursion and converting it into something more predictable, clear and manageable (Harker and King, 2004).

The role of one's neighborhood in daily living is a central one in becoming "at home with autism." Research shows that neighbors and neighborhoods can have an effect on health, emotional well-being and feelings of safety (Sampson, Morenoff and Gannon-Rowley, 2002; Farrell et al, 2004; Walker and Hiller, 2007; Weden, Carpiano and Robert, 2008). While sometimes only engaging in no more than a superficial greeting, neighbors also can be catalysts of social, instrumental and informational support: exchanging favors or watching out for each others' pets or providing information about upcoming developments in the neighborhood like a construction crew who will be out on Tuesday to fix the water lines. In times of a shared crisis – such as a hurricane hitting the community or a power line failure – neighbors can provide both social and tangible support. Neighboring can also have its drawbacks particularly when it is excessive. But design factors can help shape the extent to which residents find it easy or difficult to engage in neighboring or becoming familiar with each other. The physical siting of houses in a neighborhood, or the layout of the corridors and apartment unit entrances in a residential complex, can provide or hinder opportunities for interaction, as can the size and configuration of common areas, open spaces, porches, driveways, and bordering gardens (Unger and Wandersman, 1982; Skjaeveland and Garling, 1997; Forrest and Kearns, 2001).

Creating a good match between the residence, location and resident depends on many factors including health conditions, the appropriateness of the residence, the scope, access and prevalence of support services, and community characteristics themselves (Thorn et al, 2009). In addition, the goal of "community inclusion" goes beyond being able to walk to the local grocery store. Many adults with autism live in homes physically located within the general community where they can access goods and services, and in so doing establishing a level of self-sufficiency. But they may not be participating in activities and positive interactions with other community members. They may be physically present, but not socially included.

Community inclusion is often couched as being unidirectional – situating the residence in a neighborhood setting and having the resident shop at local stores, going to the neighborhood bowling alley, and the like. But achieving the broader goal of social inclusion is not exclusively contingent upon the individual. It also rests with neighborhood acceptance and appreciation for those who are different (Townley and Kloos, 2009). NIMBYism (not in my backyard) is practiced in many communities, expressed by challenging the building or designation of a residence for those with autism or other neurological or mental health conditions, as well as shunning or actively discouraging their presence and involvement in neighborhood activities and spaces.

The value of a supportive community cannot be underplayed in the life story of Donald Triplett, the first child diagnosed with autism by Dr Leo Kanner in 1943. In profiling his life, reporters John Donvan and Caren Zucker (2010) remark how Donald, now in his 70s, lives alone in the house where his parents raised him. It is located a few minutes' walk from the town's business district in Forest, Mississippi. During his years living there, he learned to golf, to drive, and to travel internationally, skills he developed when in his 20s and 30s. He also attended college where he was a fraternity brother and performed in the men's *a cappella* choir.

In this town of 6,000 residents and where his parents were prominent citizens (as town banker and town attorney), everyone knows and accepts Donald Triplett, recognizing his oddities as well as commonalities. Such recognition and acceptance likely evolves from the community becoming familiar not with autism in the abstract, but with this individual – his strengths, his idiosyncrasies, his passions, his fears – over time.

Community inclusion emanates not simply from Donald's residence being located in the town, but from participating in the public and shared spaces of the community:

the golf course, the grocery store, the sidewalks as he walks from his home to the business district. The reporters mention that when they were in Forest to interview Donald and others who knew him, townspeople would come up to them and advise, "'If what you're doing hurts Don, I know where to find you.' We took the point: in Forest, Donald is 'one of us'" (p 89). The town of Forest provided tranquility, familiarity, stability and security. Donvan and Zucker conclude, "Donald reached his potential thanks in large part to his community, and how it responded to the odd child in its midst" (p 84).

While the example of Triplett illustrates the value of growing up in a small cohesive and supportive community, in many cases adults with autism will be moving away from the homes and neighborhoods they grew up in. Following post action reviews of two British housing estates for adults with autism, a panel recommended that housing for those with autism be embedded in communities where residents can become known and accepted by the wider community, and where the residents themselves can easily become familiar with their surroundings (Williams and Boult, 2009). Living in a stable community where neighbors become familiar with spectrum residents helps avoid potential misunderstandings and conflicts with neighbors who may be fearful of individuals with different behavior patterns than themselves or what they are familiar with.

Community inclusion is not without its critics, however, although they do not advocate a return to the separateness of institutionalization. As Cummins and Lau (2004) point out, most people prefer associating with and living around people like them or who hold common interests and values, not with "the community" in general (Rhoades and Browning, 1977). New migrants move to neighborhoods where others live who share their culture and language. Many older adults congregate in retirement communities. Cummins and Lau ask, "[w]ould the elderly residents of a retirement village regard integration with the adolescent youth who surround their enclave as enhancing their sense of community?" The type and level of community integration that is beneficial depends upon many factors including what is optimal for the individual in his or her particular situation.

Cummins and Lau argue that the most crucial measure of community living is how people feel about themselves and their lives (Landesman, 1986). Joy of community inclusion may not have any direct relationship with the number of times a person goes shopping or uses the local bowling alley. Rather it is based on the psychological sense of community, "the feeling that one is part of a readily available, supportive and dependable structure" (Sarason, 1977, 14). This reflects a sense of community connectedness, of personal interdependency and belonging rather than simply being in the presence of a general public. For many people with intellectual disabilities, the primary community from which they derive a sense of community may not be the general community in which their residence is located. It may just as well be, if not more likely, among families or groups of people with similar interests or conditions.

In the Community Participation Project (CPP) in New Zealand – a participatory action research program of 28 adults with intellectual disability – participants spoke about where they experienced a sense of belonging (Milner and Kelly, 2009). What mattered most was not *where* but *how* they participated: that they could choose the activities to engage in; that they were known to others; that one's contribution was valued and reciprocated; where participation was expected; and when one felt a sense of psychological safety. For them, being in mainstream settings were often not valued because they tended to include discrimination, intolerance and subtle forms of personal exclusion. But when these individuals collectively engaged in their larger community, community spaces became more accessible physically and socially. Provided they could choose when, where and with whom they participated, many in the CPP felt better able to confront the social ordering of unfamiliar places in the company of other people with disabilities.

Standing apart from the philosophy of community inclusion are the "intentional" or "village communities" that have been developed primarily by independent charities or non-profit agencies for people with developmental disabilities, including autism, moving from their family homes (these are discussed further in Chapter Five). They comprise clusters of small houses, some in rural settings, some in separate subdivisions. The most recent available estimate in the United Kingdom is from 2001, and that identified 73 such communities in England (from Department of Health, 2001, as cited in Randell and Cumella, 2009).

While these intentional communities have been criticized as a return to the segregation of people with developmental disabilities, one study found that on several indicators intentional communities provided a higher quality of life than other types of supported accommodation in communities. Researchers note that it was easier for village residents to sustain friendships than would be the case with dispersed housing schemes (Emerson et al, 1999).

Straddling between intentional villages and independent housing in communities is Perry's (2009) recommendations to adults on the spectrum about to "leave the nest," that is, the parents' home. Her recommendation stems less from philosophical stances towards community integration than from affordability issues. Perry suggests that parents of adult children maximize the value of the small funds they have for their child's future living environment by forming small networks whose adult children would live together or in separate homes close to each other when they leave their parents' homes. Forming a network of several homes or apartments near one another would be key to meeting the social needs of the residents. Perry urges parents and their children to start acting on this arrangement years before the anticipated "move-out" date so children would become friends before they start establishing their "community within community."

◆

In sum, locating the residence in close proximity to services, retail, and public transportation makes it much easier for residents to access community amenities that are necessary for living more independently. And situating the residence in communities or neighborhoods where there are strongly-held values of helping, caring, and interacting with others, is also key to feelings of social inclusion. Design factors can influence the extent to which residents find it easy or difficult to engage in neighboring or in becoming familiar with each other. Locating one's home in proximity to those of others on the spectrum, whereby a mutual sense of connection and support can develop, is helpful for some individuals in advancing connections with the larger community.

FOUR
DESIGN GUIDELINES

Just as neurotypical people have strong opinions about where they would like to live and in what type of home, so, too, do people with autism. The desire for an amenity-rich neighborhood and a house that reflects individual ideas of what makes a home and is filled with features that support individual needs and preferences is similar for most people, with and without autism. As anyone who has moved recently can attest to, identifying and locating such a place often is challenging. For people with autism, this may be even more so. To facilitate the process, the following design guidelines, in conjunction with the ten quality of life goals described in Chapter Three, were created to provide a foundation for understanding the potential suitability of a home, outdoor environment and community and what modifications might be needed to increase its livability.

Covering aspects ranging from neighborhood selection to appliance recommendations, the guidelines are intended to assist people with autism, their families, housing providers, developers and designers identify residential design factors that create a rich, safe, supportive and sensory-appropriate home environment. The recommendations outlined in the following pages attempt to address all the potential areas that might affect a person with ASC and for that reason are not intended to be adopted wholesale. As with the population at large, the requirements and tastes of people with autism vary widely: what is appropriate and necessary for one autistic person may be irrelevant or even detrimental for another. For example, open shelving that permits visual access of belongings may be essential for one autistic person's well-being but would create too much visual stimulation and confusion for another.

To uncover these specific issues and create an appropriate design response, it is necessary to work closely with future residents whenever possible, using the guidelines as a tool to direct discussion and design development. Given that difficulties with communication is a hallmark of autism, it may be necessary to utilize innovative methods to understand the wishes and needs of autistic clients. Gaudion and McGinley (2012) discuss a co-design workshop strategy that brought together residents, support providers and family to formulate ideas for an outdoor living space. Photovoice is another proven strategy that promotes self-advocacy: individuals with autism and other intellectual disabilities have used it to document aspects of their environment and community that are important to them or create obstacles (Brake et al, 2012; Schleien et al, 2013). The importance of working with future residents cannot be over-emphasized: a well-designed environment that addresses the individual needs and aspirations of individual residents might not only improve their quality of life and ability to live independently, it might also minimize long-term costs associated with needing to relocate residents if the home and neighborhood are not a good fit (Wahl and Weisman, 2003; Sergeant, Dewsbury and Johnstone, 2007; Geboy, Diaz Moore and Smith, 2012; Golant, 2015).

As discussed in Chapter Two, the design guidelines are drawn from a variety of sources including conversations with and writings by autistic adults, case study research, empirically based studies and experts' assessments. As a result, the recommendations directly address an issue cited as an area of importance for people with autism. In turn, each design recommendation is linked to one or more of the ten quality-of-life design goals profiled in the Chapter Three. Relating the design guidelines with the design goals will clarify how a how a particular design feature or modification may aid an individual with ASC and facilitate use of the recommendations. The guidelines are organized spatially, beginning at the scale of the neighborhood, through various areas of the home, to features such as lighting and materials.

Neighborhood design guidelines

Selecting the right neighborhood and community often determines the overall success of any residential project and this is especially true when developing or selecting housing for adults with ASC. From locating in areas receptive to autistic people to siting residences near public transportation, shopping and employment opportunities, appropriate site selection fundamentally affects the quality of life of residents. Often it is mistakenly assumed that people with autism prefer isolation. Recent studies, however, show that autistic individuals do have a "social appetite" and "yearn for a connection with others" (Orsmond et al, 2013). Therefore choosing areas that offer opportunities to develop relationships within the community and with neighbors may positively affect the physical and mental health of people with ASC (van Alphen et al, 2009; Amado et al, 2013).

As with most people, individuals with ASC depend on community amenities such as restaurants, recreational venues, health facilities, religious and faith centers, libraries, schools and community centers to complete activities of daily living (Williams and Boult, 2009; Donvan and Zucker, 2010; Brand, 2010; Chalfont and Walker, 2013). To access these amenities, proximity to public transportation is critical. Housing located away from public transportation and amenities significantly reduces an individual's ability to determine when and where to travel, making him or her completely reliant on others to complete most or all activities (Freeley, 2009; Dudley et al, 2012).

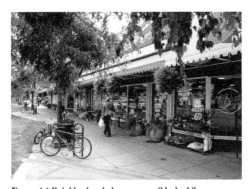

Figure 4.1 Neighborhood shops accessible by bike or walking
(photo by Dan Burden: www.pedbikeimages.org)

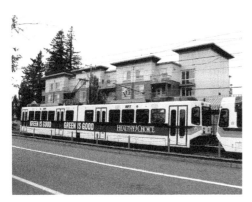

Figure 4.2 Local public transportation
(photo by Dan Burden: www.pedbikeimages.org)

PROVIDE ADEQUATE CHOICE & INDEPENDENCE

For the best outcomes, include future residents in the neighborhood selection process. Similar to most people, adults with autism prefer to have a say in where they live, what type of housing they will live in and with whom they will live. Significantly, residents who are included in the process often demonstrate increased independence and greater community inclusion (The Arc North Carolina, 2008).

Select an amenity-rich neighborhood that supports residents' activities of daily living throughout their lifespan. These amenities should be located within a 15-minute walk or a short bike ride or be easily accessible via public transportation (Abbott and McConkey, 2006; Farley et al, 2009; Williams and Boult, 2009; AIA, 2012). Amenities to look for include the following:

- Grocery stores, markets, pharmacies and other shopping venues
- Entertainment and social options
- Healthcare and social service providers
- Day programs
- Employment and volunteer sites
- Open space, parks and other recreational opportunities
- Public community spaces such as libraries and community centers
- Religious institutions and faith centers
- Public transportation (many residents do not drive)

MAXIMIZE FAMILIARITY, STABILITY, PREDICTABILITY & CLARITY

Established, stable neighborhoods with familiar surroundings suggest the best outcomes for new residents: less confusion, anxiety, stress and disruption (Williams and Boult, 2009).

ENHANCE ONE'S DIGNITY

Educating future neighbors about autism through neighborhood meetings and/or handouts works to manage expectations, reduce hostility and minimize potential conflicts between residents and neighbors (Abbott and McConkey, 2006; Williams and Boult, 2009).

Selecting a site with the appropriate zoning at the outset diminishes the potential for neighborhood opposition or NIMBYism (not in my backyard).

To increase potential for acceptance in the community, newly constructed housing should be appropriate to the context in terms of style, type and size. Alternatively, if the new housing differs from the surroundings, the difference should confer specialness and fit with residents' ideas of what home should be (Thompson et al, 1996; Harker and King, 2004).

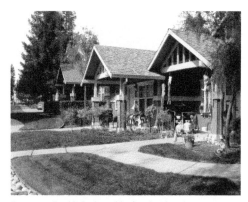

Figure 4.3 Established neighborhood with welcoming entry areas: Milagros Independent Living, San Jose, CA
(photo by Kim Steele)

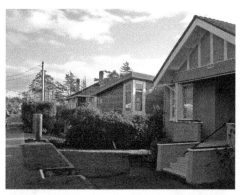

Figure 4.4 Example of new construction blending in with older homes
(photo by www.pnwra.com: Flickr CC)

FOSTER HEALTH & WELLNESS

 ## MAXIMIZE FAMILIARITY, STABILITY, PREDICTABILITY & CLARITY

Locate housing in communities near residents' families: this reduces the travel burden on families as well as increases opportunities for family involvement with residents. Higher levels of family involvement are linked to higher levels of community integration among adults with autism (Heller et al, 2007).

 ## ENHANCE SENSORY BALANCE

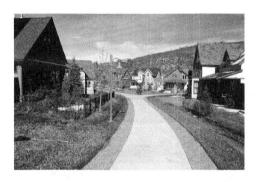

Figure 4.5 Pedestrian friendly neighborhood that minimizes vehicular interaction
(photo by Dan Burden, www.pedbikeimages.org)

Select neighborhoods with low levels of noise and pollution to minimize the potential for negative sensory reactions and health effects among residents. Given the difficulty of mitigating excessive noise and pollution through design, avoid locating housing adjacent to busy thoroughfares, highways and freeways; trains; airports; large, busy commercial districts; hospitals and fire stations; and industrial areas (Williams and Boult, 2009; Brand, 2010).

FOSTER HEALTH & WELLNESS

To encourage and support physical activity among residents, choose neighborhoods with a variety of accessible recreation opportunities. The rate of obesity among adults with autism parallels the general population; however, autistic adults tend to have higher cholesterol and triglyceride levels. Neighborhoods with options for physical recreation provide opportunities for increasing physical activity levels among residents and mitigate the onset of chronic disease (Kozma et al, 2009; Tyler et al, 2011).

Proximity to green space and the natural environment is associated with increased resiliency and greater ability to cope with stressful life events (Kaplan and Kaplan, 1989; van den Berg et al, 2010). For adults with autism this may be especially important given that many experience higher levels of stress and anxiety that may affect their ability to deal with demands of daily life (Gillott and Standen, 2007; Trembath et al, 2012; Hare et al, 2014).

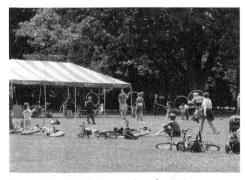

Figure 4.6 Park supporting a variety of activities
(photo by Laura Sandt: www.pedbikeimages.org)

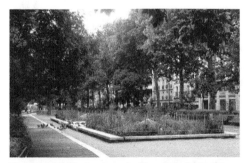

Figure 4.7 Neighborhood street with central green space
(photo: La Citta Vita: Flickr CC)

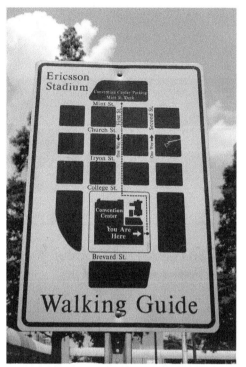

Figure 4.8 District map providing visual cues to aid wayfinding
(photo by Dan Burden: www.pedbikeimages.org)

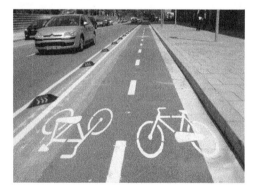

Figure 4.9 Dedicated two-way bike lane
(photo by Julia Diana: www.pedbikeimages.org)

 ENSURE SAFETY & SECURITY

 FOSTER HEALTH & WELLNESS

To minimize resident anxiety and stress and to increase resident safety and independence, locate housing in neighborhoods with well-articulated wayfinding such as signs, maps, marked pathways, lighting and landmarks (Easter Seals, 2012).

Since people with autism often lack awareness of personal safety, choosing neighborhoods with "Complete Streets" will provide a safer environment for residents when accessing public transportation, cycling or walking. Complete Streets are designed to safely accommodate all users – pedestrians, bicyclists, motorists and transit riders – of all ages and abilities by providing dedicated areas for each travel mode. For example, bike lanes are separated from vehicle traffic by a raised curb, bollards or planting strips and sidewalks are separated from travel lanes by planted boulevard strips (AAPD, 2012; National Complete Streets Coalition, nd).

CONTROLLING SOCIAL INTERACTION & PRIVACY

A neighborhood's physical form may determine opportunities for "neighboring." Therefore, select neighborhoods where the design allows for social interaction among neighbors. Design features such as front yards or gardens, driveways that abut one another and wide sidewalks create possibilities for encountering and socializing with neighbors. Also important is ensuring that there exists the possibility to avoid social interaction when it is not desired (van Alphen, 2009; Williams and Boult, 2009).

To minimize the potential for conflict, select sites that offer privacy: avoid locating housing on sites that permit residents to view neighbors and neighbors to view residents. For example, a multi-story house that overlooks the neighbor's backyard or garden could be a potential source of conflict (Williams and Boult, 2009; Brand, 2010).

To avoid conflicts with neighbors and creating traffic problems, select sites that will provide sufficient parking for families, friends and support providers (Williams and Boult, 2009).

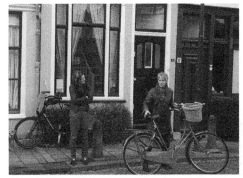

Figure 4.10 Neighbors socializing
(photo by Saxbald Photography: Flickr CC)

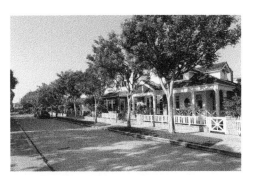

Figure 4.11 Layering of public to private spaces
(photo by Dan Burden: www.pedbikeimages.org)

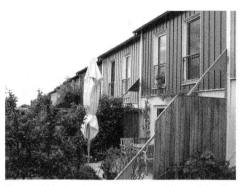

Figure 4.12 Backyard deck areas separated by partial walls allow residents to interact or maintain privacy
(photo by Tonu Mauring: Flickr CC)

 CONTROLLING SOCIAL INTERACTION & PRIVACY

 PROVIDE ADEQUATE CHOICE & INDEPENDENCE

Selecting a neighborhood where residents have the opportunity to participate in community activities when desired creates more meaningful social interaction than situations where residents must travel to events and activities that occur only occasionally (Jackson, 1997).

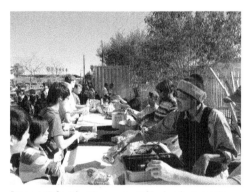

Figure 4.13 Social gathering at neighborhood community garden
(photo by Thomas Fischer)

OVERALL HOME

Similar to most people, individuals with autism often have strong preferences regarding where they live and with whom. As a consequence, consulting with residents at the outset to determine whether they would like to live alone or with a housemate, in an apartment or a house, in a city or a small town, promises the best outcomes in terms of satisfaction with accommodation, independent living potential and quality of life (Kozma et al, 2009; Brand, 2010; Zeisel, 2013). Further, the design of the home itself should reflect the preferences and needs of the resident(s) and be adaptable to meet future changes (Williams and Boult, 2009; Zamprelli, 2009).

 PROVIDE ADEQUATE CHOICE & INDEPENDENCE

Residents should be included throughout the housing selection and design process, working as members of the team. Not including residents in the process may result in conflict between how the home is used and its intended use. Also involve residents in future design changes (Scott, 2009; Williams and Boult, 2009; Zamprelli, 2009).

To assist people to make informed choices regarding what type of housing they would like to live in, provide information on various types of housing in a format (images, pictures with descriptions) that is easily accessible to all. Often family members tend to be more interested in family and group homes than are individuals with disabilities (McGlaughin et al, 2004; Zamprelli, 2009; Autism Speaks, 2013).

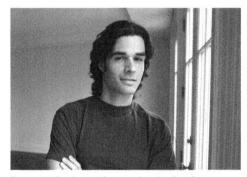

Figure 4.14 Involve residents in choosing their home (iStock)

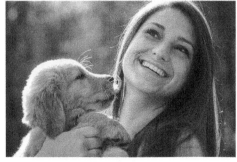

Figure 4.15 Create space for pets (photo by Bill Young: Flickr CC)

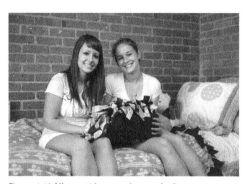

Figure 4.16 Allow residents to choose whether or not to have roommates
(photo by Tulane Public Relations: CC)

Residents not only should choose the type of housing they would like to live in but whether or not they want housemates, and they should be able to select those housemates. Allowing people to have control over important aspects of their lives improves their quality of life (Kozma et al, 2009; Brand, 2010; Lee et al, 2012).

Provisions should be made for residents to have pets and/or service animals (McGlaughin et al, 2004).

Housing design should be flexible, allowing for changes to meet individual needs and customize the home for new residents. Residents should be able to personalize their home including areas beyond their bedrooms; this makes it a home rather than a place where people are housed (Heller at al, 1998; Zeisel, 2013). Keeping a contingency fund available will make these changes possible (Williams and Boult, 2009).

To reduce the need to relocate as health circumstances change, all residences should adhere to universal design and accessibility guidelines to ensure residents are accommodated throughout the lifespan (Brand, 2010; Michael Singer Studio, 2014).

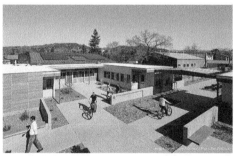

Figure 4.17 Activity area within residential community; Sweetwater Spectrum, Sonoma, CA
(Courtesy of Leddy Maytum Stacy Architects, photo by Tim Griffiths)

The house and garden or yard should invite and encourage residents to move unrestricted through them; this promotes greater independence and sense of control among residents (Zeisel, 2013).

ENHANCE ONE'S DIGNITY

In situations with roommates, keep the number of residents per residence small to avoid an institutional feel (McGlaughin et al, 2004; Williams and Boult, 2009).

 ENHANCE SENSORY BALANCE

To support residents in their daily living and to reduce potential stress and conflict, create an attractive, calming environment with high ceilings, natural light and appropriate use of color, textures and furnishings. Avoid claustrophobic, tight spaces with excess stimulation (Humphreys, 2005; Sergeant et al, 2007; Baker et al, 2008; Williams and Boult, 2009; Brand, 2010).

Single-story buildings minimize sound transmission through ceilings and eliminate the need for an elevator to accommodate people with differing mobility needs (Brand, 2010; Peter Dollard, July 2013, personal communication)

Creating sensory "neutral" spaces within the home offers residents areas where their visual, aural and/or olfactory sensitivities are not stimulated. To achieve this, the space must have natural light, muted colors, excellent acoustic dampening and good ventilation (Jones et al, 2001; Ahrentzen and Steele, 2009).

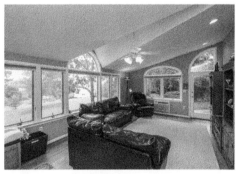

Figure 4.18 Natural light filled living space with seating options
(photo by Chris and Karen Highland: Flickr CC)

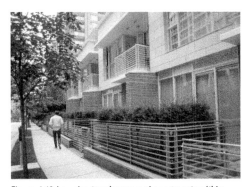

Figure 4.19 Low-rise townhomes and apartments within
established neighborhood
(photo by La Citta Vita: Flickr CC)

ENSURE ACCESSIBILITY & SUPPORT IN THE SURROUNDING NEIGHBORHOOD

ACHIEVE AFFORDABILITY

Select or design smaller homes that are integrated into the community to create a better quality physical and social environment. Not only do smaller homes avoid feeling and looking institutional, smaller homes with fewer roommates (typically three or fewer) are subject to fewer building code requirements and therefore are less costly to build (Jackson, 1997; Strouse et al, 2013).

ENSURE SAFETY & SECURITY

To ensure safety, keep pedestrian and vehicle areas separate: balance providing sufficient parking nearby for support providers, family and friends and safety for residents who may not understand issues of personal safety (Brand, 2010; Department of Family and Community Services, 2013).

To assist residents with the safe use of appliances, electrical outlets, windows, doors and other home features, incorporate visual signs into the environment. These visual elements may be in the form of pictures, words or warning colors that are understood by all residents (Ahrentzen and Steele, 2009).

FOSTER HEALTH & WELLNESS

To enable sustained interest in the environment and reduce the negative effects of boredom, create a home-like environment that offers residents variety, meaningful activity, privacy and choice (van Bourgondien and Schopler, 1996; Fleming and Purandare, 2010).

A home should not be uniform in its design and decor: environments with varied ambience – interior and exterior – have been associated with reduced levels of depression and social withdrawal (Zeisel, 2003; Fleming and Purandare, 2010).

Locate windows in public and private spaces including hallways to provide views to nature. Viewing trees and other natural features has been shown to increase focus and attention while reducing stress (Ulrich, 1999; van den Berg et al, 2007).

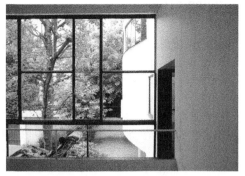

Figure 4.20 Large window overlooking plant filled courtyard (photo by Steve Cadman of Maison la Roche: Flickr CC)

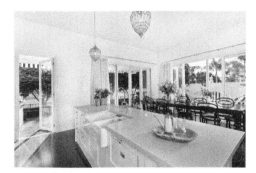

Figure 4.21 Large windows and doors allowing views to landscape (iStock)

OUTDOOR SPACE

Access to nature has been shown to provide restorative effects and improve cognitive functioning (Kaplan, 1995; Berman et al, 2008). As such, to promote resident wellness, a safe, well-designed outdoor space should be easily accessible from the home, allowing residents to enter it when they choose. The garden, yard or courtyard should offer a variety of activities, both passive and active, facilitating a range of experiences. As with most people, individuals with autism gravitate toward different environmental features, so it is important, to provide an assortment of garden elements. Along with various seating options, the yard or garden should offer opportunities for gross motor activities and sensory input. In addition to being physically accessible, the outdoor space should be visually accessible: the ability to view nature may have a calming effect while providing ample natural light.

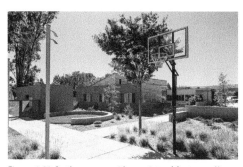

Figure 4.22 Outdoor space with a variety of features allow for exploration; Sweetwater Spectrum, Sonoma, CA (Courtesy of Leddy Maytum Stacy Architects, photo by Tim Griffiths)

FOSTER HEALTH & WELLNESS

A garden or yard should be considered an essential part of the home due to the numerous benefits associated with outdoor activity: sensory stimulation, exercise, relaxation, improved focus, verbal expression, sleep patterns and mood, and reduced levels of agitation and aggression (Gaudion and McGinley, 2012; Chalfont and Walker, 2013).

Avoid designing a risk-free garden or yard. Risk-free gardens and yards tend to be boring, under-stimulating and therefore under-utilized. Instead, design a garden or yard that includes features that may pose some risks such as including a swing, glider or trampoline (Gaudion and McGinley, 2012; Chalfont and Walker, 2013).

To encourage residents to spend time outside, incorporate a variety of spaces into the garden or yard that offer a wide range of activities and stimulating experiences:

- Vistas viewable from inside the home as well as outside
- Open communal areas with comfortable seating
- Walking paths of varying widths and lengths
- Areas near the home for physical activity
- Sheltered seating areas for one or two people
- Raised planters and in-ground beds for growing vegetables or flowers
- Sensory areas featuring different textures, colors, scents and so forth
- Interesting materials such as water, rocks, gravel, trees
- Areas with bird feeders and baths

Healing gardens positively affect people and should be included when possible. Features of healing gardens include places for privacy, settings to stimulate mental alertness, opportunities for social exchange, gathering spaces, areas for a variety of activities, comfortable seating, sense of security and full accessibility (Barnes and Cooper Marcus, 1999; Ahrentzen and Steele, 2009).

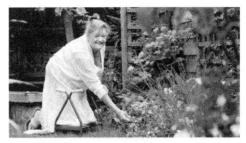

Figure 4.23 Opportunity for gardening (iStock)

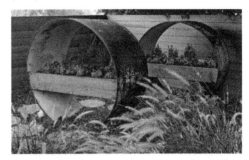

Figure 4.24 Raised planters create interest and spaces for residents to garden
(photo by Jeremy Levine: Flickr CC)

 ENHANCE SENSORY BALANCE

To avoid unexpected sensory stimulation, design neutral transitional spaces between garden/yard areas including the threshold between house and outdoors (Gaudion and McGinley, 2012).

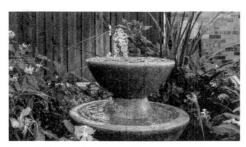

Figure 4.25 Water features provide soothing sounds
(photo by CTJ71081: Flickr CC)

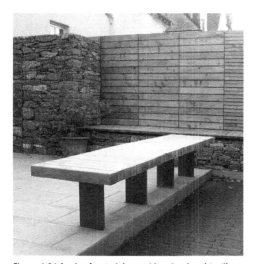

Figure 4.26 A mix of materials provides visual and tactile
interest in an outdoor space
(photo by Arya Ganesh G: Flickr CC)

Within the garden, place high sensory zones away from low sensory areas. For hyposensitive people (sensory seeking), mix textures (both plants and materials) to create visual, tactile and aural interest. For hypersensitive people (sensory avoiding), group similarly textured and colored plants and materials together and avoid lining pathways with tall grasses or other plants that might brush against legs (Gaudion and McGinley, 2012).

Include elements in the garden or yard that aid proprioception (awareness of body position in space) such as objects for lifting or areas for climbing. Many people with autism enjoy vestibular input, so consider providing trampolines, swings and hammocks (Gaudion and McGinley, 2012).

In areas with hardscape, select low reflective "cool" pavement to reduce heat gain and increase resident comfort (Maytum, 2013).

If the house is located in a noisy area, install a high, reflective acoustic fence along exposed sides to reduce sound transmission (Jones et al, 2001; Scott, 2009).

 MAXIMIZE FAMILIARITY, STABILITY, PREDICTABILITY & CLARITY

To minimize confusion and anxiety, garden and yard pathways, entries and exits should be clearly defined and visible (Zeisel, 2013).

Courtyards are a good option since they are legible, private, secure, safe and accessible (Medical Architecture, July 2014, personal communication; Ahrentzen and Steele, 2009).

Treat secured outdoor spaces as extensions of the home (Medical Architecture, July 2014, personal communication; Ahrentzen and Steele 2009).

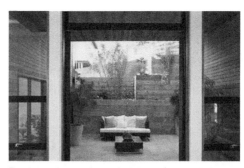

Figure 4.27 Protected courtyard viewed from inside home
(photo by JJ and Chris: Flickr CC)

 ## PROVIDE ADEQUATE CHOICE & INDEPENDENCE

Design the garden or yard so it is barrier-free and accessible: provide raised beds and smooth, level paths that are 1.2 meters (4 feet) wide. Depending on climate, stabilized decomposed granite or stabilized engineered wood fiber works well for paths (Laufenberg, 2004; Lee et al, 2012).

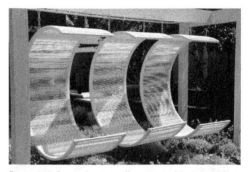

Figure 4.28 Grouped swings offer opportunities to socialize and enjoy vestibular input
(photo by Karen Roe: Flickr CC)

Install lighting in the garden or yard so that residents may enjoy it in the evening (Gaudion and McGinley, 2012). Lighting should be on timers – not motion detectors. Lighting triggered by motion sensors can be startling (Ahrentzen and Steele, 2009; Michael Singer Studio, 2014).

 ## CONTROLLING SOCIAL INTERACTION & PRIVACY

Include multiple gathering areas of varying sizes to allow residents to choose when to socialize or not and to not feel crowded. Providing small, private spaces adjacent to communal areas can help alleviate stress and allow residents to participate on their own terms (Gaudion and McGinley, 2012).

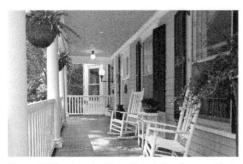

Figure 4.29 Front porch with rocking chairs allows residents to greet neighbors
(photo by Sonja Lovas: Flickr CC)

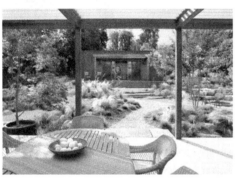

Figure 4.30 Outdoor seating, paths and varied plantings provide opportunities for different experiences
(photo by Arya Ganesh G: Flickr CC)

Provide an outdoor area where residents can visit and socialize with neighbors if they choose (Lee et al, 2011).

 ## ENSURE SAFETY & SECURITY

Maintain a degree of visual openness in the garden or yard to allow support providers to monitor residents from a distance. For screened areas, select materials or plants that are visually permeable such as lattice or bamboo (Gaudion and McGinley, 2012).

All doors connecting to the outside should have zero-step thresholds for accessibility (Ahrentzen and Steele, 2009).

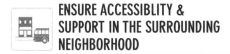 ENSURE ACCESSIBLITY &
SUPPORT IN THE SURROUNDING
NEIGHBORHOOD

Select fencing that is compatible with the neighborhood and is not fortress-like or institutional (Williams and Boult, 2009; Maytum, 2013).

 ENSURE DURABILITY

The design should specify robust landscape and hardscape materials that require minimal maintenance and are able to withstand unintended uses (Gaudion and McGinley, 2012).

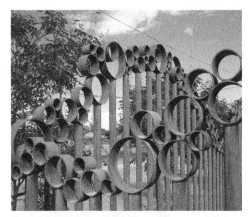

Figure 4.31 Artistic fence that allows views out to surrounding neighborhood
(photo by Ms. Phoenix: Flickr CC)

FLOORPLAN STRATEGIES

Successful wayfinding in any environment depends on clarity of layout. For people with autism, places that lack clarity can be extremely confusing and difficult or impossible to navigate. This is true within the home as well. To create a welcoming, understandable environment it is necessary to prioritize legibility and connectivity – visual and physical. A predictable environment that communicates its function may alleviate frustration and confusion and result in more effective use of all household spaces. Successful space planning will encourage choice, autonomy and independence for residents (Ahrentzen and Steele, 2009).

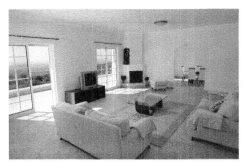

Figure 4.32 Large living area with multiple seating areas and visual access to adjoining rooms
(iStock)

 MAXIMIZE FAMILIARITY, STABILITY, PREDICTABILITY & CLARITY

Predictability in the environment, demonstrated through transparency in spatial sequencing, smooth transitions between rooms and uses, and the potential to establish routines, assists in keeping arousal levels low, minimizing stress and supporting resident independence (Harker and King 2004; Ahrentzen and Steele 2009; Brand, 2010; Mostafa, 2010; Lee et al, 2012).

The function of each space should be legible; and to limit confusion, there should be clear distinction between spaces (Sergeant et al, 2007; Michael Singer Studio, 2014; National Autistic Society, n.d).

To encourage appropriate behavior in particular rooms, ensure that rooms communicate their use through type of furnishings, materials and/or equipment. By increasing legibility, resident anxiety is reduced (Rapoport, 1990; Ahrentzen, 2002; Sergeant et al, 2007; Baumers and Heylighen, 2010; Brand, 2010).

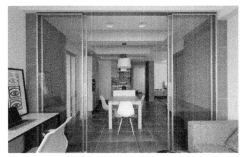

Figure 4.33 Computer nook clearly delineated from eating area by sliding glass doors
(photo by Mikhail Golub: Flickr CC)

Associating specific materials, colors or lighting (such as window shape or type of lighting fixture) with either public or private space provides residents with visual cues, orienting them to boundaries (Brand, 2010).

Within common rooms create areas that can allow the room to be used by more than one person. For example, in addition to a central seating area, a living room might have a window seat that could be used for reading or a table and chairs in one corner used for working a puzzle or doing a craft project. The room design should be flexible enough to allow a resident the opportunity to determine how they might use it (Sergeant et al, 2007; Baumers and Heylighen, 2014).

To create a home-like feel, avoid long, institutional-like hallways. Instead, connect rooms through short, wide hallways (Brand, 2010).

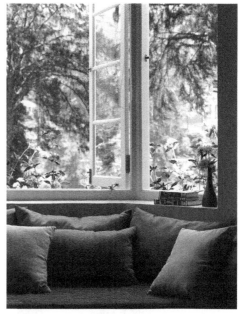

Figure 4.34 A window seat creates a spot for reading within the larger living area
(photo by Ceylon Tea Trails: Flickr CC)

 ENHANCE SENSORY BALANCE

To accommodate the preoccupation with order and the need to reduce visual stimulation that is common with autism, the design should utilize clean lines, eliminating visual and physical clutter. Avoid over-embellishing or over-furnishing (Jones et al, 2001; Ahrentzen and Steele, 2009; Elwin et al, 2012).

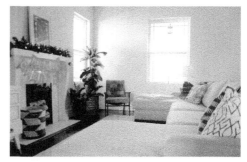

Figure 4.35 Open, clutter-free living area with natural light
(photo by Emily May: Flickr CC)

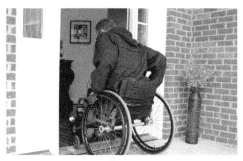

Figure 4.36 Barrier-free entry
(photo by Fairfax County Fate House: Flickr CC)

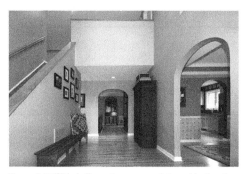

Figure 4.37 Wide hallways to accommodate resident motor activity
(photo by David Rothamel: Flickr CC)

ENSURE SAFETY & SECURITY

All entrances and exits should have zero-step thresholds to reduce tripping, accommodate wheelchair riders, and to increase accessibility over the resident's lifetime (Maytum, 2013; Michael Singer Studio, 2014).

Where possible, select or build single-story homes: eliminating stairs reduces opportunities for falls and it is easier to evacuate single-story homes (Strouse et al, 2013). If a resident has motor control issues, avoid having steps in the home (Lee et al, 2011).

Design the home to support a range of behaviors and to allow residents, support providers, family and friends to remain safe when challenging behaviors or conflict occurs. Wide halls and multiple circulation routes within and outside the home provide opportunities for retreat (Williams and Boult, 2009).

CONTROLLING SOCIAL INTERACTION & PRIVACY

In homes with multiple residents, it is important to include a preview window or sidelight in bedroom doors to allow residents to preview the hallway before entering. For privacy, a small curtain or blind can be installed (Fleming and Purandare, 2010; Sinclair, 2010; Braddock and Rowell, 2011; Smith and Sharp, 2013; Kinnaer et al, 2014; Michael Singer Studio, 2014).

The spatial layout should be easily understood by providing clear visual access into and between rooms. Use half-walls, vestibules, cutouts and sidelights to allow residents to preview a space before entering it. People will be more apt to use common rooms if they can assess the space and potential social interactions before entering them. Minimize the unknown (Ahrentzen and Steele, 2009; Fleming and Purandare, 2010; Sinclair, 2010; Braddock and Rowell, 2011; Smith and Sharp, 2013; Kinnaer et al, 2014; Michael Singer Studio, 2014).

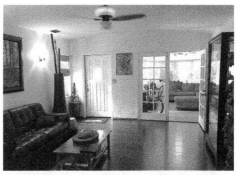

Figure 4.39 Interior glass doors provide visual access to adjacent rooms
(photo by Ines Hegedus-Garcia: Flickr CC)

To reduce resident anxiety and stress and avoid potential conflicts, it is important to provide a minimum of two exits as well as multiple ways to circulate through each room and the home. Hallways should be wide enough to allow people to pass without crowding (Williams and Boult, 2009; Brand and Gaudion, 2014; Michael Singer Studio, 2014).

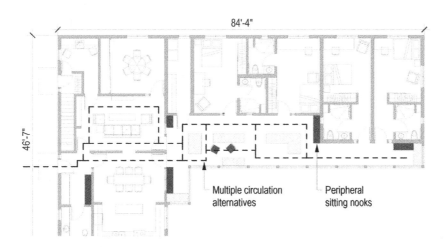

Figure 4.38 Floorplan demonstrating multiple circulation options
(Courtesy of Michael Singer Studio)

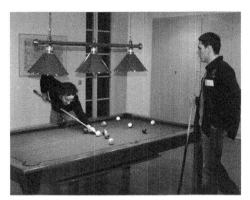

Figure 4.40 Activity rooms provide opportunities for socializing with friends at home
(photo by Nic McPhee: Flickr CC)

The physical layout of the home should support residents' ability to socialize with family, friends and neighbors without infringing on roommates' privacy. Including multiple living areas or a flexible space in the house design allows residents to have visitors (van Alphen et al, 2009).

Common rooms should include transitional spaces with seating in order to allow people to participate in social situations without being directly engaged. In homes with multiple residents, communal rooms should be large enough to accommodate multiple people without crowding. As it would be for anyone living with housemates, it is important to afford residents the ability to control their level of social interaction (Harker and King, 2004; Lee et al, 2011; Brand, 2010; Michael Singer Studio, 2014).

In living situations with roommates, the home's configuration should respect individual privacy. To ensure this occurs, establish a privacy gradient that locates common rooms together, semi-public rooms together and finally, private rooms such as bedrooms away from public and semi-public areas of the home. To maintain resident privacy, a separate office for support providers should be located near the public areas (Williams and Boult, 2009; Lee et al, 2012; Michael Singer Studio, 2014).

Include a flexible activity room for therapy, meetings, indoor exercise or structured learning. It should be located away from the private areas of the home (Michael Singer Studio, 2014).

ENHANCE SENSORY BALANCE

All areas should be generous enough to allow residents to move freely and engage in a range of movements such as jumping and pacing. Hallways, ceilings and rooms need to be larger and higher than in the average home to minimize physical harm to residents as well as the home (Sergeant et al, 2007; Williams and Boult, 2009; Fournier et al, 2010; Brand, 2010; National Autistic Society, n.d).

The home should not be void of stimulation. Rather, working with residents to determine their needs, an appropriate level of stimulation should be provided. This is achieved through the addition of color, textures and furnishings (Sergeant et al, 2007).

Create "sensory recalibration" spaces as transitions between rooms, at entrances and exits and between activity areas. These areas support residents' sensory needs as they move about their homes (Brand, 2010).

To minimize potential sensory problems, all rooms should have access to natural light, be fitted with a variety of artificial light sources (such as recessed lighting, task lighting) and be acoustically appropriate (Jones et al, 2001; Kinnaer et al, 2014).

Rooms should have doors to allow residents to control noise and visual clutter and maintain privacy from visitors (Kinnaer et al, 2014).

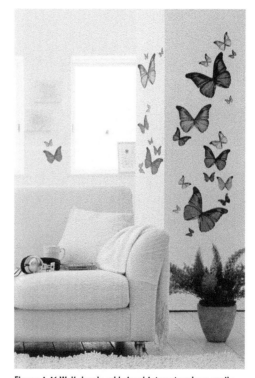

Figure 4.41 Wall decals add visual interest and are easily changed
(photo by Simon Mason: Flickr CC)

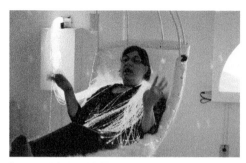

Figure 4.42 Swing with fiber optic light strings in a sensory room
(Courtesy of Linda Messbauer)

Create areas within the home where sensory stimulation can be added. This can be a designated sensory room or a portion of another space (Brand, 2010; Elwin et al, 2012).

Minimizing stimulus around the staff room is important otherwise it will become a place for residents and support providers to congregate, potentially compromising safety and privacy (Williams and Boult, 2009).

 FOSTER HEALTH & WELLNESS

To keep soiled clothes away from food preparation and eating areas, locate laundry rooms away from kitchens and dining areas (Brand, 2010).

ENTRY

As with any home, the entry should be inviting, well lit and easy to navigate. To minimize confusion, the home's entry should be readily identifiable from outside the home as well as from inside. Since it is not uncommon for many people with autism to have daily visitors – friends, family, support providers or medical providers – the entry area should be large enough to accommodate several people without overcrowding. It is also important to provide adequate visual access from the entry area into the home, allowing residents the ability to survey their home and any ongoing activity before entering. This may help reduce anxiety and promote well-being.

 ## MAXIMIZE FAMILIARITY, STABILITY, PREDICTABILITY & CLARITY

The entry should be clearly identifiable from the street and have a covered area to shelter residents and visitors (Department of Family and Community Services, 2013).

Design the entryway to be large enough to accommodate several people at a time, a bench with storage for shoes, a message board and, in a home with multiple residents, an area for resident mailboxes. The entry area should be a separate identifiable space rather than part of other hallways or living areas (Department of Family and Community Services, 2013; Michael Singer Studio, 2014).

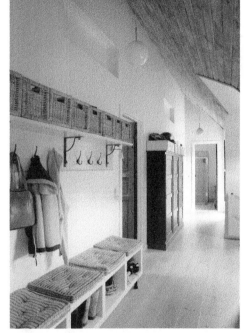

Figure 4.43 Clearly defined entry area with seating and storage
(iStock)

 ## FOSTER HEALTH & WELLNESS

Entries should have a zero-step threshold to reduce tripping potential and accommodate people with mobility conditions (Lee et al, 2012; Maytum, 2013; Michael Singer Studio, 2014).

People with autism often have difficulty with motor coordination; entryway flooring should therefore be highly durable with non-slip doormats to reduce tripping and slipping. Doormats also are important for maintaining good indoor air quality by keeping dirt from tracking into the home (Fournier et al, 2010; Michael Singer Studio, 2014).

 ENHANCE SENSORY BALANCE

A covered entryway provides a visual, spatial and physical transition into the home, creating a place for individuals with high sensory needs to prepare themselves before entering or exiting (Dohrmann, 2014).

 CONTROLLING SOCIAL INTERACTION & PRIVACY

Provide visual access from the entry area into the rest of the home; previewing allows individuals the ability to determine whether to engage with others or not (Fleming and Purandare, 2010; Sinclair, 2010; Braddock and Rowell, 2011; Smith and Sharp, 2013; Kinnaer et al, 2014; Michael Singer Studio, 2014).

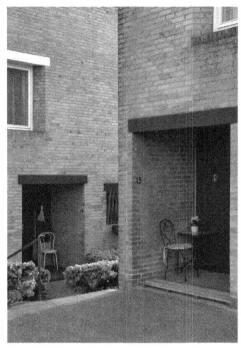

Figure 4.44 A covered entryway and a place to sit provides a calm transition space
(photo by Seier + Seier: Flickr CC)

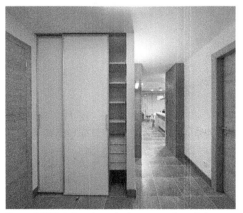

Figure 4.45 Sightlines from the front entry through the apartment
(photo by Mikhail Golub: Flickr CC)

LIVING ROOM

In most homes, living rooms need to accommodate a variety of activities. A quiet reading nook by a window, a comfortable sofa facing a television or a table for crafting or putting together a puzzle might all find space in the living room. In homes with more than one resident this variety is even more important. Research shows that people with autism often prefer to be social, so providing options for how socializing may occur is important. Living rooms, as well as other common areas, should be designed such that there are levels of participation: a peripheral seating area for observing; a middle ground for quiet conversations; and a central zone for more lively social activity.

In homes with multiple residents, provide a variety of common spaces that allow for a range of social interaction. Offering residents choices and flexibility in their living environment can reduce anxiety and conflict (Smith and Sharp, 2013; Kinnaer, Baumers and Heylighen, 2015).

Many people with autism enjoy being in the company of others although they may not want to participate directly in a group activity. Therefore, common living rooms should provide readily identifiable areas that allow multiple activities to occur simultaneously such as crafting, work, reading and watching television or listening to music. Some of these areas need to be on the periphery so that residents may retreat from main social space as necessary (Ahrentzen and Steele, 2009; Brand, 2010; Lee et al, 2012).

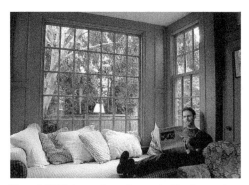

Figure 4.46 Window seats create opportunities for people to participate from the periphery
(photo by John M: Flickr CC)

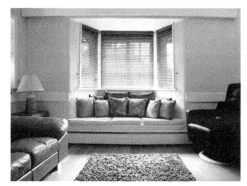

Figure 4.47 Periphery seating allows individuals to feel secure and part of the action
(iStock)

 ## ENHANCE SENSORY BALANCE

Since sensory sensitivities of people with autism often interfere with daily life activities, it is important to make living areas as sensory neutral as possible. Residents should decide whether or not to add sensory stimulation on a temporary basis (Leekam, et al, 2007; Kinnaer, Baumers and Heylighen, 2015).

Common living areas should be large enough to support different activities without crowding or creating too much sensory stimulation (Lee et al, 2012). Minimize sources of overstimulation: clutter, intercom systems, alarms, loud televisions or music, crowding, and so forth (Fleming and Purandare, 2010; Kargas, et al, 2015).

Natural light, good ventilation, effective acoustic dampening and temperature control are critical in all living areas and especially in common spaces where multiple people gather (Jones et al, 2001; Michael Singer Studio, 2014).

 ## PROVIDE ADEQUATE CHOICE & INDEPENDENCE

The careful arrangement of furniture directs movement and communicates what activities should occur where: sofas grouped together facilitate social interaction; a comfortable chair by a window encourages reading or listening to music; a computer station placed away from the main seating indicates a quiet work area; and a more centrally located table with several chairs suggests a place for group activities (Mostafa, 2010; Brand, 2010).

To ensure that all residents have full physical access to living areas, design the space and furniture arrangement to allow adequate room for wheelchair circulation (Department of Family and Community Services, 2013; Michael Singer Studio, 2014).

 ## ENSURE SAFETY & SECURITY

Design common living areas so that they are large enough to accommodate a variety of equipment as well as residents and support providers: people need to be able to safely retreat in the event of conflict or challenging behavior (Lee et al, 2012).

 ## FOSTER HEALTH & WELLNESS

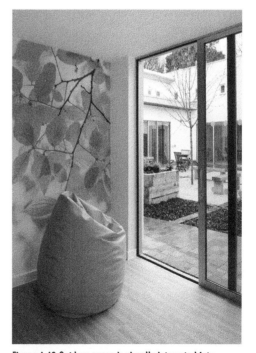

The living area should have direct access to an outdoor area, both visually and physically. Ideally, the outdoor space should be secure such that residents are able to visit it freely. For people who have a tendency to wander, creating a secure, accessible outdoor area is important (Whitehurst, 2007; Department of Family and Community, 2013).

Locate a communal bathroom in close proximity to the common areas (Ahrentzen and Steele, 2009; Michael Singer Studio, 2014).

Figure 4.48 Outdoor space is visually integrated into adjacent rooms
(Courtesy of Medical Architecture, photo by Edward Hopley)

DINING AREAS

In many homes, the dining room is not only a place to eat but also a place to read, do projects and socialize. For some people with autism, this multifunctional aspect may be confusing so it is important to understand the needs of individual residents and design the space to reflect those needs. Consideration also should be given to managing sensory aspects of food preparation and consumption: if odors and sounds are challenging, it will be necessary to provide adequate ventilation and space to mitigate the effects.

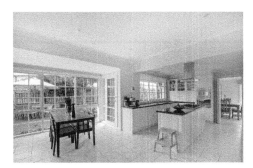

Figure 4.49 Variety of eating areas: breakfast nook, kitchen bar and dining room
(photo by Tim Collins: CC)

PROVIDE ADEQUATE CHOICE & INDEPENDENCE

Since communal dining may be difficult for some people, create a variety of eating area options. This may include eating at the kitchen island, in a breakfast nook or in a separate dining room. If there are multiple residents, design the dining area to be large enough to accommodate more than one table (Sergeant et al, 2007; Brand, 2010; Michael Singer Studio, 2014).

ENHANCE SENSORY BALANCE

For some people with autism, the textures, colors and smell of food is overwhelming. Therefore it is important to minimize sensory stimulation in the dining room and other eating areas. For some residents, dining areas and cooking areas may need to be separated. Excellent ventilation and sound mitigation along with good lighting and a calm color palette are essential (Sergeant et al, 2007; Brand, 2010).

KITCHEN

Understanding the individual needs of the resident will dictate what type of kitchen is needed. For people who cook independently, the size and layout of the kitchen may not differ significantly from other well-designed kitchens. For people who enjoy cooking but require assistance, the kitchen needs to be able to safely accommodate several cooks and independent living aides (for example, computers) operating simultaneously. In addition to size and functionality, a safe kitchen will incorporate non-toxic materials and appropriate, durable appliances.

PROVIDE ADEQUATE CHOICE & INDEPENDENCE

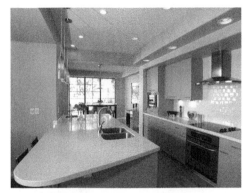

Figure 4.50 Kitchen with multiple work areas to accommodate several people
(photo by Nancy Hugo: Flickr CC)

The kitchen layout should facilitate resident participation in food preparation: provide multiple work areas including areas with seating and adjustable height countertops; specify more than one sink; and ensure ample circulation space to eliminate crowding (Zamprelli, 2009; Brand, 2010; Lee et al, 2011; Lee et al, 2012; Michael Singer Studio, 2014).

FOSTER HEALTH & WELLNESS

If any residents have obsessive food behaviors then some kitchen cabinets as well as the refrigerator should be lockable. If needed, consider installing moveable kitchen cabinets/islands (on lockable casters) that can be used to block circulation through the kitchen. This type of island also adds flexible workspace (Williams and Boult, 2009; Michael Singer Studio, 2014).

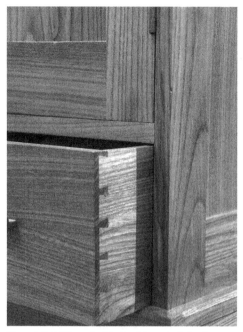

Figure 4.51 Solid wood cabinets with non-toxic finishes are a healthy and durable choice
(photo by Jordanhill School D&T Dept: Flickr CC)

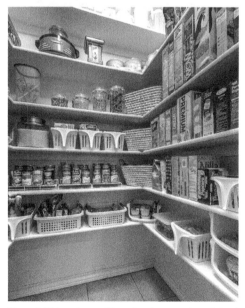

Figure 4.52 A pantry provides extra storage and good visual access
(photo by Bill Wilson: Flickr CC)

Avoid specifying cabinets constructed of pressed woods such as particleboard, medium-density fiberboard (MDF), melamine over particleboard or hardwood plywood as all of these emit formaldehyde. Green Cabinet Source (http://greencabinetsource. org) lists cabinet manufacturers and brands certified by the Environmental Stewardship Program (ESP) in the United States. Solid wood cabinets – including end panels, backs, shelves and drawer bottoms and sides – with a non-toxic finish are the healthiest choice. If residents are not sensitive to odors, Medex fiberboard (www. sierrapine.com/green-products/mdf/) is a formaldehyde-free option (Healthy House Institute, 2014; NKBA, 2014; Michael Singer Studio, 2014).

 MAXIMIZE FAMILIARITY, STABILITY, PREDICTABILITY & CLARITY

Provide sufficient kitchen storage to minimize clutter. If there are multiple residents, storage should be provided such that individuals may have their own cupboards. Avoid using nameplates to identify individual resident storage areas; instead consider aesthetically appropriate icons or colors. This will create a more home-like rather than institutional feel (Williams and Boult, 2009; Ahrentzen and Steele, 2009; Michael Singer Studio, 2014).

For garbage, recycling and compost, designate a clearly marked area that is easily accessible (Michael Singer Studio, 2014).

Design the kitchen to resemble a typical kitchen in a typical home; avoid an institutional quality. Include appliances found in typical kitchens but specify models appropriate for residents. For example, wall-mounted ovens with side-swing doors are barrier free and accessible, and safer to use than freestanding ovens or wall-mounted ovens with pull-down doors (Zamprelli, 2009).

Provide a variety of countertop heights or install adjustable counters: work areas should be provided at heights of 42 inches, 36 inches and 30 inches (seated prep area). This allows residents to choose what is most comfortable for them at any particular time (Ahrentzen and Steele, 2009; AARP Livable Communities, 2014).

To ensure visibility and access to contents, select cabinets with pullout shelves or drawers and corner cabinets with Lazy Susans. Cabinets and drawers should close automatically (Ahrentzen and Steele, 2009).

 ## ENSURE SAFETY & SECURITY

Some people with autism may experience unusual sensitivity to pain or may have difficulty discerning what is causing pain. Therefore, to minimize accidental injury from touching a hot pan, isolate stovetop/cooking hob away from primary work areas.

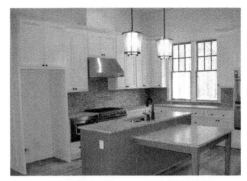

Figure 4.53 Different height work areas allow residents to sit or stand
(photo by Atlanta Scott: Flickr CC)

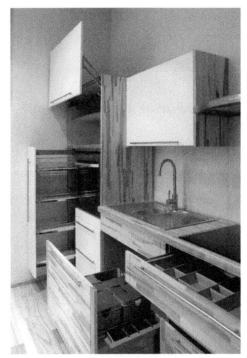

Figure 4.54 Pull-out cabinets and drawers with inserts provided are accessible and easy to organize
(iStock)

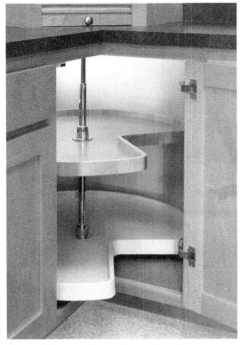

Figure 4.55 Corner cabinets with rotating shelves increase accessibility
(iStock)

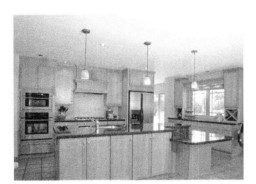

Figure 4.56 Wall-mounted oven is separate from stovetop
(photo by Nancy Hugo: Flickr CC)

Install under-cabinet task lighting to ensure that there is adequate light during meal preparation (Michael Singer Studio, 2014).

Many people with autism are fascinated by water and enjoy playing with it. To alleviate the possibility of leaving the water running unattended, which may lead to flooding, install low-flow faucets with a motion sensor automatic shut-off switch (Michael Singer Studio, 2014).

Since some people with autism may experience unusual responses to pain, reduce the possibility of scalding by installing single-handle faucets fitted with a temperature sensor.

To avoid inadvertent injury, do not install a garbage disposal in the kitchen sink. Instead, install a drain trap and ensure the sink has a captive plug (Ahrentzen and Steele, 2009).

Install waterproof, slip-resistant flooring in the kitchen (Michael Singer Studio, 2014).

Food storage areas should be placed away from the cooking surface to reduce accidents related to reaching and crowding (Ahrentzen and Steele, 2009).

 ENHANCE SENSORY BALANCE

Good lighting is essential: provide a mix of artificial and natural lighting (Department of Family and Community Services, 2013).

Excellent (and quiet) kitchen ventilation will allow people with sensitivities to smell to participate in meal preparation. Proper product selection and installation is imperative: select range hoods and fans that minimize sound and install a duct attenuator or silencer in the steel or aluminum duct (HVAC Quick, 2014).

To help reduce slamming noise, install cabinet door dampeners and bumpers (Michael Singer Studio, 2014).

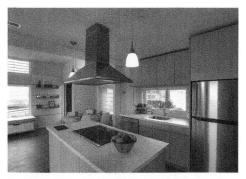

Figure 4.57 Utilize natural and mechanical ventilation
(photo by Jason Flakes: Flickr CC)

 ## FOSTER HEALTH & WELLNESS

 ## ENSURE DURABILITY

Countertop materials should be hygienic, non-toxic and able to withstand significant wear and tear including stains, cutting, heat and impact. While there is no perfect countertop material – impervious to damage, antibacterial, no off-gassing and low to no maintenance – some choices are better than others. (Bower, 2000; Ahrentzen and Steele, 2009; Brand, 2010; Michael Singer Studio, 2014).

Engineered stone (quartz) rates highly in all categories as does granite, although granite is more susceptible to staining and there are some concerns regarding radon emission (Health Physics Society, n.d.).

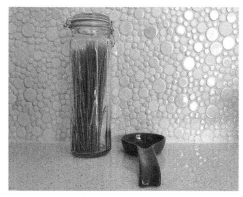

Figure 4.58 A visually interesting and durable backsplash adds texture without being too busy
(photo by Leelooshka: Flickr CC)

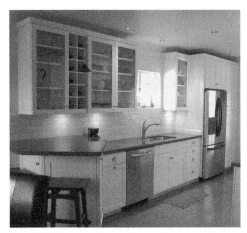

Figure 4.59 Engineered quartz (such as Caesarstone) countertops are a durable choice
(photo by Nancy Hugo: Flickr CC)

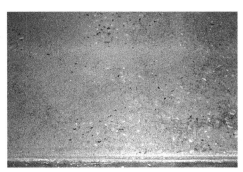

Figure 4.60 Although concrete requires some maintenance, it also is a good countertop choice
(photo by Bay Dragon: Flickr CC)

Recycled paper countertops also are a good choice and since the material is formaldehyde- and petroleum-free, it works well for people with chemical sensitivities (www.paperstoneproducts. com/ and www.richlite.com/).

Other choices include concrete (requires regular sealing with a non-toxic sealer), large porcelain tiles (more durable than regular ceramic tile and as stain and scratch resistant as quartz) and stainless steel (use thicker gauge to minimize denting and to eliminate the need to laminate it to a plywood base).

If choosing plastic laminate countertops, replace the particleboard substrate with formaldehyde-free particleboard or construction-grade plywood adhering it with a water-based, low-toxicity contact adhesive. To fully encase the substrate material and trap any residual wood odors, encase it on all four sides (rather than the typical two) with the laminate. Durability may be an issue: laminate countertops scratch easily and pooling water causes delamination (Healthy House Institute, 2014).

Helpful online sources include the Countertop Guide (2014), Consumer Reports (n.d), and the Healthy House Institute (2014).

HALLWAYS, STAIRS, RAMPS & DOORWAYS

Treat hallways as multi-functional zones: they offer opportunities for impromptu socializing and areas to engage in gross-motor activities such as jumping. To accommodate these uses, hallways need to be wide with high ceilings. If possible, limit residences to one-story to reduce the possibility of falls and to accommodate residents throughout their lifespan. All doorways should be zero-threshold to minimize tripping and to allow wheelchair access when necessary.

MAXIMIZE FAMILIARITY, STABILITY, PREDICTABILITY & CLARITY

In homes with several residents, keep hallways short, wide and bright with good visibility to facilitate navigation and maintain a home-like feel. Long, narrow, windowless corridors with multiple doors and no windows convey an institutional-like quality and do not encourage residents to engage in social exchanges or to sit and relax (Brand, 2010; Lee et al, 2012; Michael Singer Studio, 2014).

Gently curving walls and corners create a more inviting, less visually rigid space that may be more appealing and welcoming to many residents (Beaver, 2006; Whitehurst, 2006; Brand, 2010).

Minimize "blind" corners since they introduce unpredictability (Department of Family and Community Services, 2013).

Each floor should be accessible to all residents. Including a ramp and/or elevator is preferable: a ramp facilitates social interaction and eases resident anxiety in event of a power outage (Ahrentzen and Steele, 2009; Mikiten, 2008).

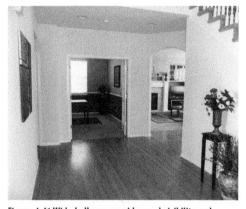

Figure 4.61 Wide hallways provide good visibility and accommodate resident activity
(photo by Brian & Rita Burke: Flickr CC)

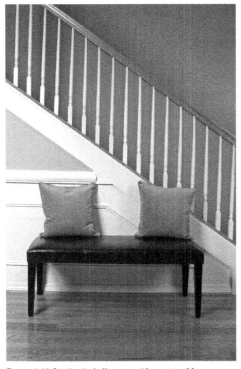

Figure 4.62 Seating in hallway provides a transition space and opportunity for socializing
(iStock)

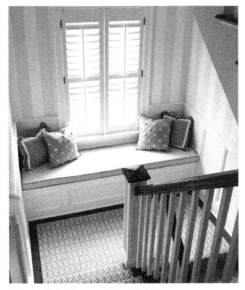

Figure 4.63 Seating area at top of stairs
(photo by Homestilo: Flickr CC)

 CONTROLLING SOCIAL INTERACTION & PRIVACY

Treat hallways as integral living space, places for residents to occupy rather than just pass through. Include features that provide opportunities for social interactions such as benches, chairs and window seats, mailboxes, activity calendars and community event boards (San Francisco, CA, 2009, personal communication; Brand, 2010; Braddock and Rowell, 2011; Manager, Mission Bay Senior Housing, Lee et al, 2012).

In homes with stairs, provide seating at landings to create opportunities for socialization and to allow for previewing of common areas (Ahrentzen and Steele, 2009).

 FOSTER HEALTH & WELLNESS

Opt for single-loaded hallways with windows or doors opening onto shared spaces or a courtyard. This allows for cross-ventilation, natural light and views to nature (van den Berg et al, 2007; Ahrentzen and Steele, 2009; Lee et al, 2012; Medical Architecture, July 2014, personal communication).

To facilitate access and accommodate residents' gross motor movements as well as mobility changes throughout the lifespan, doorways should be 1 meter or 36 inches wide (Department of Family and Community Services, 2013).

ENHANCE SENSORY BALANCE

Wide hallways with tall ceilings provide residents with space to move, jump, pace and so on. The ability to engage in gross motor movements helps some people with autism reduce stress and anxiety and control negative reactions (Baker et al, 2008; Williams and Boult, 2009 Braddock and Rowell, 2011; Fournier et al, 2010;).

Install well-secured carpet runners on stairs to reduce noise. Carpet runners are economical to replace or clean when soiled (Ahrentzen and Steele, 2009).

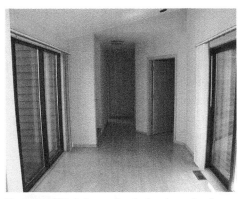

Figure 4.64 Wide hallways allow for jumping and pacing (photo by Nicolas Will: Flickr CC)

 ## ENSURE SAFETY & SECURITY

Where there are stairs, closed risers and continuous handrails on both sides with spacious landings are safest (Livable Housing Australia, 2012).

BEDROOMS

To enhance the quality of life and dignity of adults with autism, in homes with more than one resident, a private bedroom with an ensuite bathroom should be provided for each resident. Private bedrooms with ensuite bathrooms are integral to resident wellbeing, sense of security and quality of life, allowing residents opportunities to personalize and have control over personal space. Being able to retreat to a private sanctuary also provides residents with the possibility of avoiding unwanted interactions with others. In homes where bedrooms and bathrooms are shared, there are more interpersonal conflicts, less resident satisfaction and poorer outcomes (Barnes and Design in Caring Enviroments Caring Group, 2002; Williams and Boult, 2009; Braddock and Rowell, 2011; Lee et al, 2012; Zeisel, 2013).

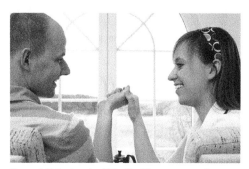

Figure 4.65 Design should be flexible to accommodate couples
(iStock)

 ENHANCE ONE'S DIGNITY

 CONTROLLING SOCIAL INTERACTION & PRIVACY

Similar to most people, many people with autism seek lifetime partners. Therefore, bedrooms should be large enough to accommodate a couple. (Farley et al, 2009; Brand, 2010; Wedmore, 2011; Lee et al, 2012; Michael Singer Studio, 2014).

Bedrooms should be designed to include substantial storage, a desk or sitting area and, for some residents, a small kitchenette with a microwave and small refrigerator (Zamprelli, 2009).

Including a small sidelight adjacent to the bedroom door permits residents to view the hallway before entering, thereby controlling potential social interactions (Lee et al, 2012; Michael Singer Studio, 2014)

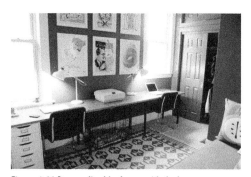

Figure 4.66 Personalized bedroom with desk space
(photo Emily May: Flickr CC)

MAXIMIZE FAMILIARITY, STABILITY, PREDICTABILITY & CLARITY

Private areas of the home where bedrooms are located should be clearly distinguished from communal areas. This can be accomplished through changes in wall color, flooring, and/or lighting style (Williams and Boult, 2009; Michael Singer Studio, 2014).

Bedrooms should look like regular domestic bedrooms not like hospital or institutional rooms (Lee et al, 2012).

Consult residents to determine if cabinets should have transparent or opaque doors: some people with autism need to see belongings (Anonymous architectural clients, June 2014, personal communication).

Closets should be internally lit and outfitted with a built-in organization system to assist residents with their daily dressing and grooming tasks (Ahrentzen and Steele, 2009).

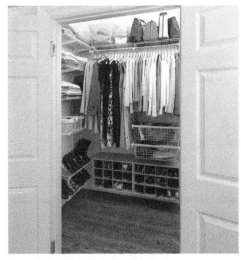

Figure 4.67 Closet with built in organization system (photo by Rubbermaid Products: Flickr CC)

 FOSTER HEALTH & WELLNESS

Each bedroom should have a window with a view to nature. The window should be operable to allow for ventilation and contact with the outdoors (Ulrich, 1999; Kaplan, 2001; Brand, 2010; Lee et al, 2012; Michael Singer Studio, 2014).

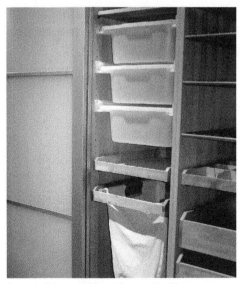

Figure 4.68 Open shelving with organizing bins (iStock)

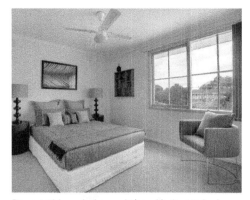

Figure 4.69 Large bedroom window with views to landscape (photo by Tim Collins: CC)

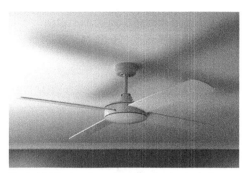

Figure 4.70 Unobtrusive, quiet ceiling fan for the bedroom (photo Russell Street: Flickr CC)

For many people with autism, sleeping through the night is a challenge. To control light intrusions, install external louvers or 'blackout' shades on bedroom windows. Incorporating excellent sound insulation into floors, ceilings, walls, doors and windows is essential (Oyane and Bjorvatn, 2005; Vanderbilt Sleep Disorders Center, 2013).

Installing individual thermal controls and ventilation fans in each bedroom improves resident comfort and sleep, and reduces overall energy consumption (Ahrentzen and Steele, 2009; Vanderbilt Sleep Disorders Center, 2013; Department of Family and Community Services, 2013; Michael Singer Studio, 2014).

CONTROLLING SOCIAL INTERACTION & PRIVACY

PROVIDE ADEQUATE CHOICE & INDEPENDENCE

Wireless internet connection, a media center with television and music, and movable storage should be incorporated into each bedroom. For residents who wish to have a television in their bedrooms, it may be necessary to install a protection screen to protect it from accidental damage (Brand, 2010; Department of Family and Community Services, 2013).

ENSURE SAFETY & SECURITY

 ENSURE DURABILITY

For some residents, built-in furniture, especially bookshelves, is necessary to prevent it from tipping and falling. This will also prolong the life of the furniture (Department of Family and Community Services, 2013).

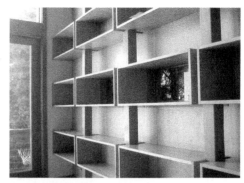

Figure 4.71 Wall of built-in shelves
(photo Jeremy Levine: Flickr CC)

BATHROOMS

To ensure privacy and enhance dignity, in homes with multiple residents each resident should have a private bathroom adjacent to his or her bedroom. Since some people with autism may have issues with incontinence and require assistance, each bathroom should be able to accommodate a support provider. It is important to provide an additional, accessible bathroom in proximity to common living areas for use by guests and other visitors.

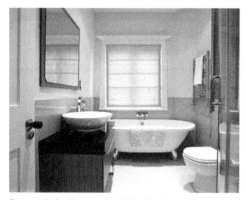

Figure 4.72 Inviting, non-institutional style bathroom (photo by Holland & Green Architecture: Flickr CC)

MAXIMIZE FAMILIARITY, STABILITY, PREDICTABILITY & CLARITY

Where it is the cultural norm, toilets should be separate from the bathtub, shower and sink. This will reduce confusion and chance for misuse (Sergeant et al, 2007; Brand, 2010).

Decorative wall and floor tiles help create a home-like quality rather than an institutional feel (Department of Family and Community Services, 2013).

Design bathrooms to be large enough to accommodate a wheelchair and support provider with the door opening inward. Outward opening doors convey an institutional atmosphere (Brand, 2010; Michael Singer Studio, 2014).

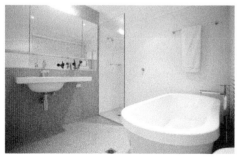

Figure 4.73 Accessible bathroom with roll-in shower and wall-hung sink (iStock)

PROVIDE ADEQUATE CHOICE & INDEPENDENCE

Bathrooms should be designed to accommodate a wheelchair rider. Install a roll-in shower (if possible, bathtub as well) and wall-hung sink and toilet with adequate surrounding space (Brand, 2010; Department of Family and Community Services, 2013; Michael Singer Studio, 2014).

FOSTER HEALTH & WELLNESS

Provide a communal bathroom in the common living area for visitors. To ensure resident privacy, the bathroom door should not open directly onto a living area (Brand, 2010; Michael Singer Studio, 2014; Department of Family and Community Services, 2013).

In multistory residences include a main floor bathroom for accessibility for residents and guests (Ahrentzen and Steele, 2009; AARP Livable Communities, 2014).

Reduce moisture buildup, potential mold growth and unpleasant odors by installing non paper-faced backing materials such as cement board or fiber cement board (Enterprise Green Communities, 2011).

The bathroom should have access to natural light and ventilation: install frosted glass windows, transom or clerestory windows and/or skylights/solatubes (Michael Singer Studio, 2014).

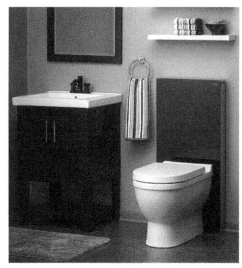

Figure 4.74 Communal bathroom or powder room for visitors
(photo by Design Milk: Flickr CC)

 ENHANCE SENSORY BALANCE

To minimize noise, select an ultra-quiet bath fan with a remotely mounted motor. The fan should not come on with the light as this can be startling (Beaver, 2010; Brand, 2010).

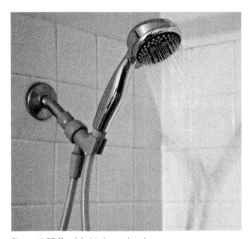

Figure 4.75 Hand-held showerhead
(photo by Geoffrey Fairchild: Flickr CC)

 ENSURE SAFETY & SECURITY

Provide built-in wet location lighting for shower, sink and bathtub (Michael Singer Studio, 2014).

Telephone or hand-held showerheads typically are easier for many people to use; however in some cases it might be necessary to install anti-ligature shower fixtures (Zamprelli, 2009; Brand, 2010).

To prevent the bathtub (or sinks) from overflowing, install a water-level monitor such as MagiBath or Nova-Flo (Sensorium, n.d.; www.nova-flo.com).

Consider installing a flood detector near the bathtub, toilet or sink to alert residents and support providers of water on the floor (Tunstall Solutions, 2014).

The shower should feature a built-in shower seat to assist people with motor coordination and mobility issues (Enterprise Green Communities, 2011; Bryant and Bryant, 2012).

Handrails should be installed in the bathtub, shower and adjacent to the toilet. Walls need to be reinforced to accommodate heavy use. It is wise to reinforce walls under towel racks since these might be used as grab rails (Zamprelli, 2009; Department of Family and Community Services, 2013; Michael Singer Studio, 2014).

To minimize tripping and ensure accessibility, design the shower stall to have a zero-threshold entry (Zamprelli,

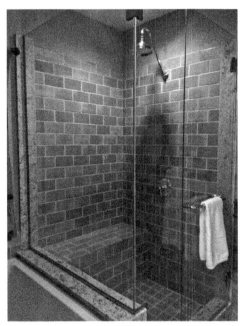

Figure 4.76 Spacious shower with built-in seat
(photo by Memphis CVB: Flickr CC)

2009; Department of Family and Community Services, 2013; Michael Singer Studio, 2014).

Bathrooms should be large enough to comfortably accommodate two people. This allows a support provider to accompany a resident safely if needed (Brand, 2010; Braddock and Rowell, 2011; Michael Singer Studio, 2014).

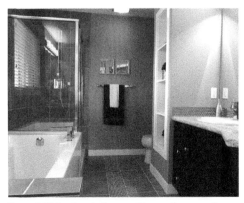

Figure 4.77 Spacious bathroom with room for support provider if needed

Similar to kitchen and laundry sinks, consider fitting bathroom sinks as well as showers and bathtubs with auto shut-off motion sensors. It is important that sensors are not too sensitive and only turn off after resident is out of the shower or has stepped away from the sink (Michael Singer Studio, 2014).

ENSURE SAFETY & SECURITY

ENSURE DURABILITY

Design bathrooms to be as waterproof and slip proof as possible: often people with autism enjoy playing with water. Floors and walls should be well sealed and a floor drain should be installed in the shower and main area (Brand, 2010; Lee et al, 2012; Maytum, 2013; Michael Singer Studio, 2014).

Select non-slip, non-toxic waterproof materials for floors and walls such as tiles and non-toxic grout; avoid toxic epoxy floor coatings (Hello Housing, 2009, personal communication; Maytum, 2013; Michael Singer Studio, 2014).

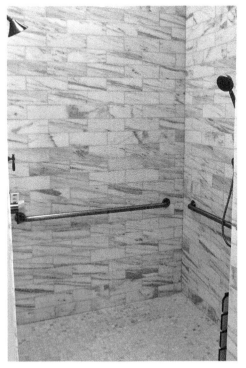

Figure 4.78 Handrail in the shower
(photo by Heritage: Flickr CC)

Additional options for non-slip, bacteria resistant, waterproof, 'wet room' solutions for floors, walls and shower liners include Granit Multisafe waterproof vinyl flooring and Aquarelle Wall HFS by Tarkett/Johnsonite (http://professionals.tarkett.com/) or Safestep Grip by Forbo (www.forbo-flooring.com/). These products may off-gas; therefore procedures for thoroughly ventilating fumes after installation need to be followed carefully.

When using any of these products, it is important to ensure that the bathroom does not appear institutional.

 ENSURE DURABILITY

Toilets should have concealed cisterns and use a push panel flush system for durability and ease of use (Ahrentzen and Steele, 2009; Brand, 2010).

Select heavy-duty toilet seats and bowls to accommodate heavy wear such as bouncing (Sergeant et al, 2007; Peter Dollard, The Center for Discovery, June 2013, personal communication).

Incorporate extra wall reinforcing to support toilets, sinks, shower heads and towel racks as fixtures often are subjected to excessive wear. Avoid specifying showerheads that can be used for swinging (Beaver, 2010; Braddock and Rowell, 2011; Michael Singer Studio, 2014).

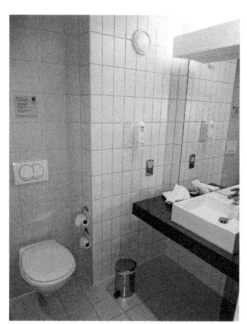

Figure 4.79 Concealed cistern toilet with push panel flush (photo by Sean MacEntee: Flickr CC)

To simplify removing clogs from toilets, sinks, showers and bathtubs, install over-sized clean-outs and debris traps. Brand (2010) suggests installing "a large bore toilet waste pipe with inspection chamber behind the toilet pan" (see also, Michael Singer Studio, 2014).

All pipework should be concealed (Beaver, 2010; Michael Singer Studio, 2014).

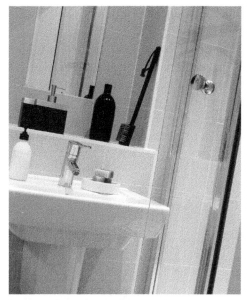

Figure 4.80 Sink with concealed pipework (iStock)

MULTI-SENSORY ENVIRONMENTS

Most people with autism experience unusual sensory responses (Crane, Goddard and Pring, 2009; Cascio et al, 2012; Elwin et al, 2012). To assist people to manage sensory input, provide a separate room fitted with elements that residents can manipulate and control. Multi-sensory environments may help reduce stress and anxiety and assist in modifying behaviors. For the greatest benefit, it is important that the room be large enough to accommodate movements such as bouncing, jumping and pacing.

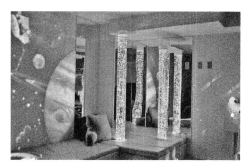

Figure 4.81 Sensory room with lighting, cushions and wall-projections
(Courtesy of Linda Messbauer)

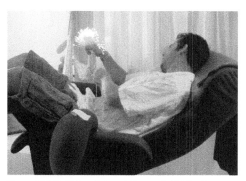

Figure 4.82 Reclining chair and fiber optic lighting in sensory room
(Courtesy of Linda Messbauer)

 ENHANCE SENSORY BALANCE

To assist autistic residents in modulating their sensory needs and stereotypic behaviors, provide a dedicated room or space that contains a range of equipment and sensory tools that residents may manipulate. The room should be painted white, allowing the user to determine what colors to add and what equipment to use (Messbauer, 2009).

Equipment for the room should address all sensory modalities: tactile, visual, olfactory, auditory, vestibular (movement and balance) and proprioceptive (understanding position of body in space). This equipment may include rocking chairs and swings, bean bag chairs, vibrating floor mats, a sound system, aromatherapy oils, mirror light balls and bubble columns and a projection system (Cuvo et al, 2001; Messbauer, 2012).

For the room to be functional it needs to be fairly large: a room that is too small will not be used because it will be too confining, limiting the use of the equipment (Messbauer, 2012).

The room should have individual thermal controls to allow residents to adjust the temperature to meet their needs (Messbauer, 2008).

The room should be acoustically contained such that outside noises do not intrude and sound generated within does not escape (Ahrentzen and Steele, 2009).

Snoezelen Rooms (Dutch for "sniff" and "doze") are an established sensory room model that can be referenced (Ahrentzen and Steele, 2009).

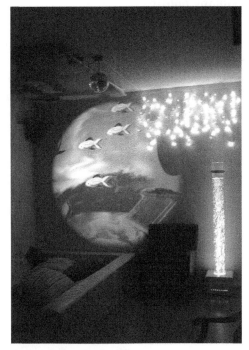

Figure 4.83 Snoezelen Room
(photo by Ciell: CC)

LAUNDRY ROOMS

Each home should include a dedicated laundry room that is bright and with adequate ventilation. Since some people with autism may have issues with incontinence, to preserve their dignity and maintain hygienic standards it is best to provide a separate room where soiled clothing and linen can be kept separate from other areas of the home. Incorporate into the space adequate room for sorting and folding.

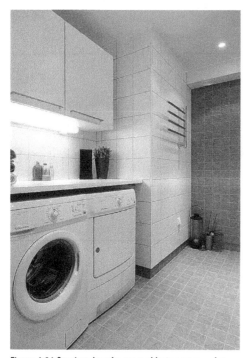

Figure 4.84 Spacious laundry room able to accommodate resident and support provider if needed
(photo by Maegan Tintari: Flickr CC)

 ENHANCE ONE'S DIGNITY

Providing private laundry facilities in the home is important for maintaining the dignity of people who are incontinent as well as promoting independence (Zamprelli, 2009; Williams and Boult, 2009).

 FOSTER HEALTH & WELLNESS

To minimize the possibility of soiled clothing coming in contact with food, place the laundry room in proximity to bedrooms and bathrooms and away from kitchen and dining areas (Brand, 2010).

Locate the laundry room on an exterior wall to ensure excellent ventilation and to allow the dryer to be exhausted directly outdoors: minimizing the duct run helps avoid moisture and particle buildup. In some homes it may be necessary to install a sterile air purifier to destroy any airborne bacteria or viruses (Enterprise Green Communities, 2011; JTM, 2014).

A door connecting the laundry room to the outside will provide easy access to an outdoor clothesline facilitating hanging clothes out to dry (Brand, 2010).

To improve hygienic washing for residents and support providers, consider including a sluice washing machine (handles solids) in addition to the regular washing machine. Miele Professional and Electrolux Laundry Systems make front load sluice machines (Brand, 2010; Careinfo, 2014).

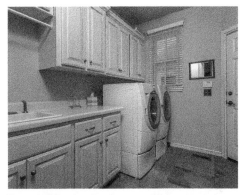

Figure 4.85 Spacious laundry room with door to exterior (photo by Bill Wilson: Flickr CC)

Incontinence is not uncommon among autistic individuals; therefore, include a macerator for disposing of incontinence pads. A macerator reduces odor and potential for contamination (Brand, 2010; Haigh Hygienic Solutions, 2014).

Include a utility sink or commercial hopper to contend with heavily soiled items (Ahrentzen and Steele, 2009; Michael Singer Studio, 2014).

 FOSTER HEALTH & WELLNESS

 MAXIMIZE FAMILIARITY, STABILITY, PREDICTABILITY & CLARITY

Establish a color-coded laundry bag/ trolley system to assist residents in keeping soiled and clean clothes and linens separate (JTM, 2014).

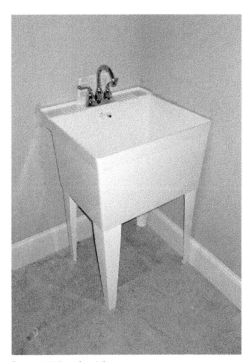

Figure 4.86 Laundry sink (photo by Jesus Rodriguez: Flickr CC)

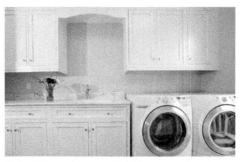

Figure 4.87 Laundry room with folding area and ample storage
(iStock)

The room should be large enough to include clearly identified, separate areas for soiled and clean clothes and linens as well as ample multi-level counter space to accommodate sorting, stain prep, folding and ironing. The space should be large enough for a resident and support provider to work simultaneously (Brand, 2010; Michael Singer Studio, 2014; JTM, 2014).

To eliminate clutter, provide adequate storage for laundry supplies (Michael Singer Studio, 2014).

PROVIDE ADEQUATE CHOICE & INDEPENDENCE

Front load washing machines and dryers installed at the appropriate height are most accessible for residents and support providers. If necessary, raise the appliance to accommodate wheelchair riders (Michael Singer Studio, 2014).

ENHANCE SENSORY BALANCE

To reduce odors from detergents and soiled clothes or linens, provide adequate ventilation through inclusion of an ultra-quiet ventilation fan and operable windows. The fan should not come on with the light as this can be startling (Ahrentzen and Steele, 2009; Beaver, 2010; Michael Singer Studio, 2014).

Laundry room insulation must be robust to contain machine noise. Install shake absorber pads under appliances and an ultra-quiet ventilation fan for the room (Ahrentzen and Steele, 2009; Michael Singer Studio, 2014).

 ENSURE DURABILITY

Install durable, waterproof flooring with a floor drain to accommodate spills and accidental flooding (Ahrentzen and Steele, 2009; Michael Singer Studio, 2014).

Cabinetry and countertops should be durable; use the same materials as those in the kitchen (Michael Singer Studio, 2014).

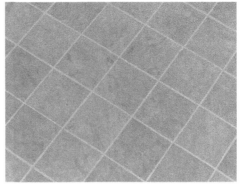

Figure 4.88 Textured, vitreous porcelain tile is a durable, non-slip flooring option
(photo by PJM: CC)

 ENSURE SAFETY & SECURITY

Include a fold-down ironing board with sufficient room surrounding it to reduce the possibility of residents inadvertently bumping into a hot iron (Ahrentzen and Steele, 2009).

Similar to kitchen and bathroom sinks, consider fitting the utility sink with an automatic shut-off motion sensor. It is important that sensors are not too sensitive and only turn off after a resident has stepped away from the sink (Michael Singer Studio, 2014).

Consider installing a flood detector to alert residents and support providers of water on the floor (Tunstall Solutions, 2014).

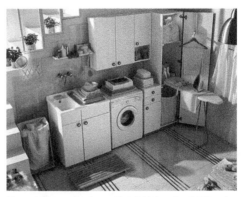

Figure 4.89 Laundry room with a fold-down ironing board
(photo by Maegan Tintari: Flickr CC)

STORAGE

To minimize clutter, integrate storage solutions throughout the house. Understanding the specific needs of the residents is particularly important when it comes to organizing belongings: some people prefer visually calm environments where everything is out of sight where others rely on viewing their things in order to know what is available to them. A storage solution that does not respond to these specific needs can result in significant frustration and anxiety for residents.

MAXIMIZE FAMILIARITY, STABILITY, PREDICTABILITY & CLARITY

Storage solutions should accommodate wheelchair riders and individuals using walkers (Zamprelli, 2009).

Storage in both public and private areas should have a variety of compartments to support individual routines and needs (Ahrentzen and Steele, 2009; Mostafa, 2010).

Integrate storage into bench seating and other built-in elements; this will reduce visual clutter and create a sense of order. Provide built-in lighting to enhance visibility (Michael Singer Studio, 2014).

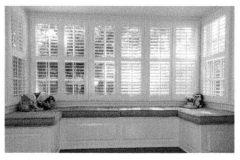

Figure 4.90 Bench seat with integrated storage
(photo by Stephen Harris: Flickr CC)

ENHANCE SENSORY BALANCE

Storage solutions should take into account the individual needs of the residents: some people with autism need to have visual access to their belongings while others need to minimize visual stimulation (Anonymous architectural client, June 2014, personal communication).

Strategically placed built-in storage can function as an acoustic buffer between rooms (Michael Singer Studio, 2014).

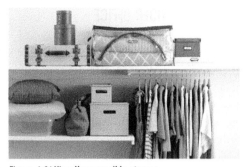

Figure 4.91 Visually accessible storage
(photo by Rubbermaid Products: Flickr CC)

 PROVIDE ADEQUATE CHOICE & INDEPENDENCE

Storage should be accessible to residents, allowing them to retrieve their belongings when they choose (Michael Singer Studio, 2014).

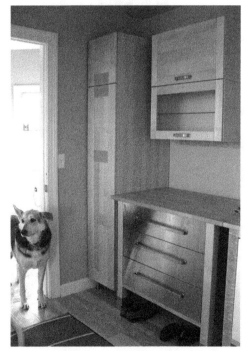

Figure 4.92 Mudroom with storage doubles as transition space
(photo by FD Richard: Flickr CC)

SUPPORT PROVIDER OFFICE

In homes with multiple residents where support provision is required, it is necessary to provide a dedicated support provider office. In addition to the functional aspects of a dedicated office space – maintain client privacy, safely store and disseminate medications – it also provides a space for support providers to retreat to and take breaks. In homes with round-the-clock support, the office should include a bed and bathroom so that providers may rest and shower.

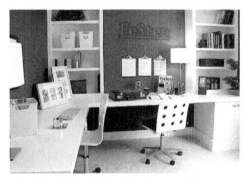

Figure 4.93 Dedicated office with adequate workspace
(photo by FE Group Bangkok: CC)

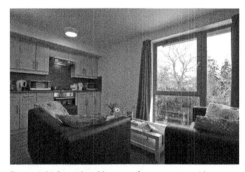

Figure 4.94 A comfortable space for support providers to take breaks and do paperwork is essential
(photo by University of Exeter: Flickr CC)

 FOSTER HEALTH & WELLNESS

To create a healthy work environment, provide a clearly defined office space for support providers where they may retreat to do paperwork in private, prepare medications and, importantly, take breaks (Hello Housing, personal communication, 2009; Brand, 2010).

The lockable office should include a desk, lockable file storage, shelving and a sink and secure medication cabinet. In homes with 24-hour support provision, the office should include a bed and bathroom with shower for sleep-in support staff (Hello Housing, 2009; Brand, 2010; Michael Singer Studio, 2014).

The support provider office should have excellent acoustic insulation to ensure conversations are private and to reduce noise flow at night when residents are sleeping (Department of Family and Community Services, 2013).

ENSURE SAFETY & SECURITY

Not only must the office be lockable, but also the sightlines from the office to the common living areas need to be good. This allows support providers to observe from a distance without routinely intruding on residents (Lee et al, 2011; Department of Family and Community Services, 2013).

VENTILATION

For residents who are hypersensitive – experience heightened sensory reactions to environmental stimuli – spaces that accumulate odors can be overwhelming. To mitigate any potential problem, ventilation should be carefully considered at the outset and a variety of solutions should be incorporated into the design.

 ENHANCE SENSORY BALANCE

To reduce ambient noise, select passive ventilation over extractor fans when possible (Sergeant et al, 2007).

For better control of indoor air quality and reduced noise, install a central ventilation system with acoustical insulation. Specify acoustic duct board rather than traditional ducting systems (Brand, 2010; Michael Singer Studio, 2014).

Ultra-quiet ventilation fans should be specified for bathrooms, laundry room and kitchen. Fans and lights should be on separate switches (Beaver, 2010; Michael Singer Studio, 2014).

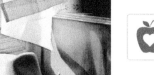 **FOSTER HEALTH & WELLNESS**

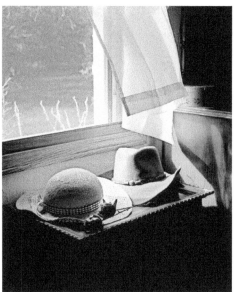
Figure 4.95 Operable windows for good ventilation (iStock)

Include operable windows in all living areas. For ideal ventilation, design to promote cross ventilation wherever possible: air entering a low placed window will be pulled out of a window placed high on the opposite wall. Include secure, operable windows in all living areas (Ahrentzen and Steele, 2009; Beaver, 2010).

For the best indoor air quality, install a whole home HVAC system with an integrated HEPA filter (Ahrentzen and Steele, 2009; Hirshberg, 2011; Michael Singer Studio, 2014).

Installing an inadequate ventilation system has a negative impact on indoor air quality, potentially leading to the build-up of moisture, chemical fumes from cleaning supplies, dust particles and heat. The Home Ventilation Institute (www.HVI.org) provides guides for selecting ventilation systems appropriate for the project type: products and manufacturers are listed for Canada and the US.

To prevent contaminants from the garage from entering the house, install a continuous air barrier between the living space and garage. On doors connecting the garage and living space, include auto-closer or spring hinges with airtight weather stripping. Do not install air-handling equipment in the garage (Emmerich et al, 2003; Enterprise Green Communities, 2015).

To reduce dirt and allergen buildup, select blinds enclosed between windowpanes rather than curtains. If this is not an option, select washable curtains made of cotton or washable roller-type shades (Ahrentzen and Steele, 2009; Mayo Clinic, 2014).

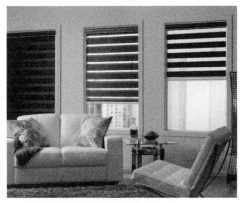

Figure 4.96 Adjustable, integrated window blinds
(photo by Blinds Online: Flickr CC)

HEATING AND COOLING

Since individuals with autism often have divergent sensory experiences, in homes with multiple residents providing individual climate controls in private bedrooms allows people to adjust the temperature of the environment to meet their needs. Individual autonomy fosters independence, control and wellbeing and may reduce conflict and overall resident dissatisfaction.

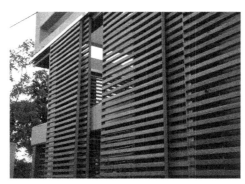

Figure 4.97 Mobile sun shades provide passive heating and cooling
(photo by Jeremy Levine: Flickr CC)

FOSTER HEALTH & WELLNESS

To maximize passive heating and cooling potential and reduce overall costs, optimize the building's solar orientation and if possible, consider including a solarium or atrium for passive solar heating (Mostafa, 2010; Michael Singer Studio, 2014).

ENSURE SAFETY & SECURITY

Underfloor, radiant heating systems provide consistent heat, are quiet, efficient and because the elements are not exposed there is no risk of damage or harm to residents. Selecting the proper system is important, as some systems may be too complicated for residents to operate (Whitehurst, 2006; Sergeant et al, 2007; Williams and Boult, 2009; Beaver, 2010; Brand, 2010; Deidre Sheerin, 2013, personal conversation).

ENHANCE SENSORY BALANCE

Specify a HVAC system with an ultra-quiet air handler and condenser; be sure to locate the air handler and condenser away from the bedrooms because of the noise (Michael Singer Studio, 2014).

 ENHANCE SENSORY BALANCE

 ACHIEVE AFFORDABILITY

Installing individual climate controls in bedrooms not only increases comfort, it may also reduce overall heating and cooling costs. At a minimum, provide a centralized programmable thermostat with controls for multiple zones (Brand, 2010; Department of Family and Community Services, 2013; Michael Singer Studio, 2014).

To reduce heating and cooling costs, install a sensor system that alerts when either a door or window is open. For ease of use, consider specifying an integrated thermostat/sensor system that automatically adjusts when a door or window is opened (Michael Singer Studio, 2014)

For long-term affordability and reduced environmental impact, investigate the feasibility of using solar, wind, geothermal or other renewable energy sources for heating and cooling (Michael Singer Studio, 2014; SCGH, 2014; NREL, 2014).

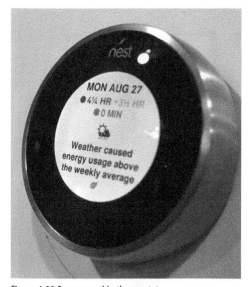

Figure 4.98 Programmable thermostat

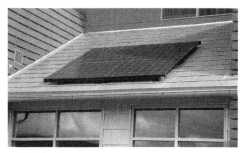

Figure 4.99 Solar panels
(photo by Dave Dugdale: Flickr CC)

LIGHTING

For people experiencing visual perceptual problems, poor lighting often exacerbates the situation. To mitigate potential difficulties, a variety of lighting options should be provided throughout the home. For the best outcomes, include windows with integrated blinds that allow residents to control natural light. Avoid overhead lighting as this can be harsh and over-stimulating. Instead, provide moveable task lighting that residents can adjust as necessary.

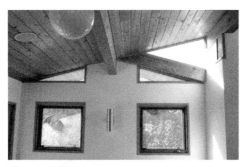

Figure 4.100 Clerestory windows provide indirect, natural light
(photo by Jeremy Levine: Flickr CC)

 ENHANCE SENSORY BALANCE

Provide natural light in all living areas. For indirect, natural light, put in clerestory and transom windows and skylights where possible (Ahrentzen and Steele, 2009; Williams and Boult, 2009; Brand, 2010; Mostafa, 2010).

Avoid standard fluorescent bulbs because of the noise and flicker many of them produce. If compact fluorescent bulbs are specified, verify that they do not flicker or buzz (Beaver, 2010; Mostafa, 2010).

Install buzz-free dimmer switches on all recessed and wall-mounted lighting to allow for greater control over lighting levels. For cost effectiveness and optimal lighting, specify warm spectrum, energy efficient, LED bulbs (Sergeant et al, 2007; Ahrentzen and Steele, 2009; Beaver, 2010; Mostafa, 2010; Michael Singer Studio, 2014).

To create the appropriate level of visual stimulation, when designing lighting for the home, be cognizant of light color, luminance ratios, and light levels (van Hoof et al, 2010; Smolders and de Kort, 2012).

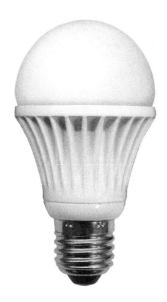

Figure 4.101 LED bulb
(photo by Team EarthLED: Flickr CC)

To avoid lighting glare, especially for people who use wheelchairs, be careful of under cabinet lighting or lights that are angled down as these often shine directly in their eyes. Instead install lights at a lower level and select reduced glare fixtures (IES, 2014).

 FOSTER HEALTH & WELLNESS

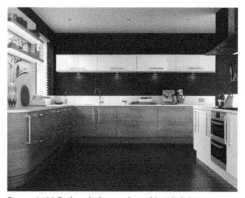

Figure 4.102 Reduced glare under cabinet lighting (photo by Steve Larkin: Flickr CC)

To enhance healthier living conditions, vary the size, number and orientation of windows and also the location and levels of artificial lighting (Smolders and de Kort, 2014).

 ENSURE SAFETY & SECURITY

Use wet location fixtures for all bathroom lighting in case of excessive water play. Also use wet-area fittings on all portable lighting and wall outlets (Ahrentzen and Steele, 2009; Michael Singer Studio, 2014).

Avoid using high-heat tungsten and halogen light bulbs (Ahrentzen and Steele, 2009).

 MAXIMIZE FAMILIARITY, STABILITY, PREDICTABILITY & CLARITY

For best results, involve a lighting consultant in the design. A consultant will ensure that lighting solutions for each room are properly scaled with the right fixtures.

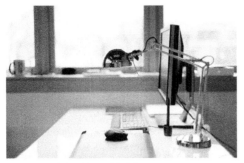

Figure 4.103 Adjustable task lighting
(photo by Aurimas: Flickr CC)

In addition to overhead adjustable recessed LED lighting, rooms should have adjustable task lighting. This creates a warm, efficient, home-like atmosphere and allows residents to control lighting. Recessed LED lighting is necessary in hallways as well (Ahrentzen and Steele, 2009; Brand, 2010; IES, 2014; Michael Singer Studio, 2014).

Bathrooms should have bright, uniform, shadow-free light. For bath and shower, specify energy efficient, recessed LED lights and for the mirror, specify a high color rendering light mounted at head height to eliminate shadows while shaving and applying make-up (Ahrentzen and Steele, 2009; IES, 2014).

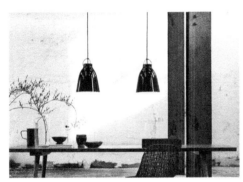

Figure 4.104 Durable pendant lamps
(photo by Lightyears.dk: Flickr CC)

To create a warm atmosphere, in addition to recessed lighting install a durable pendant lamp over the dining room table. If there is a kitchen island, place a pendant lamp there as well (IES, 2014).

In kitchens, a skylight provides energy efficient, glare-free lighting. To illuminate countertop work areas and eliminate shadows cast by ceiling lighting, use under-cabinet, dimmable LED lighting that can double as a nightlight (IES, 2014; Michael Singer Studio, 2014).

To minimize frustration, provide built-in lighting in closets and storage areas (Michael Singer Studio, 2014).

Consider installing recessed lighting on the front and back porches. Up-lighting trees, bollards, post-top lanterns and a shielded light fixture on the garage illuminates the walkway without causing neighborhood light pollution (IES, 2014).

Use timers rather than motion sensors to turn outdoor lights on in the evening. Do not install outdoor lighting near bedrooms (Williams and Boult, 2009; Michael Singer Studio, 2014).

For ease of use, light switches should be installed 36 inches high and not at the back of counters or other inaccessible areas (IES, 2014).

 ENSURE DURABILITY

Include ample electrical outlets in all rooms to accommodate portable task lighting needs and to avoid outlet overloading (Ahrentzen and Steele, 2009).

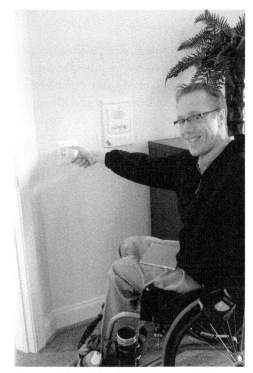

Figure 4.105 Accessible height light switches
(photo by Fairfax County Fate House: Flickr CC)

APPLIANCES

With the technological sophistication of appliances changing daily, selecting the most appropriate appliance requires research combined with a thorough understanding of the resident's needs and capabilities. In general, it is important to consider an appliance's safety features, especially since some people with autism may be inattentive, have sensory responses that may make them susceptible to injuries, or be unable to recognize a problem. Also important to consider is whether the appliance is designed for durability, quietness and ease of use (Ahrentzen and Steele, 2009).

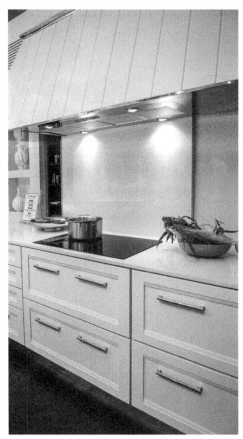

Figure 4.106 Induction cooktop with cookware (photo by Susan Serra: Flickr CC)

 ENSURE SAFETY & SECURITY

Since people with autism may not recognize the danger associated with high heat, minimize the risk of burns by specifying induction cooktops and cool-touch small appliances such as griddles, toasters, fryers and small cookers (Brand, 2010; Maytum, 2013; Wurlitzer, 2014).

Small appliances should have an automatic shut-off feature or should be plugged into an auto shut-off safety outlet (Ahrentzen and Steele, 2009).

To prevent someone from inadvertently turning on an appliance or to keep an appliance door from opening, include a lockout or override feature (Ahrentzen and Steele, 2009).

Appliances with front or side controls minimize reaching across hot surfaces (Ahrentzen and Steele, 2009).

Install intake alarms on sinks and toilets: if a leak or overflow is detected, the water is automatically shut off (Ahrentzen and Steele 2009).

To help minimize water play, excessive water use and reduce stress caused by waiting for warm water, either install hot water heaters near bathrooms or consider installing an on-demand/smart hot water recirculation system. Smart systems monitor hot water use and adjust pump cycling to meet user demand (Flopro SmartPlus, n.d.; Brand, 2010)

 PROVIDE ADEQUATE CHOICE & INDEPENDENCE

Separate the oven and stove to create opportunities for multiple people to cook at the same time (Brand, 2010).

For accessibility and greater safety, select an oven with side-swing doors (Brand, 2010; Katz, 2013).

Front load washing machines and dryers installed at the appropriate height are most accessible for residents and support providers (Ahrentzen and Steele, 2009; Michael Singer Studio, 2014).

 MAXIMIZE FAMILIARITY, STABILITY, PREDICTABILITY & CLARITY

For the most flexibility and to reduce need to replace appliances to meet a resident's evolving needs, select accessible appliances (Ahrentzen and Steele, 2009).

Select appliances that are simple to operate with controls that are easy to see, read and turn. Letters and numbers should be large and nonreflective and knobs or buttons should be

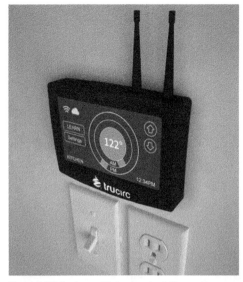

Figure 4.107 On-demand hot water circulation system (photo by Scott Lewis: Flickr CC)

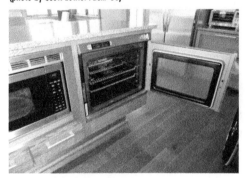

Figure 4.108 Side-swing door oven (photo by Joffre Essley: Flickr CC)

distinguishable from background surface (Ahrentzen and Steele, 2009).

If possible, select appliances that provide both visual and audible alerts (Ahrentzen and Steele, 2009).

Handles on appliances, drawers and doors should be lever-style allowing for the use of the whole hand. Knobs can be difficult for some people to use (Ahrentzen and Steele, 2009; AARP Livable Communities, 2014).

Wall-hung sinks provide the greatest flexibility for accommodating resident mobility needs. Since residents might lean, bounce and sit on sinks, it is necessary to use heavy duty anchoring methods for proper support (Ahrentzen and Steele, 2009; Beaver, 2010; Michael Singer Studio, 2014).

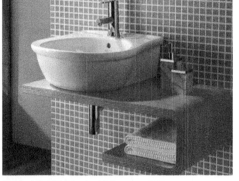

Figure 4.109 Wall-hung sink for accessibility (photo by Architecture, Food & One: Flickr CC)

 FOSTER HEALTH & WELLNESS

Appliances should be easy to clean and maintain: racks and drawers should be removable (Ahrentzen and Steele, 2009).

ACOUSTICS

For many people with autism, environmental noise poses a significant problem. To accommodate individuals with hypersensitivity to sound it is necessary to design all aspects of the home with acoustics in mind. Everything from materials and appliances to how the joints are constructed affects the acoustical performance of a building. Therefore, for the best results, it is highly recommended that an acoustical consultant be involved from the beginning (Marsha Maytum, July 2014, personal communication).

 ENHANCE SENSORY BALANCE

For the best acoustical performance, engage an acoustical consultant at the outset; a consultant will develop the best system for the specific project. The National Council of Acoustical Consultants (www.ncac.com/) provides information on how to select an expert (Maytum, 2013).

With exposed brick or stone, deeply raked masonry joints help break up sound waves (Beaver, 2006; Ahrentzen and Steele, 2009).

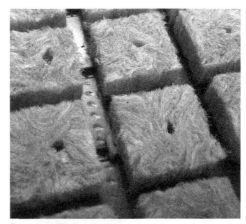

Figure 4.110 Rockwool cubes
(photo by D-Kuru: CC)

There are a variety of soundproofing options. To work effectively it is imperative that they are properly installed (Ahrentzen and Steele, 2009):

Rockwool (www.rockwool.com/) is a highly sustainable product that provides excellent acoustics and is fire resistant. It has received Quiet Mark Solutions status (ISO Store, 2014).

Acoustikblok, when properly installed, provides sound reduction equivalent to 24 inches (61 centimeters) of concrete;

for increased thermal insulation, pair Acoustiblok with Thermablok (www. acoustiblok.com/).

QuietRock, a form of sheetrock, also reduces noise transfer (www.quietrock. com/).

To maximize acoustic performance, it is best to decouple the ceilings and walls and add dampening to both; and install a rubber underlayment on floors and seal door bottoms and frames (Brand, 2010; ISO Store, 2014; Phakos, 2013).

In sensitive areas such as bedrooms, consider staggered or double wall assemblies and thicker wall sections. Environmental noise is associated with poor sleep and health, distraction and agitation (van Hoof et al, 2010; Michael Singer Studio, 2014).

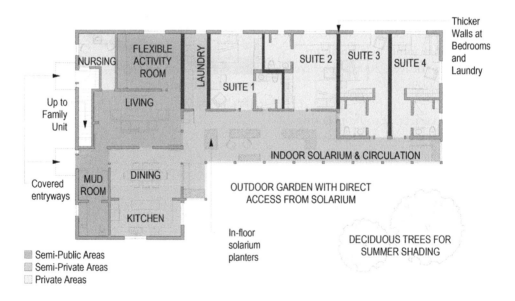

Figure 4.111 Thicker walls are incorporated into sensitive areas such as bedrooms and laundry area
(Courtesy of Michael Singer Studio)

Noise-proofing clips help reduce noise transfer by isolating walls from studs (City Quiet, 2014).

Utilize natural materials, such as wood, within the home to absorb noise (Mostafa, 2010).

To reduce environmental noise, select quiet rated home systems and appliances. Eliminating high-pitched sounds is especially important as these can trigger stress responses in some individuals (Sergeant et al, 2007).

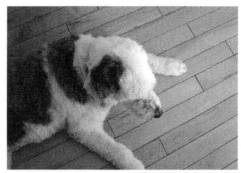

Figure 4.112 Wood flooring and other natural materials help absorb noise
(photo Alex Kehr: Flickr CC)

TECHNOLOGY

The growing interest in smart home technology combined with the expanding population of older adults who wish to live independently for as long as possible has lead to the creation of a sophisticated array of sensor and other assistive technology systems for the home. Today, a home can be outfitted with sensors that monitor resident health and activity levels; indicate whether someone has fallen, is wandering at night or is making an unusual number of trips to the bathroom; or if a window has been opened or the bath water is too hot. While many sensor systems operate as part of a telehealth service or other monitoring program, others may be configured strictly as in-home reminders or alerts. Choosing the type of sensors and other assistive technologies to install in the home depends on the needs and desires of the resident: systems should be selected in consultation with the resident to support him or her in daily life without intruding unnecessarily on his or her privacy or usurping a resident's autonomy. Care should be taken not to over-rely on home sensor technology. As noted by one support provider, "use of sensors can place too much emphasis on the medical model of disability. In this model, participants are treated primarily as patients and all behavioral-psycho-social issues tend to be dealt with from a medical perspective. In short, people are treated as though they are sick when in fact they are simply living with a disability" (quoted in Wolbring and Leopatra, 2013, p. 28).

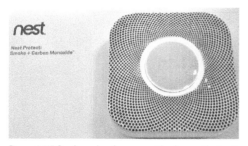

Figure 4.113 Smoke and carbon monoxide alarm with visual and spoken notification
(photo by Raysonho: CC)

 ENHANCE SENSORY BALANCE

 ENSURE SAFETY & SECURITY

For many people with autism loud sounds are incapacitating; therefore, select detectors with alarms that feature both visual signals and spoken directions (Ahrentzen and Steele, 2009).

Install property exit sensors on exterior doors and windows. Select systems that provide a calm, audible warning when doors or windows are opened (Laberg et al, 2005; Sergeant et al, 2007; Ahrentzen and Steele, 2009).

ENSURE SAFETY & SECURITY

Install detectors for smoke, carbon monoxide, natural gas, radon and propane. Detectors should be capable of contacting outside assistance. Sensorium (www.sensorium.co.uk/), Redi-Exit Egress Systems (www.redi-exit.com/talking-smoke-alarm-p-10.html), Hearmore (www.hearmore.com/categories/17/Carbon-Monoxide-and-Smoke-Detectors.html) and Tunstall (http://uk.tunstall.com/solutions/products) are good sources for these types of products (Ahrentzen and Steele, 2009; Brand, 2010).

To monitor possible flooding in bathrooms, kitchens and laundry rooms, install flood and water level detectors. Sensorium (www.sensorium.co.uk/Products/Assistive-Technology/Assistive-Tools/Magiplug.aspx), Byretech (www.byretech.com/acatalog/overflow-protectors.html) and Tunstall (http://uk.tunstall.com/solutions/flood-detector) provide a range of water damage prevention solutions (Ahrentzen and Steele, 2009; Brand, 2010).

Install lockable fuse boxes to prevent tampering (Ahrentzen and Steele, 2009).

Entry/exit systems should be easy for residents to operate. Keyless locks, card, biometric or proximity systems all are options. To avoid leaving the door unlocked, select a system that locks automatically (Ahrentzen and Steele, 2009; Sergeant et al, 2007).

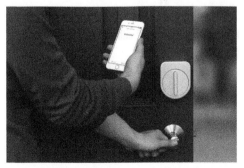

Figure 4.114 Keyless smart lock with lever-style handle for accessibility
(photo by Scott Lewis: Flickr CC)

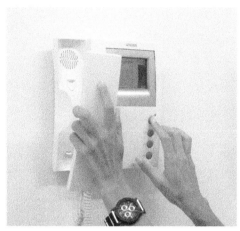

Figure 4.115 Entry system with telephone and camera for previewing
(iStock)

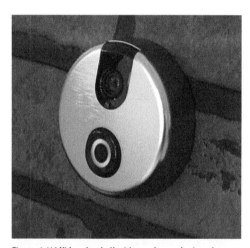

Figure 4.116 Video doorbell with speaker and microphone
(Scott Lewis: Flickr CC)

Entry/exit systems should feature a camera and intercom/telephone so that residents are able to preview visitors before opening the door (Laberg et al, 2005; Michael Singer Studio, 2014).

All locks on internal doors must have the ability to be opened externally in case of emergency (Ahrentzen and Steele, 2009).

 ## PROVIDE ADEQUATE CHOICE & INDEPENDENCE

Select technologies that assist an individual to live the way he or she wants to live; avoid installing sensors that are not needed at this stage of a resident's life. Instead choose sensors, daily activity monitors and task prompting systems that support residents in having greater control over their lives (Wehmeyer et al, 2012; Wolbring and Leopatra, 2013).

Avoid installing a core package of assistive technologies in a home. For assistive technologies to be used and be effective, they must be selected and designed to meet the needs of each individual (Berry et al, 2009).

Subscribing to a Telehealth or Telecare system may be appropriate for some individuals. HomeLink Support Technologies (http://homelinksupport. com/about-us/) and SimplyHome (http://simply-home.com/index.html) are two models that provide home services to people with disabilities in the U.S. The National Health Service offers information on available Telecare and Telehealth services in the U.K.

and maintains a list of providers on its website (National Health Service, n.d.; Dewsbury and Ballard, 2012; Strouse et al, 2013).

 ## CONTROLLING SOCIAL INTERACTION & PRIVACY

In homes with multiple residents, technologies installed to assist one person must not intrude on the privacy of the other residents (Berry et al, 2009).

 ## MAXIMIZE FAMILIARITY, STABILITY, PREDICTABILITY & CLARITY

To minimize resident stress, install a silent, battery-powered backup system to maintain seamless power during power outages (Laberg et al, 2005; Hello Housing, 2009, personal communication).

Consider using RFID (radio frequency identification) or Bluetooth location sensors on items that are easily misplaced (Ahrentzen and Steele, 2009).

To simplify maintenance and installing upgrades, locate technology hardware in a single, accessible place.

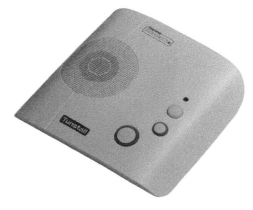

Figure 4.117 Telecare telephone prompt service (Tunstall: CC)

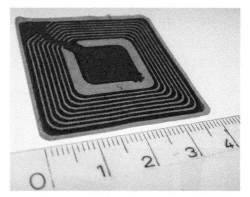

Figure 4.118 RFID sensor tag (photo by Maschinenjunge: CC)

FOSTER HEALTH & WELLNESS

If it is determined that sensors are warranted, select the least invasive type possible.

Include an emergency call system for residents and support staff. Consider installing panic alarms in the kitchen and bathrooms (Ahrentzen and Steele, 2009; Zamprelli, 2009; Dewsbury and Ballard, 2012).

Seizure disorders and/or epilepsy occur more frequently in individuals with autism, therefore it may be necessary to install an epilepsy sensor (Gillberg and Neville, 2010; Berg and Plioplys, 2012; Tunstall Solutions, 2014).

Bed occupancy sensors may be appropriate for some residents and are available from Tunstall Healthcare, which has offices worldwide (www.tunstall. com/).

To reduce condensation and the possibility of mold and mildew, consider installing a humidity sensor that is able to activate a ventilation fan.

 ENHANCE ONE'S DIGNITY

Installing the appropriate assistive technologies such as sensors and monitoring systems allows residents to live with less direct observation from support providers (Brand, 2010).

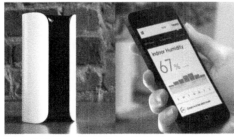

Figure 4.119 Home monitoring system
(Scott Lewis: Flickr CC)

To minimize the stigma associated with using assistive technologies, always consider the aesthetics of any device or sensor system. Those that reflect the size and aesthetics of devices used by the general public or by technology-savvy individuals diminish a sense of "impairment" in using the device (Berry et al, 2009).

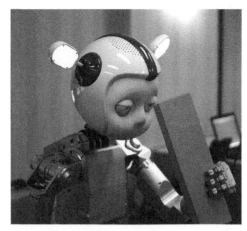

Figure 4.120 Simon, the humanoid robot
(Jiuguang Wang: Flickr CC)

MATERIALS

Often people with autism experience sensitivities to environmental chemicals and many have underlying health conditions that are exacerbated by exposure to these chemicals. To minimize negative health reactions and prevent chronic exposure to indoor air pollutants, select zero-VOC (volatile organic compounds), nontoxic building materials and finishes. Many of these building materials are extremely durable, making them cost-effective in the long-term.

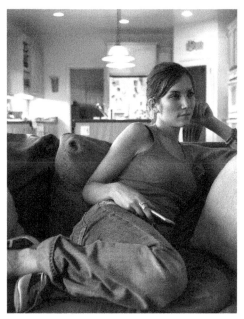

Figure 4.121 Comfortable, personalized furnishings (iStock)

 PROVIDE ADEQUATE CHOICE & INDEPENDENCE

To help residents feel a sense of ownership of their home, encourage them to choose materials and finishes such as paint colors whenever possible (Hello Housing, 2009, personal communication; Zamprelli, 2009).

Ensure that some furniture throughout the house is moveable so that residents can customize the environment according to their needs and interests (Baumers and Heylighen, 2014).

 ENHANCE ONE'S DIGNITY

Balance the robustness of the materials with their home-like qualities to prevent an institutional-like feeling; institutional and commercial materials should be used sparingly, if at all (Brand, 2010; Mostafa, 2010).

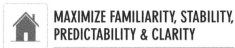

MAXIMIZE FAMILIARITY, STABILITY, PREDICTABILITY & CLARITY

Use contrast (tonal value vs. bright color) to highlight light switches, electrical outlets and other pertinent features that need to stand out (Ahrentzen and Steele, 2009).

ENSURE SAFETY & SECURITY

All window glass should be laminated or tempered for both inner and outer panes to minimize potential injury (Brand, 2010).

If elopement is a concern, install window stops on operable windows to constrain the size of the opening (Brand, 2010).

For all corded window coverings – blinds, curtains and shades – replace cords with a remote control operating system. The Window Covering Safety Council (www.windowcoverings. org/) provides free cord-retrofit kits for existing window coverings and safety and design information (Beaver, 2010; Brand, 2010).

FOSTER HEALTH & WELLNESS

To minimize indoor air pollution, select materials with zero VOCs (volatile organic compounds) and no added urea formaldehyde. Be aware, the label "low VOCs" simply indicates that the

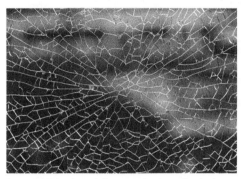

Figure 4.122 Laminated glass stays in place when broken (photo by Conan: Flickr CC)

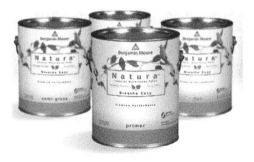

Figure 4.123 Zero VOC Paint (photo by Scott Lewis: Flickr CC)

product does not "promote pollution in the outdoor environment." It does not mean it is necessarily safe or healthy (Hirshberg, 2011).

To reduce environmental toxins, avoid specifying materials that contain VOCs such as laminate, particleboard, melamine, medium-density fiberboard (MDF) or plywood cabinets; standard drywall or greenboard drywall; sheet vinyl flooring; standard paints, stains, adhesives, grouts and sealants. Instead, consider solid wood for cabinetry, cement board and magnesium oxide wallboard, and zero-VOC products. The United State Environmental Protection Agency provides information on green products and eco-labeling programs. In the United Kingdom, the Green Building Council provides information on healthy materials, responsible sourcing and a rating system for specifying green materials. (EPA(c), n.d.; Green Building Council, n.d.).

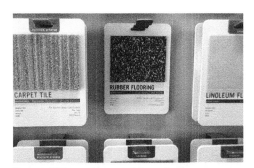

Figure 4.124 Low toxicity material samples
(photo by Ted Eytan: Flickr CC)

It is important to select non-toxic, zero VOC finishes – paints, sealants, primers, caulks, grouts, stains – since some people might lick surfaces or lick their hands after excessively touching and rubbing walls and be at risk of ingesting chemicals or aggravating existing health conditions. If finishes contain VOCs and other toxins, mixing them on top of one another can create new chemicals and magnify the problem (Scott, 2009; Enterprise Green Communities, 2015; Maytum, 2013).

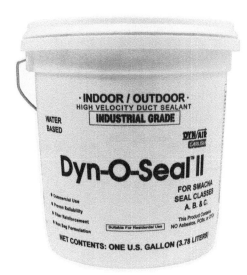

Figure 4.125 Non-toxic, water-based sealant available in different grades and applications
(photo by Carlisle HVAC: Flickr CC)

Avoid epoxy-based paints, sealants and caulks – including those that comply with VOC standards – as they contain

Bisphenol A (BPA), identified by
the U.S. Environmental Protection
Agency (EPA(a), n.d.) in 2010 as a
chemical of concern (Enterprise Green
Communities, 2015).

Materials and finishes should be easy
to clean and maintain but should not
appear institutional or commercial. Use
non-toxic, fragrance-free, biodegradable
cleaners. The Environmental Working
Group (www.ewg.org/) provides an
excellent consumer guide for healthy
cleaning products (Ahrentzen and Steele,
2009; Brand, 2010).

Sealing the concrete slab or sub-floor
prevents odors from penetrating. Since
some residents may be incontinent
or may become so as they age, it
is important to address this during
construction (van Hoof et al, 2010).

Opt for hypoallergenic materials such
as Marmoleum (www.marmoleum.
com) for floors and wainscoting. Since
carpet readily harbors allergens, it is best
to avoid using it (Ahrentzen and Steele,
2009; Hello Housing, 2009, personal
communication).

Avoid using pesticides and insecticides
indoors and outdoors since many
persist in the environment long after
application. Regular maintenance
and cleaning will help keep problems
in check, however, if pests become a
problem, Beyond Pesticides (www.
beyondpesticides.org) provides
information on controlling pests in the
home and garden using the least toxic
methods (Ahrentzen and Steele, 2009).

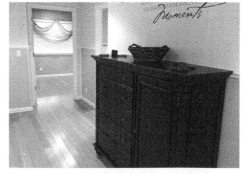

Figure 4.126 Marmoleum wainscoting
(Courtesy of Hello Housing)

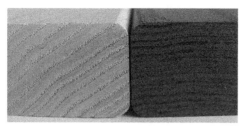

Figure 4.127 Untreated European Ash on left and thermally modified European Ash on right
(photo by Anubis100: CC)

For outdoor decks, select thermally modified wood rather than pressure treated wood. Pressure treated wood contains inorganic arsenic which can be absorbed by the skin and can contaminate food and other surfaces. The U.S. Environmental Protection Agency ((EPA(b), n.d.)) is a good source of information on pressure treated wood.

 ## ENHANCE SENSORY BALANCE

To reduce noise transmission, install a rubber underlayment under flooring. Foam underlayment lacks sufficient density to be effective (ISO Store, 2014).

To minimize glare, specify non-reflective surfaces wherever possible (van Hoof et al, 2010).

In areas with high levels of exterior noise, install windows with high acoustical performance. The Glass Education Center provides information on the sound transmission properties of different types of glass (Glass Education Center, n.d.; Brand, 2010; Maytum, 2013).

Select window coverings that allow residents the ability to control light transmission: in common living areas, window coverings should allow 70 percent light transmission and bedrooms should be fitted with blackout shades or louvers to promote sleep (Michael Singer Studio, 2014).

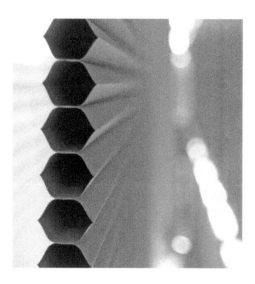

Figure 4.128 Honeycomb blinds control light and are energy efficient
(photo by Blinds Online: Flickr CC)

ENSURE DURABILITY

Materials and finishes need to be able to withstand heavy use. Resilient materials, fixtures and finishes help keep residents safe and reduce maintenance and replacement costs (Wahl and Weisman, 2003; Harker and King, 2004; Brand, 2010; Golant, 2012; Geboy et al, 2012).

Select hard, continuous surface flooring such as high quality vertical grain bamboo, hardwood, natural linoleum or Marmoleum (Hello Housing, 2009, personal communication; Michael Singer Studio, 2014).

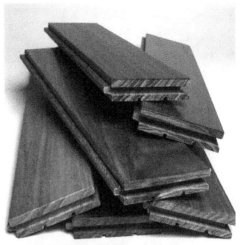

Figure 4.129 Hardwood flooring
(photo by Mauroguanandi: Flickr CC)

If using carpet, opt for carpet tiles over rolled carpet to simplify replacing damaged sections. Flor Modular Floorcovering by Interface (www.interfaceglobal.com/Products/Flor.aspx) uses recycled materials and non-toxic adhesives (Ahrentzen and Steele, 2009).

Wainscoting, chair rails and tall baseboards protect walls in high traffic areas. Marmoleum, tile and stone are all durable choices (Ahrentzen and Steele, 2009).

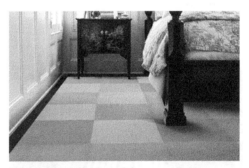

Figure 4.130 Interface floor tiles
(photo by Rosenfeld Media: Flickr CC)

Use solid doors and heavy-duty hinges such as piano hinges hung within reinforced doorframes to accommodate heavy and unintended use (Brand, 2010; Michael Singer Studio, 2014).

Encased window blinds operated via remote control will minimize wear and tear, increasing the longevity of the product (Ahrentzen and Steele, 2009; Zamprelli, 2009; Beaver, 2010; Brand, 2010).

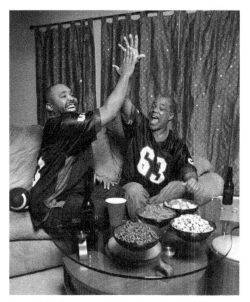

Figure 4.131 Homey, non-toxic environment in which to entertain friends
(iStock)

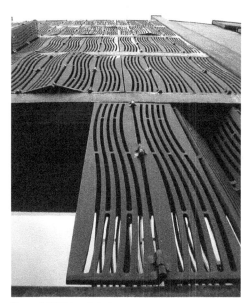

Figure 4.132 External shutters
(photo by Detlef Schobert: Flickr CC)

Selecting washable, hard-wearing materials and finishes will help them withstand damage from excessive touching, rubbing and licking from sensory-seeking residents (Sergeant et al, 2007; Brand, 2010).

Furniture and other furnishings should be durable but not institutional or commercial: create a warm, inviting, homey environment. To prolong life of furnishings, select well-made furniture that can handle bouncing and is upholstered in moisture-resistant non-toxic fabrics (Sergeant et al, 2007 Brand, 2010).

 ## ACHIEVE AFFORDABILITY

In addition to employing passive solar design strategies to enhance heating, cooling and lighting, install high performance insulated windows. In some climates it might be necessary to install awnings or external shades to reduce energy leakage. The United States Department of Energy (http://energy.gov/) and the Energy Saving Trust in the United Kingdom (www.energysavingtrust.org.uk/) provide helpful information on energy saving strategies including tips for passive solar design (Ahrentzen and Steele, 2009; Maytum, 2013).

FIVE
ON THE HORIZON

Introduction

The policy of deinstitutionalization – replacing complete institutions of long-term care with residences and services in the community – was first articulated in the late 1960s and early 1970s, but it took decades to see noticeable, widescale changes on the landscape (Campaign for the Mentally Handicapped, 1972; Kugel and Wolfensberger, 1969; Mansell, 2006). In North America, Europe, Australia and New Zealand, this transition from large residential institutions to networks of community-based living with support services is steadily progressing. Sweden and Norway are the leaders in this transition, where all institutional provision has been replaced and where the law now provides the right to community services (Mansell, 2006).

Nonetheless, many critics believe that the progress is much too slow, and that initiatives for creating and supporting residences that meet the growing numbers and needs of adults on the spectrum – as well as others whose health and capabilities are not being met by current housing market or government practices and policies – are too few. Our efforts in this book have been to provide guidance – grounded in available research and experts' reflective practice to date – of design features and spatial characteristics that can advance a generation of homes and residential developments that resonate with the aspirations of those on the spectrum.

Attention to adults with autism is relatively fledgling within research arenas as well as service programs, including housing provision. For parents and for those aging out of the school system, the time for laser-focused attention on issues affecting the lifespan – not just the childhood and adolescence of autism – is *now*, not for some distant future. And it is finally happening – likely too glacial a movement for many who are desperate for immediate solutions – but with a vigor and commitment that has not been witnessed before.

What we have profiled in the previous chapters was gleaned from current practices, thinking and research. But there are applications and approaches on the horizon that we believe will further guide the next generation of environmental design and development for those on the spectrum – not only in terms of what is built or renovated, but also in terms of how residential spaces are used and how individuals can advocate for what works best for them. We have divided these into three categories: housing types; smart technologies for independent living; and self-advocacy approaches for housing choice.

New visions of housing types and models

The early attempts to replace institutional living for those with disabilities initially resulted in relatively large residential homes, such as the intermediate care program in the U.S., the Wessex experiment in England, and the residential home program in Sweden. These larger-scale homes of 12 to 20 residents were still characterized by much institutional living and care. They gradually became less popular with families, residents and even policymakers, and new efforts arose to target smaller, residential-scale housing. Group homes then gained increasing prominence in the 1980s, where anywhere from four to eight people live together with extensive and pervasive – often 24/7 – paid assistance from trained support staff, who may or may not live in the same residence. While the group home model does not refer to a particular housing style *per se*, many are single-family homes or converted estate homes given that three or four bedrooms are sometimes necessary to accommodate the number of roommates with dedicated space for staff. They are typically located in residential neighborhoods and designed to serve individuals with autism, intellectual disabilities and other chronic health conditions. Staff typically assist residents both in the residence and when they leave home to use community-based settings (Clement and Bigby, 2010). Aside from family co-residence, group homes are becoming the dominant model of deinstitutionalized residence for those with developmental disabilities in North America, Europe, Australia and New Zealand (Mansell, 2006).

Innovations beyond the group home are appearing in numerous cities and communities in recent years, however, and we expect them to flourish in the next decade. A useful overview of both conventional and emerging types of housing is one developed by The Bureau of Autism Services of the State of Pennsylvania (Myers and Associates, 2010). Table 5.1 outlines their classification of seven different housing settings or arrangements, with numerous models or versions of each type (see Table 5.1). The names of these arrangements may vary across countries and regions. Each housing arrangement can vary by characteristics of the structure, size, number of people in the household, and location.

Table 5.1: Seven housing settings and affiliated models

- Remaining at home
  - House donated by the family
  - Elder cottage housing opportunity (ECHO)
  - Accessory apartment
- Family living
  - Lifesharing
  - Domiciliary care
- Renting an apartment or home
  - LLC owned
  - Non-profit owned
- Purchasing a home
  - Ownership by an individual
  - Tenants in common
  - Limited equity cooperative
- Shared housing
  - Group shared residence
  - Shared housing – Match up
  - Fairweather Lodge
  - L'Arche
- Intentional communities
  - Intergenerational community as intervention (ICI)
  - Collaboration with a college or university
  - Farmsteads
  - Co-housing
- Licensed facilities
  - Private licensed facility
  - Intermediate care facility for people with mental retardation (ICF/MR)
  - Community living arrangement (CLA)

Source: Bureau of Autism Services, State of Pennsylvania, 2010

In this section, we profile a number of housing models we expect to see increasing in our communities in the near future.

◆

Increasing criticism of group homes, or group shared residences, is based on ideological grounds and on recent research demonstrating that even smaller housing arrangements are associated with better resident outcomes (Lakin and Stancliffe, 2007). Critics point out that in many group home settings, residents usually have very limited choice of with whom they live, where they live, and even how they spend their time at home or outside. These concerns have fostered in part the "supported living model" in which an individual rents or purchases a residence, lives alone or with roommates or companions they choose (and typically a small number such as one or two others), and receives needed support and assistance from service and health providers on their own terms (Mansell, 2006). These supported living models are increasing in numbers, resident favor, and in policy directives in communities in North America, Europe and Australia.

Critics also warn, however, that not everyone can live in supported living arrangements, which often demand significant and fairly independent living skills and experience. They may be models that many persons with autism strive towards; but because of one's current capabilities as well as financial resources, these housing models may not be appropriate at a present moment. So in all likelihood, group shared residences will continue to remain in our residential landscapes – but in new forms.

One version of the group home model, at a smaller scale and emulating more of family-living than service-living model, draws from the decades-old practice of Community Living Option's (CLO) *Family Teaching Model* (Kirigin, 2001; Strouse et al, 2013). In these cases, a duplex is created or used whereby a family teaching couple (with or without children) live in one unit. They provide most of the support for three or four housemates with disabilities who live in the other unit. This has been a successful model operating in Kansas since the 1970s, and has emerged in other states in recent years. The Center for Discovery (TCFD) is developing an example of this model in a rural area of New York State.

For several decades, TCFD in Harris, NY, has provided medical care, treatment and residential services for children and adults with disabilities and complex medical conditions. Where previously the Center worked with a small population of individuals with autism, now nearly 90 percent of new residents have autism (Dr. Terry Hamlin, July 2013, personal communication). The majority of autistic individuals come to TCFD as children and adolescents to participate in therapeutic services and attend the residential school program. Until recently, the long-term goal has been for these individuals to move back to their hometowns and families upon graduation. However, TFCD has realized that many of these young people have become embedded in the Center and the neighboring community and moving away no longer is a desirable option. Inspired by the success of the Family Teaching Model, TCFD sees the shared living model as a way to provide housing and independent living support to adults with ASC and to create meaningful employment and housing opportunities for TCFD staff and spouses who relocate to upstate New York.

Much of the work and practice at TCFD involves expanding healthy living and eating among participants, residents and employees. A large, multi-site organic farm provides much of the Center's food and all recent new construction follows U.S. Green Building Council LEED (Leadership in Energy and Environmental Design) standards. Following this approach, the *TCFD Duplex Model* prototype builds on CLO's Family Teaching model by integrating sustainable design practices into housing tailored to meet the needs of autistic adults. By implementing autism specific and sustainable design elements, the goal is not only to create a supportive, healthy environment for residents but also to study whether these design features lead to lower long-term care and support costs. The Family Teaching service model already has been shown to reduce service provision costs through a significant decrease in staff turnover (Strouse et al, 2003); determining to what extent physical design reduces resident stress, conflict and/or injury thereby reducing costs for monitoring and/or medical treatment has yet to be definitively determined (Michael Singer Studio, 2014).

Working with architects from Michael Singer Studio and a team of autism specialists (including the authors), TCFD developed a duplex prototype to be constructed within a new neighborhood located adjacent to the main street of the small town of Hurleyville. The selected site is in a new housing development and within walking distance of shops and, possibly, jobs, offering residents opportunities to participate in activities outside TCFD. Over time additional duplexes may be added to create a village-like setting.

The two-story Duplex Model provides housing for autistic adults on the first floor and for a teaching family on the second with both spaces connected through an interior door (Figure 5.1). The first floor design addresses the complex needs of future residents through a series of carefully considered factors: the need to mitigate sensory issues, the need to create a gradient of privacy and social interaction, and the need to enhance wellness, safety and quality of life. The floor plan unfolds along a south-facing solarium that serves as the home's primary circulation space. The solarium not only allows ample natural light to permeate into the living spaces, it provides passive solar heating in the winter and a year-round interior garden space. The public (living room and kitchen) and private spaces (bedrooms) are accessed from the solarium; a series of thresholds in the form of seating nooks and informal seating areas intervene between each space creating buffers as well as layers for potential engagement. To lower resident anxiety stemming from unwanted encounters, each of the public rooms include at least two options for entering and exiting. Complementing this, each space, including bedrooms, has a glazed wall that allows for previewing.

Flexibility is built into the design of the first floor unit. An activity room employs a "second skin" system creating a storage cavity to house foldout elements such as tables and individual seating as well as items for physical or creative activities. In the kitchen, moveable islands may be configured to temporarily change circulation or to create individual workstations. The bedroom wing features four one-bedroom suites, each with a sitting area and an en-suite bathroom. In some situations, two of the bedroom suites may be combined to create a one-bedroom apartment within the larger unit. This apartment could be used by a cohabitating couple or as a transitional apartment

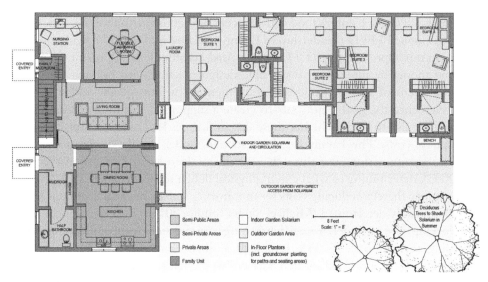

Figure 5.1: First floor of TCFD Model Duplex for residents with ASC
(Courtesy of Michael Singer Studio)

for an individual preparing to move out into more independent living. Further, the first floor is completely accessible, allowing residents to age in place.

Beyond layout considerations, the architects incorporated a wide array of sensory mitigation features, state-of-the-art technology and durable, environmentally sensitive materials into the design. Walls, ceilings and floors are acoustically insulated with select key walls, such as those in bedrooms and the laundry area, designed to be 12 inches (30 cm) thick to accommodate additional sound proofing. Where possible, storage is built into wall cavities, providing an acoustic buffer as well as reducing clutter. To minimize odors and improve indoor air quality, windows are operable, an integrated HEPA air filtration system is used, and durable, non-toxic materials and finishes are specified throughout. There is also the option to install a green roof to increase acoustic and thermal insulation.

◆

In many cases, housing or service providers, as well as families and individuals, acquire individual homes – often apartment units but also condominiums, townhouses, or single-family homes – in existing communities. The housing or service provider typically owns the unit (for condominiums or single family homes) or has an extended, multi-year lease (in case of rental units in an apartment complex), and then rents or leases the home to adults with developmental disabilities or autism, either a single individual or two to three roommates who choose to live together (whereas in the group home model roommates are typically paired by the agency, not the individuals).

One example is ESPA in the U.K. whose extensive portfolio in Sunderland, Durham and North Tyneside includes not only group homes but also cases of supportive living arrangements for adults with autism (ESPA, n.d.). *Beechwood*, for example, is a renovated single detached residence that was converted into four large apartments. Each unit has assistive technology for supporting more independent living activities as well as for security. In addition, Beechwood has a common space within the building where residents can get together if desired, a space intended to encourage residents to spend time out of their flats, socialize and minimize social isolation.

Another example but one of new construction is *Orchard Commons* in the borough of Allendale, New Jersey (Bergen County's United Way, n.d.). Newly constructed within walking distance of a vibrant downtown district, this single-story apartment complex houses four two-bedroom units (approximately 900 square feet each) and two one-bedroom units (approximately 550 square feet each). All residents are low-income individuals with developmental disabilities, some who work in the area, and each resident selects his or her own support providers to assist them to live independently in the community. Like Beechwood, there is a community room at the front of the complex that residents can use for get-togethers – or simply to get away from their home and roommate when desired. The scale, materials and architecture of the complex fits into the surrounding older established neighborhood. The curving site plan on the lot minimizes the scale of the project when driving by. The property lot itself was strategically selected to be in close proximity to the business district with small shops and services, public transportation, recreation and employment in some of the local businesses. Orchard Commons is also across the street from the police station, ambulance corps and two houses of worship.

The development was spearheaded by Allendale Housing, Inc., in partnership with Bergen County's United Way, the Madeline Corporation and the New Jersey Community Development Corporation. Multiple funding sources, including state trust fund accounts dedicated to housing for people with special needs, were necessary to keep the rents affordable to residents, many of whom are employed at least part time in low-wage positions.

◆

While Orchard Commons and Beechwood are apartment complexes exclusively for residents with autism or developmental disabilities, there are also examples of apartment complexes being developed that have only a small number of units as designated set-asides for adults with developmental disabilities including autism. As in Orchard Commons, Beechwood and other supportive living models, each resident chooses support providers who provide assistance with health conditions and living in the community.

Willakenzie Crossing in Eugene, Oregon, is a recent model of this type which includes a total 56 units of affordable housing, all dedicated to those whose income is between 30 and 51 percent of the area median income (which is $59,255 as of 2015).

Within this complex, 16 units of studios and one-bedroom apartments are designated for occupancy of adults with developmental disabilities. Developed by a non-profit housing developer, Cornerstone Community Housing, the development is next to a public park, within two blocks of a shopping center that includes a bank, a couple of grocers and other shops, and within a block of a major bus route. Within the complex is a shared community garden, a playground and a community center (Figure 5.2). The residential services for everyone at Willakenzie – distribution of excess food from food banks, nutrition workshops, continuing education classes – reside in the community center. The center also services the larger community as it brings in neighbors for a summer lunch program for neighborhood children who qualify for free or reduced-price meals during the school year. A LEED-certified structure, the two-story building reflects the forested surroundings of the city of Eugene with tall windows, wood siding and high-pitched roofs. Willakenzie Crossing strives towards many of the quality of life goals emphasized in this book: access and support in surrounding neighborhood, dignity, familiarity and clarity, and affordability in particular. Its affordability lies with government assistance from a combination of federal programs (such as Community Development Block Grants funds, HOME funds, low-income housing tax credits) as well as state and local programs, such as Oregon's affordable housing tax credit and property tax waivers for 20 years (Cornerstone Community Housing, n.d.).

According to the operations director of Willakenzie Crossing, the success of this community – and perhaps the key in reproducing a similar effort – lies in its partnership with SAIL Housing (Cady, 2014). SAIL housing helps to provide additional services and connections to personal support agents for the best interest of the resident. An on-

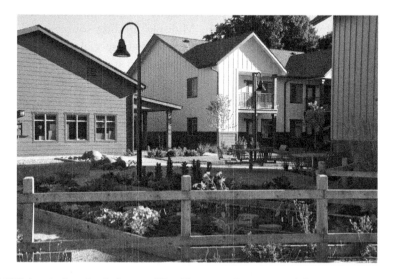

Figure 5.2: Willakenzie Crossing in Eugene, OR, with community center at left
(Courtesy of Cornerstone Community Housing)

site resident liaison works to develop connections in the community and ensure that this collaborative model is a success for residents, parents and the entire community.

An innovative example of set-asides is *29 Palms* in Phoenix, Arizona, an affordable housing property with 15 units of housing for seniors and six units for adults with autism. Utilizing a mix of public and private funds, 29 Palms was developed by the Foundation for Senior Living (FSL) in collaboration with First Place and the Southwest Autism Research and Resource Center (SARRC). The development brings together 22 seniors who have received training to understand the potential needs of their autistic neighbors who are 12 adults transitioning to more independent living. As part of the larger First Place Academy (profiled later in this chapter), 29 Palms is home to adults participating in their second year at the academy, preparing them for their eventual move into apartments within the larger Phoenix community. SARRC, a long-time leader in autism research and education, will provide on-going independent living skills training and support to the 12 residents.

The apartment complex, chosen for its proximity to shopping and public transportation, was completely renovated by Dohrmann Architects to meet the needs of the new tenants. The one-and-a-half acre development features four single-story buildings grouped around a large landscaped courtyard. A community center that includes laundry facilities, a computer room, a full-service kitchen, offices, bathrooms and a large covered outdoor patio, anchors the south side of the site. Each apartment has

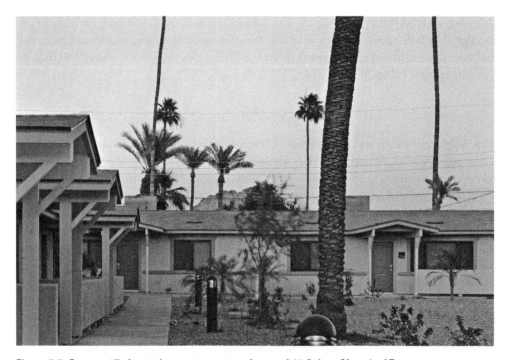

Figure 5.3: Entry vestibules and common courtyard area of 29 Palms, Phoenix, AZ
(Courtesy of Dohrmann Architects, Inc.)

a well-defined covered entry flanked by a patio enclosed by a half-wall and overlooking the central courtyard. This semi-public outdoor room not only extends the living space, it also provides opportunities for informal socializing (see Figure 5.3). The six two-bedroom apartments specifically designed for autistic residents are each 900 square feet and include a spacious shared bathroom, an open concept living–dining–kitchen space and a large storage closet. Built-in units in the bedrooms, bathroom and hallway allow for plenty of additional storage. Even though the apartments are not large, the layout conveys a sense of spaciousness, providing residents room to move without crowding one another.

Cognizant of the many sensory issues common to people with autism, the architects specified products that promote a peaceful living environment ranging from ductless HVAC systems, quiet ventilation fans and kitchen appliances to acoustic windows and doors. To further reduce noise, discrete sound absorption panels were installed in the bedrooms and the living room. Formaldehyde-free cabinets and doors, low VOC paints and adequate ventilation and air circulation promote good indoor air quality and work to reduce health problems associated with chemical sensitivities. Materials also were chosen for their durability: solid surface countertops in the kitchen, bathroom, and on top of storage units and bedroom desks resist chipping and scratching; safety glass for windows; and solid core doors. For ease of use, the entry lock opens either with a key or a key fob.

For the Foundation for Senior Living and First Place, 29 Palms is a pilot project. Working with SARRC researchers, FSL and First Place are developing an assessment strategy that will allow them to evaluate the effectiveness of the residential program and use that information to guide future housing developments. Residents began moving into 29 Palms in Fall 2014.

◆

The supported living model typified in the variations above (29 Palms, Willakenzie Crossing, Orchard Commons, Beechwood) is not an exclusive residential solution for everyone with autism. Some critics and researchers question its affordability, appropriateness and even proclivity towards social isolation for many individuals on the spectrum. Since it requires a certain level of independent living skills, motivation and affinity for getting out in the community, it may be a housing model that some individuals gradually work towards but is not necessarily appropriate for one's first residence after leaving the parental home.

Straddling the gap between supported living models and group homes are an increasing number of residences that provide accommodation for a relatively small number of housemates (between four and six in a single residence), but are organized and structured to provide choice and meaningful personal living spaces within support networks of the resident's choosing, in their homes and communities. One example is *Sweetwater Spectrum* in Sonoma, California.

In 2009, a group of families with autistic children, autism professionals, and community leaders founded the nonprofit organization Sweetwater Spectrum with the intent to create a high-quality residential community for adults with autism (Sweetwater Spectrum, n.d.). The architects, Leddy Maytum Stacy of San Francisco, drew upon the design goals and guidelines produced in the report *Advancing Full Spectrum Housing* (Ahrentzen and Steele, 2009), a precursor to this book. They also incorporated a number of sustainable design elements for water conservation, energy efficiency and indoor environmental quality such that the development qualified for LEED Gold certification.

The Sweetwater Spectrum organization acquired a 2.8 acre, vacant midblock parcel in the town of Sonoma, several blocks away from the historic town square, but immediately close to public transit, bicycle trails, a movie theatre and three grocery stores. The fenced site includes four 3,260-square foot residential buildings; each building with four separate en-suites for the four residents living there, and shared living room and kitchen. There is also a separate room near the front entry that support providers can use while visiting residents. These residences were intentionally designed to mitigate sensory overload through simple furnishings and a palette of natural colors with minimal patterning; uncluttered sight lines; soundproof walls between living areas; separation of high-stimulus areas; wood acoustical ceiling panels; wide hallways for easy access and movement; lighting on timers, not motion detectors; and quiet, individually controlled radiant heating and cooling systems. The architects also situated hallways and windows so that residents had the opportunity to preview activities and people in rooms and outdoor spaces before entering. A number of places of retreat for quiet and calm – both inside and outside – are also provided (Figure 5.4). Safety features were also key, including window stops, unobtrusive sensors on doors and windows, talking smoke/carbon monoxide detectors, and induction stovetops. In addition to ensuring accessibility through a variety of universal design strategies, the architects deliberately selected building materials and systems to promote healthy

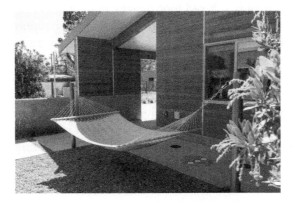

Figure 5.4: Hammock in quiet courtyard area, Sweetwater Spectrum, Sonoma, CA
(Courtesy of Leddy Maytum Stacy Architects; photograph by Tim Griffiths)

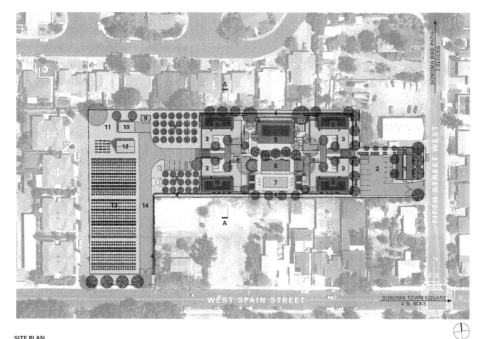

SITE PLAN
1 WELCOME BUILDING 2 PARKING 3 HOUSE 4 STORMWATER TREATMENT BIO-SWALE 5 COMMUNITY CENTER 6 THE COMMONS: PLAZA & LAWN
7 THERAPY POOL & SPAS 8 ORCHARD 9 TRASH 10 STORAGE BUILDING 11 IRRIGATION WELL 12 GREENHOUSE 13 ORGANIC FARM 14 FIRE ACCESS ROAD

Figure 5.5: Site plan of Sweetwater Spectrum, Sonoma, CA

(Courtesy of Leddy Maytum Stacy Architects)

indoor air quality, acoustical control, and comfortable, energy-efficient heating/ cooling/ventilation systems.

The four residential buildings surround the community spaces that are in the center of the property (Figure 5.5). A community building includes a fitness room, a fully equipped professional teaching kitchen, a library alcove, and a community room intended for groups to watch movies or engage in other group activities. Across from the community building is a 20x48 foot therapy pool; and at the end of the property is a 1.25 acre urban farm with fruit orchards, crops and a greenhouse.

Sweetwater Spectrum opened in Fall 2013. With an interest not only in the effectiveness of this complex in enriching residents' lives but also with an eye towards building other residential developments for adults with autism in the future, the Sweetwater Spectrum organization has engaged local university faculty and students to conduct pre- and post-occupancy evaluations. Results from these evaluations will help target which design features and social/education programs are most efficacious and popular, which ones are not, and for whom. Such insight will help guide future developments in selecting and prioritizing design and programmatic features, particularly when capital funds may not be as available as those of this US$10.5 million development.

On the other side of the U.S., in Ramsey, New Jersey, is *Airmount Woods* (Figure 5.6). It, too, reflects the middle ground between traditional group home and supportive

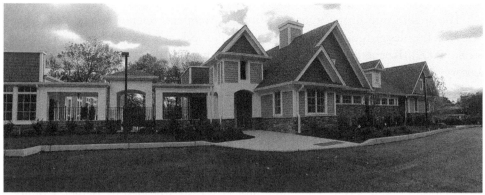

Figure 5.6: Street front of Airmount Woods, Ramsey, NJ
(Courtesy of Bergen County's United Way)

living (Bergen County's United Way, n.d.). With public funding from the state of New Jersey, it is affordable to a larger pool of adults with ASC with limited financial resources.

Airmount Woods provides nine small one-bedroom units in two identical two-story buildings that are connected by an outdoor patio. Adults with autism occupy eight of the units, and one unit is designated for supervising staff. Each resident has his/her own unit with a bedroom, bathroom, and efficiency kitchen, and shares the common living and dining areas and full kitchen (Figure 5.7).

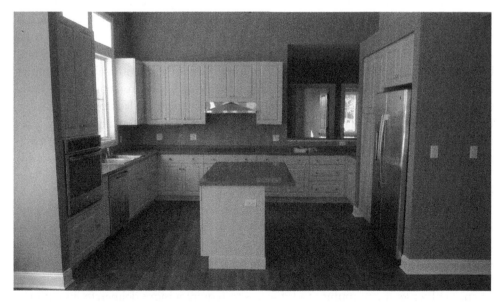

Figure 5.7: Accessible kitchen, Airmount Woods
(Courtesy of Bergen County's United Way)

The architecture firm Virgona + Virgona Architects referenced and drew upon many of the design guidelines of *Advancing Full Spectrum Housing* (Ahrentzen and Steele, 2009). Recognizing that some residents may be highly sensitive to different sensory experiences and also for the need for building durability, the building's design incorporated soundproof insulation, high-impact resistant drywall, tempered glass windows, fully tiled bathrooms, solid surface countertops and a number of energy and water efficient features. The exterior and massing of Airmount Woods reflects the residential character of the neighborhood. It is also within walking distance to a large commercial parkway, with connections to bus lines (Figure 5.6).

Supportive services are provided by New Horizons in Autism, a not-for-profit organization in New Jersey. The entire project was spearheaded by Bergen County's United Way who in the last few years has developed an extensive and growing portfolio of newly constructed and renovated housing for adults with developmental disabilities, sensitive to many of the design goals and issues profiled in this book.

◆

An "intentional community" is a planned residential community intended to have a high degree of social cohesion and teamwork. While some intentional communities hold a common social, political, religious, or spiritual vision, that shared vision can also be nothing more than a strong mutual proclivity to promote community feeling and support, and realized by shared responsibilities and resources. Many farmstead and homestead communities in the U.S. developed for people with autism (Agricultural Communities for Adults with Autism, n.d.), and the village communities in the U.K. mentioned in Chapter Three are examples of intentional communities. Since many of these farmsteads and village communities are situated on large acreage in rural communities, they are relatively isolated from neighbors and often lack the sense of being a community within a larger community. Recently intentional communities exclusively occupied by adults with developmental disabilities are appearing in non-urban settings as gated subdivisions, such as *The Arc Village* in Jacksonville, Florida. Located near a commercial corridor but enclosed by a formal fence and entry gate, this 97-unit community will consist of one- and two-bedroom rental units, in two- and three-unit villas. Each village has a variety of accessible floor plans and elevations. The residential villas ring a community center. Ground breaking for The Arc Village occurred in Spring 2015 (The Arc Jacksonville, n.d.).

Critics often portray the remote location or gated insular nature of these intentional communities as a retreat from the community living tenets fostered by the disabilities rights movement. An exception is cohousing. Many people believe – and regret – that the notion of "community" has been lost in the modern era (for example, Putnam, 1993). While communities may have grown organically in the past, fostering an engaged sense of community today seems to require a more deliberate, intentional effort among dedicated individuals and households who are so inclined toward more interdependent or interconnected living with those in their immediate neighborhood.

These inclinations – coupled with a strong desire to live in a supportive, sharing neighborhood while still maintaining one's household privacy and identity – lie at the heart of the cohousing model.

This movement began in Denmark and Netherlands in the 1960s to1970s, gradually emerged in other European countries afterwards, and transmigrated to North America in the early 1990s. Cohousing allows for people to maintain a sense of private ownership but within a residential development whose neighborhood design and organization encourages people to interact in shared common spaces, such as gardens and kitchens, and avoids those design practices that isolate owners (such as a private garage with an interior door connected to the home, allowing a resident to drive to and from home without ever stepping outside the residence). Cohousing neighbors may share meals together in the common house; delegate or rotate daily living tasks, such as babysitting or grocery shopping, among residents; and establish a cohousing governance structure that encourages participation from most if not all members of the cohousing effort. Cohousing's core principles are: a participatory process, neighborhood design, common facilities, resident management, non-hierarchical structure and decision-making, and no shared economy (McCamant and Durett, 1988).

Private, individually owned or rented homes are generally downsized to allocate more space to shared community spaces, such as gardens, workshops, communal kitchen and dining room, guest rooms and playgrounds. Residences are typically clustered, leaving undeveloped land for environmental preservation or community recreation. Each person participates in the design and management of the cohousing community, with a vote in how the community is structured and coordinated. Residents do not pool their finances. Role-sharing of childcare, grocery-shopping, home maintenance, and the like, recognizes that one person cannot do everything well.

The foundation of cohousing is therefore in its embrace of *interdependence*, which soundly resonates with the spirit of disability rights. "Rather than seeing only people with disabilities as needing 'special' help, communities that acknowledge interdependence de-stigmatize the expectation of assistance for and from every community member" as noted by legal scholar Carrie Griffin Basas (2010, 693).

A few thousand people in North America live in nearly 120 cohousing developments, with the size ranging between 15 and 35 households (cohousing.org). The cohousing movement is more pervasive in Europe: more than one percent of the Danish population live in cohousing (Lietaert, 2009).

There are a few examples of cohousing communities in the U.S. where at least one of the units is occupied by persons with developmental disabilities. While typical units in a cohousing development are owned by individuals and families, the one unit dedicated to residents with disabilities in *Jackson Place Cohousing* in Seattle is owned by a community organization – Parkview Services – who rents the three-bedroom unit to three men with disabilities, each with his own lease with Parkview. Two residents have federal housing vouchers that augment their private funds to afford rent (Jackson Place Cohousing, n.d.). *CoHo Ecovillage* in Corvallis, Oregon, is a cohousing community of 34 homes with a large common house. A mixed-income community, eight homes are set aside for low or moderate home buyers including one four-bedroom unit for residents with developmental disabilities (CoHo Ecovillage, n.d.).

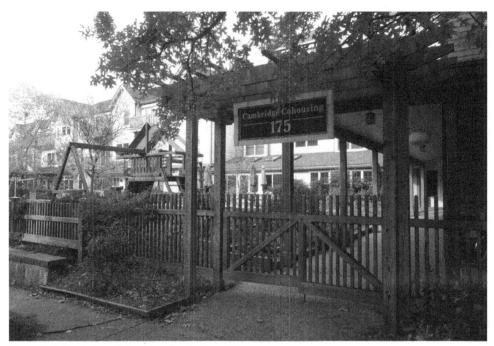

Figure 5.8: Cambridge Cohousing, Cambridge, MA
(Courtesy of Cambridge Cohousing)

Situated on a 1.5 acre site within walking distance to schools, parks, shopping and public transportation, there are 41 units in the *Cambridge Cohousing* complex in Cambridge, Massachusetts (Figure 5.8) The units range in size and configuration – studios, flats, townhouses – which allows for a mix of residents of different ages, backgrounds, incomes and abilities (Cambridge Cohousing, n.d.). Of the 41 homes, two are affordable housing (subsidized by local public housing authority) and one is a four-bedroom supported independent living unit occupied by four adults. (While the local housing authority also subsidizes this unit which makes it more affordable to these residents, it is more expensive than living in a group home.) Accessibility features such as wider doors were incorporated in this unit, but otherwise there are no special design treatments for this four-bedroom unit.

Across the hall from this unit is a two-bedroom flat occupied by support providers of these residents, a family who has lived and worked in that role for the past 12 years.

According to one of the cohousing residents who is also mother of one of the men living in the supported residence, the cohousing community is supportive of this residential option (Anonymous, 2014). She and her husband have lived in the cohousing community from its initial opening in 1998, and they felt that their son Matt (pseudonym) would be more independent living in a unit in cohousing located in Cambridge – with its dense network of transit, services, employment opportunities, and activities – than a group home located in a more suburban community. Cambridge is a very active, relatively dense community adjacent to the city of Boston, with a wide assortment of health, medical and care services. The public transit stop is a seven-minute walk away, and Matt uses transit to go to both of his jobs, medical appointments, and other places where he meets friends.

Cambridge Cohousing operates like most other cohousing communities: decisions are made by consensus, there is a high degree of self-sufficiency, turnover is minimal and residents tend to stay, even age in place. Many of the regular community tasks – taking out the trash to the curb, preparing common meals, tending to gardens and landscapes – are done on a rotational basis among all members of the cohousing development. As members, Matt and his roommates participate in those community activities which they are able to perform.

At Cambridge Cohousing, common meals are not stipulated. There are three common meals: a takeout pizza and potluck combination on Mondays, a home-cooked meal on a mid-week evening, and another home-cooked meal over the weekend. Throughout the community, some residents attend almost every meal and

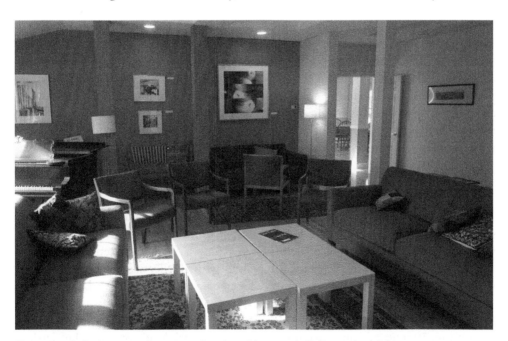

Figure 5.9: Gathering space in common housing with entry to dining room at right, Cambridge Cohousing

(Courtesy of Cambridge Cohousing)

cook regularly; a few attend only one or two meals per year; and the rest fall in between. There are also special events like St. Patrick's Day parties. On occasion, Matt and his housemates attend meals and these special community events as well. But when he wants to go to movies or out to dinner, he usually goes with friends from his peer group who live outside the cohousing community,

Thus, Cambridge Cohousing provides opportunities for different levels and scales of socializing. Matt and others engage with cohousing neighbors for the occasional social event or community meal in the development's common house located in a prominent central location of the development (Figure 5.9). With members cooperatively involved in maintaining the common house and grounds, Cambridge Cohousing also affords opportunities to connect with neighbors in a mutually functional manner. Its proximity to an extensive public transit network in the activity-rich Boston metropolitan area allows Matt and his friends outside the cohousing community to meet and go to movies, sporting events or simply hang out together.

In writing about her proclivity toward "hermit-like behavior" but still with longings for a friendly crowd around – but one slightly removed – blogger Margaret Massey (2012), an associate member of a cohousing residence profiles cohousing as "all about options, preserving the individual with separately owned units, while nurturing community with common spaces and shared decision making, optional group meals, and cooperative events."

While few adults with autism live in cohousing, it is a housing model in which people can perform some of the tasks at which they excel (for example, cleaning, gardening) and trade off the tasks which they may not be able to do (for example, driving, home repair) because of physical, cognitive/neurological, or economic capabilities (Basas, 2010). Urban cohousing's emphasis on equal, participatory citizenship within the community, the layering of community within a larger resource-rich community, and the intentional construction of shared living spaces and shared lives, along with independent and interdependent living, may, as Basas (2010, 680) suggests, "hold the greatest potential for realizing the vision of *Olmstead* and its plaintiffs."

◆

Finally, an emerging model in the United States encompasses integrated–continuum settings offering post-secondary educational opportunities and vocational training to young adults who, at 22 years old, are out of the secondary school system. While there are a growing number of programs for people with intellectual disabilities (Think College, n.d.), those developed specifically for people with autism are relatively few.

First Place in Phoenix, Arizona, is an example of this model aimed at adults with autism. Slated for groundbreaking in 2015, First Place integrates three programs in one setting: 50 units of supportive housing, a Transitional Academy, and a Leadership Institute. As a mixed-use development located in downtown Phoenix one block from the light rail line, First Place offers residents and Transitional Academy students easy access to neighborhood amenities and services. Aimed at adults moving out of the family home for the first time, the First Place Apartments consist of fifty units of one- and two-bedroom apartments for residents who may choose to live on their own or with a roommate or with an aide or support provider. First Place provides a wide range of services and amenities tailored to meet the individual interests and needs of residents. Services and amenities available to choose from include peer mentoring; meal planning, shopping and preparation assistance; stress management and crisis intervention; technology assistance; money management; health related assistance; and recreational and social opportunities. Apartment residents will be supported by staff members who oversee the property and the various programs. Residents requiring additional supports not offered on site may elect to hire outside service providers (Denise Resnik, personal communication)

The First Place Transition Academy is a two-year independent living program operated by the Southwest Autism Research and Resource Center (SARRC). Closely modeled after a California program – the Taft Community College Transition to Independent Living Program – the First Place program provides vocational and life skills training to 16 students annually. First-year students live on-site in one of the four, four-bedroom-bedroom apartments where each student has his or her own room and en-suite bathroom. In year two, students move to transitional off-campus housing, sharing a two-bedroom apartment with a roommate.

The third piece of First Place is the Leadership Institute. With a focus on research and training, the Institute will bring together autism experts to educate support providers, advance public policy and create national housing and service provision standards including training and continuing education requirements for providers. A primary goal is to substantially increase the number of well-trained support providers as well as re-make the field into a valued career choice.

Funding for First Place comes from a mix of private, public and non-profit sources.

Smart technologies for independent living

Technology increasingly is viewed as a resource for supporting people to live longer and more independently in their homes. Devices and programs that assist individuals complete activities of daily living, enhance safety and promote health all are seen as valuable tools for increasing and maintaining this autonomy. Fueled by the rapidly growing number of older people and in particular those with dementia, much of the current research and prototype development focuses on solutions for this population. Responding to both the desire expressed by older adults to remain in their homes as well as the cost effectiveness of doing so, researchers are creating a range of assisted living technologies that may make this possible. At a lesser rate, there are various new technologies under development that focus expressly on assisting individuals with intellectual or cognitive disabilities including autism. However, since both groups experience some of the same challenges when living independently, there exists considerable opportunity to implement technologies designed for older people in homes for people with autism. This section is intended to provide a brief overview of the future of smart home technologies as well as a selection of some of the specific products and systems now being tested.

Today, creating a smart home typically involves installing a variety of networked devices and appliances that automate various environmental features and can be controlled by residents either on-site or remotely. These smart devices and appliances often include lighting and audio systems, thermostats, door lock and security systems, as well as refrigerators, beds and even toilets. At this stage of design evolution, most of these objects act passively, requiring routine user interaction to adjust automation schedules or to input information for the device to work "smartly." The next iteration of these technologies seeks to facilitate a more seamless and unobtrusive relationship between the user and technology through the creation of Ambient Intelligent environments. According to Augusto and colleagues (2013), for an environment to be intelligent, it must be able to function in several critical domains: it must be able to recognize individual users and learn from them; it must be able to understand the context of an event; it must be able to function autonomously; and it must be able to reason such that it is able to determine when to assist a user and when not to.

The success of an intelligent environment stems from its ability to adapt its behavior to the user (Aztiria et al, 2012). To do this, an intelligent environment needs to be context-aware such that it "learns" by unobtrusively collecting data on the user and the environmental aspects through a network of embedded devices such as wireless sensor networks, distributed computing and RFID (radio-frequency identification) installed throughout the house without requiring input from the user. It then uses that information to adapt to the present situation and provide an appropriate level of support. The resulting system assists the resident rather than replaces him or her: it knows when to offer a prompt (food in the refrigerator is expired or possible meals based on refrigerator content) and when not to (when someone is on the phone) (Olivier et al, 2009; Hayes et al, 2009; Augusto et al, 2013). As Wobbrock and colleagues (2011) point out in their discussion of ability-based design, the success of any assistive technology hinges on understanding what an individual can do and creating a system that is person-centric rather than system-oriented such that it is able to adapt to users without requiring people to alter their behavior, bodies or acquire special knowledge to use it.

The intelligent environment scenario describes the most comprehensive model of this evolving technology. Components of intelligent environments including smart materials, interactive smart spaces, ambient assisted living environments, artificial intelligence, pervasive and ubiquitous computing, and smart environments. Along with a growing number of mobile applications, these are all aspects of the broadening array of computing applications designed to enhance occupants' experiences of particular environments and assist with activities of daily living. Falling within this array of technologies are several systems and programs in testing or prototyping phase that either are targeted toward or applicable for autistic individuals.

Given the challenges and potential dangers associated with cooking, it is unsurprising that many systems focus on assisting people in the kitchen. *Smart Kitchen* is a smart environment utilizing ambient assisted living technologies to support elderly people and people with disabilities with kitchen activities. The system merges various technologies including RFID, wireless sensor networks, distributed computing and artificial intelligence to create a context-aware environment managed by an "e-Servant." As a learning system gathering information from the appliances, sensors and interfaces, the e-Servant is able to "detect and compensate the behavior, habit changes and loss of abilities of the user" (Blasco et al, 2014, 1635) as well as provide information regarding the functioning of the appliances. If changes are observed in a user's abilities, e-Servant reports that data to support providers and/or relatives so that the user's profile can be updated. Blasco and colleagues (2014) note that the purpose of the e-Servant is to supervise and assist the user not to take over daily living tasks. To date, 63 end-users and 31 support providers at two labs in the UK and Spain have positively evaluated the Smart Kitchen; additional studies are planned.

The Ambient Kitchen and Kitchen As-A-Pal also are whole kitchen systems designed to assist people to prepare meals. Developed at Newcastle University in 2009, the Ambient Kitchen integrates a variety of sensors and display technologies into a state-of-the-art kitchen to provide support to individuals with food planning, preparation and cooking (Olivier et al, 2009). Through the use of cameras, RFID tags and readers, pressure sensors, accelerometers and projected displays, the system assesses where the user is and what display he or she is viewing and adjusts the display content to reflect what is needed at that moment (Dong et al, 2009). Information displayed may include recipes or cooking instructions. Kitchen As-A-Pal, located at MIT-Huset, Umeå University, Sweden, also offers cooking and meal preparation support to people based on their individual needs. Using RFID technology embedded in surfaces and containers and a sonar network able to determine proximity relationships, this interactive kitchen recognizes individual users, ascertains the specific support level needed and provides the appropriate guidance (Surie, Baydam and Lindgren, 2013). Privacy concerns may arise with Kitchen As-A-Pal as it employs facial recognition technologies to identify users. Another promising technology is FoodBoard, a food identification system that uses optical fibers and a camera embedded in a custom chopping board to identify unpackaged foods (Pham et al, 2013). Where other systems use RFID technology to recognize packaged food or require microphones or cameras to record the environment, FoodBoard is capable of recognizing fresh, unpackaged foods with a high degree of accuracy and without raising privacy concerns. FoodBoard is envisioned as a building block of a total kitchen activity monitoring system.

In addition to intelligent environments, there are a variety of smart technologies and objects under development that focus on a particular task. Two technologies developed by the Ubiquitous Computing Group at the Georgia Institute of Technology are the Social Mirror and Hydrostream. Targeted specifically at adults with autism, the Social Mirror employs an individual's online social network to promote and support independence (Hong et al, 2012). Through the mechanism of an interactive mirror, individuals are able to consult with family members, support providers and friends for assistance with self-help activities such as dressing and grooming and other activities of daily living. As well as being located in the home, the Social Mirror is designed to be accessible via smart phones and tablets, allowing users to access it throughout the day. Hydrostream is a monitoring system using infrastructure-mediated sensing to record water usage related to various activities of daily living (Thomaz et al, 2012). By assessing water usage associated with activities such as brushing teeth, cooking or washing dishes, it would be possible to understand if an individual is maintaining good hygiene or eating well without the need for numerous environmental sensors and the associated privacy concerns.

The Intelligent Assistive Technology Systems Lab (IATSL) at the Toronto Rehabilitation Institute is developing a prompting system using robots to help people complete daily living tasks around the home. COACH (Cognitive Orthosis for Assisting aCtivities in the Home) is an intelligent environment that uses artificial intelligence and a video camera to assess how an individual is completing a particular task, offering prompts when needed (Mihailidis et al, 2008; Czarnuch and Mihailidis, 2011). Designed to assist older people with dementia and children with autism with hand washing, COACH observes and prompts individuals to complete the various repetitive steps of the activity, relieving family members or support providers of the need to routinely intrude. The COACH system features a small robot located on the sink that models hand washing gestures along with verbal coaching (Young, 2014). IATSL also is developing a tele-operated robot capable of socially interacting with people with dementia while assisting them with daily tasks (Begum et al, 2013). Standing upright with a monitor for a face, the robot is equipped with two cameras, two speakers and a microphone and is able to move through the house. When speaking with residents the monitor's screen displays an animated face. If a resident needs support, the display converts to visual images that correspond with the verbal prompts. Currently the robot, nicknamed 'Ed' only has assisted users with making a cup of tea.

Designed both to assist older people at home and to provide a social connection to family and friends, the GiraffPlus system consists of a network of environmental and physiological sensors and a movable robot (Coradeschi et al, 2013). The system not only monitors an individual's activities to assess any changes in abilities and to determine if any support is needed, it also provides social interaction through the robot itself. The monitor 'head' of the robot facilitates communication with family members, friends, support providers and others through a "Skype-like" interface, giving a sense of actual presence. Developed by a consortium of European universities, organizations and businesses (GiraffPlus, n.d.), the GiraffPlus system uses affordable, commercially available components and currently is being evaluated in homes in Sweden, Italy and Spain. Although not designed specifically for individuals with autism, GiraffPlus may be appropriate for some autistic people, especially those who experience seizures or epilepsy or other specific health issues.

While there are many exciting possibilities suggested by intelligent environments and other smart technologies, there also are several challenges including ethical issues pertaining to privacy and questions regarding how to utilize the potentially vast quantities of collected data (Berry, Beyer and Holm, 2009). Significantly, as these technologies assist residents with activities of daily living, many also collect data on individual users documenting different aspects of, users' abilities and actions. The data may be used for a range of purposes; however, most developers intend it to be used to adjust the different systems to better meet users' needs as their abilities evolve. As these new technologies reach the market and become commercially available to consumers, residents, in discussion with their support providers, medical providers and family members, will need to determine what level of personal oversight and intrusion on their privacy they are comfortable with. This is especially important when considering whether or not to install activity and health monitoring systems that rely on a combination of sensors, microphones and video cameras; where possible, residents should have control over the data collected on them including how it will be stored, accessed and used (Augusto et al, 2011).

New directions in self-advocacy for housing choice

The underlying current running through the pages of this book is that of *informed and viable choice*. We have structured our book not as a directive but as a friendly guide that one can take on a journey to a new place – a new residence, perhaps – to gauge the terrain of possible routes and destinations depending upon the inclination, interest, and companions on that journey. The essence and beauty of informed choice is not the chosen product *per se*, but the process. This concept of choice undergirds prevailing policies and philosophies of independent and community living, although it is often labeled under the terms of "person-center planning" or "self-determination" (there are hundreds of documents on these, but a few that represent both governmental and service provision perspectives include: O'Brien and O'Brien, 2000; Program Design, 2005; Vatland et al, 2011).

As described at the beginning of this book, choice is a multifaceted endeavor that goes beyond methods to assess statements of "preference." While they can be somewhat informative, efforts such as surveys to gauge preferences – of an individual or of a community of individuals – are fraught with challenges and potential biases. This applies to all populations. National and multinational, high-profile survey research firms such as Pew, Gallop, Ipsos MORI and many others invest hundreds of thousands of dollars and employ sophisticated sampling and modeling techniques to gauge people's preferences – and are known to get only part of the story right, or even, at times, entirely wrong.

Assessment methods that require verbal or written responses can be inappropriate for many persons with autism given communication mismatches between those assembling the assessment tool and those using it. Questionnaires – even those that rely on checklists – assume an individual's language skills can process the content and intent in the same manner as those writing and assembling those questionnaires.

It is also more than simply a matter of communication mismatches, however. Gauging preference is difficult when one is not familiar with many of the options, or concepts, posed. Cohousing, for example, is rarely mentioned as a preferred living arrangement – but then again, in many countries or regions few people have even heard of cohousing, let alone seen one in their neighborhood. Even if one was familiar with a particular housing type or arrangement, it can be difficult to make an informed judgment if one has never experienced living in that setting or arrangement. *Informed choice* then implies a process: being engaged, becoming informed of possibilities and what each of those may mean in one's life, taking the initiative and movement towards realizing that choice – with or without assistance from others in one's support circle.

Self-determination and self-advocacy tools that go beyond expressing preferences to engaging in such processes are increasingly being developed and used, and some of these are quite thorough (for example, Fisher et al, 2007). These "tools" are often administered or managed by supportive living coaches or other service providers; and as such, they strongly depend upon the coach's knowledge and acceptance of a range of options, as well as recognition of what options *could* be chosen if in the future they became more available. In Virginia, for example, the state's Department of Behavioral Health and Developmental Services plans to increase the availability of independent living options for individuals with intellectual and development disabilities. With advice and assistance of national housing experts of the Technical Assistance Collaborative in Boston, Department staff concluded that only face-to-face and person-centered planning processes could ascertain people's preferences for housing or residential services. Virginia has thus begun collecting data on each individual's choice and housing need gathered from case managers as they work with individuals in developing annual person-centered plans. Aggregated later, this data will be used to provide projections of types of housing desired and needed for future years, starting in 2015 (Fletcher, 2013).

While a commendable strategy that goes beyond ill-formed results from an online survey, for Virginia's plan to be successful and truly representative, case managers will need to be well versed in the range of residential alternatives on the landscape – not only those currently existing, but also those on the horizon that may be better matches for the needs and aspirations of clients, both of today and in the near future.

A means to increase engagement in the decision-making process are participatory strategies. Such techniques are increasingly being advocated for in the autism community (Wright et al, 2014). For example, AASPIRE (Academic Autistic Spectrum Partnership in Research and Education) advocates community based participatory research (CBPR) or participatory action research (PAR). In these situations, professionals and community members work together as equal partners in the development, implementation, and dissemination of research that is relevant to the community (AASPIRE, n.d.). Some groups have used AASPIRE's approach for research and intervention proposals for healthcare, social support and violence victimization.

Given that the focus of this book is on residential living and housing choices, the community participatory design field has much to offer. The decades-long work of Henry Sanoff (1991; 2000), Randy Hester (2006), and others in this field have produced a number of visually-based participatory design strategies whereby communities and individuals explore, test, envision and decide on the shaping of the built environment – schools, parks, neighborhoods, housing – in their lives. This approach seems immensely applicable to those with autism. Indeed, designers and researchers of the Helen Hamlyn Centre for Design of the Royal College of Art in London have already made steady and exemplary progress in advancing participatory design efforts that can serve as a model for others to consider.

While the portfolio of projects of the Helen Hamlyn Centre for Design encompasses a range of settings and populations with social needs, for the last several years they have been involved in action research and participatory design projects with people with autism, focusing on housing design, sensory preferences, green spaces and household objects for everyday activities at home, such as vacuuming (Brand, 2010; Brand and Gaudion, 2012; Gaudion and McGinley, 2012; Gaudion, 2013; Gaudion, 2014).

They use a myriad of methods – participatory observation, co-design workshops, trialing and assessment, interviewing, visual profiling, visual questionnaires, digital tools, mapping, prototyping and piloting design concepts, to name a few (see Figure 5.10 for one example). There is much to learn from these leaders in the field.

Part of the success of the efforts of Gaudion, Brand, McGinley and others at the Helen Hamlyn Centre is the extended engagement of those with autism in the design

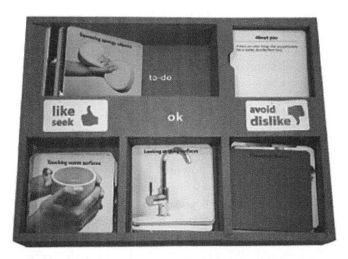

Figure 5.10: Visually-oriented cards for eliciting participation in housing preference, developed and used by Helen Hamlyn Centre for Design

(Courtesy of Helen Hamlyn Centre for Design, Royal College of London)

research process. Another way to help make informed housing choice is through direct experience of alternatives. Experience with and exposure to situations enable people to make decisions about what they like and dislike (Greenbie, 1981). Unfortunately, most autistic adults – and even their support providers – are exposed to a rather limited number of residential options. If people are not familiar with or do not experience different living options, it becomes difficult to make informed choices by comparing what might work best. This may be exacerbated by efforts to prevent imaginative thinking including visualizing new environments and placing themselves in those settings (Murray, 1996). Thus, if exposure is limited, then it would follow that one's ability to choose is also limited.

Increasing exposure to possibilities has been advanced by a number of self-advocates in the disability rights movement. Take, for example, "Welcome HOME" in Newburg, Wisconsin. This development was the brainchild of Diane Miller who acquired adult-onset polio as a young adult. Facing how to remodel her home to better suit her condition, she was perplexed with the myriad different home and accessibility features profiled in catalogs, showrooms, and stores. Options were numerous, but seeing them alone did not allow her to judge which would work best for herself.

Miller recognized that others faced the same predicament: of being exposed – even overwhelmed at times – to numerous accessibility devices and housing features but not knowing *from experience* if and how those features would be suitable for her particular situation at home. In the 1990s, she developed and built a uniquely designed bed and breakfast, with different accessibility features and spatial arrangements in each bedroom, bathroom, and in the various eating and lounging areas. Guests can visit for a few days or a week, stay in different rooms, and try out different fixtures, lighting, flooring materials, furnishings, gadgets and the like, to see what might later work best for them in their own homes (Ahrentzen, 2002).

Since Welcome HOME was developed over 20 years ago, this can hardly be considered an innovation on the horizon. But its intent to create opportunities to experience living in different spaces to better inform one's own housing choices is being explored in today's computer environmental simulation and virtual reality technology. A number of software designers in the user-design field are developing and refining these technologies to advance participatory design efforts whereby persons can "experience" different environmental conditions and situations. One example is the commonSENSE platform being developed by Vardouli and colleagues (2012) that allow individuals to explore the potential of their own living space and actively engage them in its design and remodeling or rearrangement. While not targeting individuals with autism *per se*, its application and other computer-based participatory design techniques to the autism community is considerable.

Going beyond conventional software architectural design systems such as Sketch-Up, the CommonSENSE platform provides what the software developers/ researchers call "environment intelligence" that allows user control, collaboration and participation; they describe it as a convergence of the digital and the physical. While the details of the monitors, technologies, software, and online design engine are described elsewhere (Vardouli et al, 2012), the prototype comprises a sensor kit that allows users to collect space use and occupancy data by installing the kit in their apartments and communal spaces. From the collected space-use data, users can then later watch how they use the spaces where they live. Design alternatives or spatial scenarios can be simulated, and residents can use these as a basis to discuss, keep or alter these alternatives – and eventually test them in physical space. CommonSENSE and other interactive technologies that use actual and simulated scenarios may provide a new approach to design decision-making.

While these innovations in participatory decision-making and informed choice range from prop-based approaches to sophisticated computer simulation of actual and altered settings, most central is the emphasis on process-oriented goals, a mainstay of the neurodiversity and self-advocacy movement. These approaches are not trying to help people with autism "pass" or become somehow more "normal" or "typical" in their choice of settings. Rather they are intended to provide a greater range of approaches to developing skills for learning about and advocating for the type of residential setting in which each individual might choose to live. This empowers the individual, resulting in not only decreased dependency on support providers but also affording greater opportunity for life fulfillment through active participation in shaping and making the decisions affecting one's life (Murray, 1996) – and a more suitable and desirable place to be at home with autism.

REFERENCES

AAPD. 2012. *Equity in Transportation for People with Disabilities.* [online] Available at: <http://www.aapd.com/resources/press-room/press-releases/people-with-disabilities.html> [Accessed 13 May 2014].

AARP Livable Communities. 2014. *What is Universal Design?* [online] Available at: <http://www.aarp.org/livable-communities/info-2014/what-is-universal-design.html> [Accessed 8 March 2014].

AASPIRE (Academic Autistic Spectrum Partnership in Research and Education). n.d. *CBRP.* [online] Available at: <http://aaspire.org/?p=about&c=cbpr> [Accessed 18 July 2015].

Abbott, S. and McConkey, R. 2006. The barriers to social inclusion as perceived by people with intellectual disabilities. *Journal of Intellectual Disabilities,* 10, 275-287.

Acoustiblok. 2014. *Acoustiblok: quieting the world.* [online] Available at: <http://www.acoustiblok.com/> [Accessed 10 June 2014].

Adler, T. 2003. Aging research: The future face of environmental health. *Environmental Health Perspectives,* 111(14), A761-A765.

Agricultural Communities for Adults with Autism. n.d. *Community.* [online] Available at: <http://ac-aa.org > [Accessed 18 July 2015].

Ahrentzen, S. 2002. Socio-behavioral qualities of the built environment. In Dunlap, R.E., and Michelson, W., eds. *Handbook of Environmental Sociology.* Westport, CT: Greenwood Press.

Ahrentzen, S. 2007. Actionable knowledge: A research synthesis project for affordable housing design practice. In American Institute of Architects, eds. *2006 Report on University Research.* Washington DC: American Institute of Architects.

Ahrentzen, S. and Steele, K. 2009. *Advancing Full Spectrum Housing: Designing For Adults With Autism Spectrum Disorders.* [pdf] Phoenix, AZ: Arizona Board of Regents. Available at: <http://stardust.asu.edu/docs/stardust/advancing-full-spectrum-housing/full-report.pdf> [Accessed 18 July 2015].

Ahrentzen, S., Jue, G.M., Skorpanich, M.A. and Evans, G.W. 1982. School environments and stress. In Evans, G.W., ed. *Environmental Stress.* New York: Cambridge University Press. (224–255).

AIA. 2012. *Local Leaders: Healthier Communities through Design.* New York: American Institute of Architects (AIA).

Algase, D.L., Antonakos, C.,Beattle, E.R., Beel-Bates, C.A. et al. 2009. Empirical derivation and validation of a wandering typology. *Journal of American Geriatrics Society.* 57(11), 2037-2045.

Altman, I. 1976. *Environment and Social Behavior.* Belmont, CA: Brooks/Cole.

Altman, I. and Chermers, M.M. 1980. *Culture and Environment.* Belmont, CA: Brooks/Cole.

Amado, A.N., Stancliffe, R.J., McCarron, J. and McCallion, P. 2013. Social inclusion and community participation of individuals with intellectual/developmental disabilities. *Intellectual and Developmental Disabilities*, 51(5), 360–375.

American Psychiatric Association. 2013. *Diagnostic and statistical manual of mental disorders.* Fifth edition. New York: American Psychiatric Association.

American Psychological Association. 2001. *Publication Manual of the American Psychological Association.* 5th edition. Washington DC: American Psychological Association.

Amlet, C., Gourfinkel-An, I., Bouzamondo, A., Tordjman, S., Baulac, M., Lechat, P. et al. 2008. Epilepsy in autism in associated with intellectual disability and gender: Evidence from a meta-analysis. *Biological Psychiatry,* 64, 577–582.

Anderson, C., Law, J.K., Daniels, A., Rice, C., et al. 2012. Occurrence and family impact of elopement in children with autism spectrum disorders. *Pediatrics,* 130, 870-877.

Anderson, K.A., Shattuck, P.T., Cooper, B.P., Roux, A.M. et al. 2013. Prevalence and correlates of postsecondary residential status among young adults with an autism spectrum disorder. *Autism.* doi: 10.1177/1362361313481860.

Anderson, L., Larson, S., Lakin, K.C. et al. 2002. *Children with Disabilities: Social Roles and Family Impacts in the NHIS-D, DD Data Brief.* Volume 4. Minneapolis, MN: Rehabilitation Research and Training Center on Community Living, University of Minnesota.

Anonymous. December 2014. Personal communication.

Archea, J. 1977. The place of architectural factors in behavioral theories of privacy. *Journal of Social Issues,* 33(3), 116–137.

Armitage, R. 2013. *Crime Prevention Through Housing Design: Policy and Practice.* London: Palgrave Macmillan.

Armstrong, T. 2010. *Neurodiversity: Discovering the Extraordinary Gifts of Autism, ADHD, Dyslexia, and Other Brain Differences.* Cambridge, MA: De Capo Press.

Arnaiz Sánchez, P., Segado Vázquez, F. and Albaladejo Serrano, L. 2011. Autism and the built environment. In Williams, T. ed. *Autism Spectrum Disorders – From Genes to Environment*. Rijeka, Croatia: InTech.

Arnett, J. 2000. Emerging adulthood: A theory of development from the late teens through the early twenties. *American Psychologist,* 55, 469-480.

Arnett, J. 2001. Conceptions of the transition to adulthood: Perspectives from adolescence through midlife. *Journal of Adult Development*, 8, 133-143.

Aubry, T., and Myner, J. 1996. Community integration and quality of life: A comparison of persons with psychiatric disabilities in housing programs and community residents who are neighbors. *Canadian Journal of Mental Health,* 15, 5-20.

Augusto, J.C., Callaghan, V., Cook, D., Kameas, A. and Satoh, I. 2013. Intelligent environments: A manifesto. *Human-centric Computing and Information Sciences*, 3(12), 1-18.

Augusto, J.C., McCullagh, P.J. and Augusto-Walkden, J.A. 2011. Living without a safety net in an intelligent environment. *ICST Transactions on Ambient Systems*, 11(10-12), 1-9.

Augusto, J.C., Nakashima, H. and Aghajan, H. 2010. Ambient intelligence and smart environments: a state of the art. In Nakashima, H., Aghajan H. and Augusto, J.C. eds. 2010. *Handbook of Ambient Intelligence and Smart Environments*. New York: Springer. (3-31).

Autism Society of Delaware. n.d. *Best Practices for Serving Adults with Autism: Results of the Study on Services and supports for Adults on the Autism Spectrum Across the United States.* [pdf] Available at: <http://www.delautism.org/wp-content/uploads/2015/01/Adult-Best-Practices.pdf> [Accessed 16 April 2015].

Autism Speaks. 1 April 2011. *The 10 best places to live if you have autism.* [online] Available at: <www.autismspeaks.org/about-us/press-releases/10-best-places-live-if-you-have-autism> [Accessed 22 August 2013].

Autism Speaks. 2013. *National Housing and Residential Supports Survey: An Executive Summary.* [pdf] Available at: <http://www.autismspeaks.org/sites/default/files/docs/2013_national_housing_survey.pdf> [Accessed 10 January 2014].

Ayres, K., Mechling, L., and Sansosti, F. 2013. The use of mobile technologies to assist with life skills/independence of students with moderate/severe intellectual disability and/or autism spectrum disorders: considerations for the future of school psychology. *Psychology in the Schools*, 50(3), 259-271.

Aztiria, A., Augusto, J.C., Basagoiti, R., Izaguirre, A. and Cook D.J. 2012. Discovering frequent user-environment interactions in intelligent environments. *Personal and Ubiquitous Computing*, 16(1), 91-103.

Bagatell, N. 2010. From cure to community: Transforming notions of autism. *ETHOS,* 38(1), 33-55.

Bågenholm, A. and Gillberg, C. 1991. Psychosocial effects on siblings of children with autism and mental retardation: A population-based study. *Journal of Intellectual Disabilities Research,* 35, 291-307.

Baio, J. 2014. Prevalence of autism spectrum disorder among children aged 8 years: Autism and Developmental Disabilities Monitoring Network, 11 sites, United States, 2010. *Morbidity and Mortality Weekly Report,* 63(SS02), 1-21.

Baker, A.E.Z., Lane, A., Angley, M.T. and Young, R.L. 2008. The relationship between sensory processing patterns and behavioural responsiveness in autistic disorder: a pilot study. *Journal of Autism and Developmental Disorders,* 38, 867-875.

Baker, D.L. 2006. Neurodiversity, neurological disability and the public sector: Notes on the autism spectrum. *Disability and Society,* 21(1), 15-29.

Balfe, M. and Tantam, D. 2010. A descriptive social and health profile of a community sample of adults and adolescents with Asperger syndrome. *BMC Research Notes,* 5(3), 300-306.

Ballabum-Gil, K., Rapin, I., Tuchman, R. et al. 1996. Longitudinal examination of the behavioral, language, and social changes in a population of adolescents and young adults with autistic disorder. *Pediatric Neurology,* 15, 212-223.

Barnes, M. and Cooper Marcus, C. 1999. *Healing Gardens: Therapeutic Benefits and Design Recommendations.* New York: John Wiley & Sons.

Barnes, S. and Design in Caring Environments Study Group. 2002. The design of caring environments and the quality of life of older people. *Ageing & Society,* 22, 775-789.

Baron-Cohen, S., and Belmonte, M.K. 2005. Autism: A window onto the development of the social and the analytic brain. *Annual Review of Neuroscience,* 28, 109-126.

Baron-Cohen, S. and Wheelwright, S. 2003. The friendship questionnaire: An investigation of adults with Asperger syndrome or high-functioning autism, and normal sex differences. *Journal of Autism and Developmental Disorders,* 33(5), 509-517.

Baron-Cohen, S. and Wheelwright, S. 2004. The empathy quotient: An investigation of adults with Asperger syndrome or high functioning autism, and normal sex differences. *Journal of Autism and Developmental Disorders,* 34(2), 163-175.

Baron-Cohen, S., Ashwin, E., Ashwin, C., Tavassoli, T. et al. 2009. Talent in autism: Hyper-systemizing, hyper-attention to detail and sensory hypersensitivity. *Philosophical Transactions of the Royal Society, B,* 364, 1377-1383.

Barrett, P. and Barrett, L. 2010. The potential of positive places: Senses, brain and spaces. *Intelligent Buildings International,* 2, 218-228.

Basas, C.G. 2010. *Olmstead's* promise and cohousing's potential. *Georgia State University Law Review,* 26(3), 663-704.

Baum, A., Singer, J.E. and Baum, C.S. 1982. Stress and the environment. In Evans, G.W., ed. *Environmental Stress.* New York: Cambridge University Press. (15-44)

Baumers, S. and Heylighen, A. 2010. Beyond the designers' view: How people with autism experience space. *Design and Complexity. Proceedings of the Design Research Society Conference. 2010.* [pdf] Available at: <http://www.drs2010.umontreal.ca/data/PDF/008.pdf> [Accessed 7 May 2014].

Baumers, S. and Heylighen. 2014. Performing their version of the house: Views on an architectural response to autism. In D. Maudlin and M. Vellinga, eds. *Consuming Architecture: On the Occupation, Appropriation and Interpretation of Buildings.* London: Routledge.

Bauminger, N., Shulman, C., and Agam, G. 2004. The link between perceptions of self and of social relationships in high-functioning children with autism. *Journal of Developmental and Physical Disabilities,* 16(2), 193-214.

Beaver, C. 2006. Designing environments for children and adults with ASD. London: The National Autistic Society, [online] Available at: <http://www.autism.org.uk/ working-with/leisure-and-environments/architects/designing-environments-for-children-and-adults-with-asd.aspx> [Accessed 14 September 2009].

Beaver, C. 2010. Autism-friendly environments. *The Autism File,* 34, 82-85.

Begum, M., Wang, R., Huq, R. and Mihailidis, A. 2013. Performance of daily activities by older adults with dementia: the role of an assistive robot. In: *13th International Conference on Rehabilitation Robotics.* Seattle, USA 24-26 June 2013.

Ben-Sasson, A., Hen, L., Fluss, R., Cermak, S.A. et al. 2009. A meta-analysis of sensory modulcation symptoms in indivduals with autism spectrum disorders. *Journal of Autism and Developmental Disorders,* 39, 1-11.

Benos, D.J., Bashari, E., Chaves, J.M., Gaggar, A., et al. 2007. The ups and downs of peer review. *Advances in Physiology Education,* 31, 145-152.

Berg, A.T. and Plioplys, S. 2012. Epilepsy and autism: Is there a special relationship? *Epilepsy & Behvarior,* 23(3), 193-198.

Bergen County's United Way. n.d. *Orchard Commons.* [online] Available at: < http://www.bergenunitedway.org/howwehelp/housing-works-2/orchard-commons. php> [Accessed 18 July 2015].

Berman, M.G., Jonides, J. and Kaplan, S. 2008. The cognitive benefits of interacting with nature. *Psychological Science,* 19(12), 1207-12.

Berry, J., Beyer, S. and Holm, S. 2009. Assistive technology, telecare and people with intellectual disabilities: Ethical considerations. *Journal of Medical Ethics,* 35(2), 81-86.

Beyers, E.S., Nichols, S., Voyer, S.D. and Reilly, G. 2012. Sexual well-being of a community sample of high-functioning adults on the autism spectrum who have been in a romantic relationship. *Autism,* 17(4), 418-433.

Bhat, A.N., Landa, R.J. and Galloway, J.C. 2011. Current perspectives on motor functioning in infants, children and adults with autism spectrum disorders. *Physical Therapy,* 91, 116-1129.

Bigby, C. and Wiesel, I. 2011. Encounter as a dimension of social inclusion for people with intellectual disability: Beyond and between community presence and participation. *Journal of Intellectual Disability,* 36(4), 259-263.

Biklen, D., Attfield, R., Bissonnette, L., Blackman, L., Burke, J., Frugone, A. et al. 2005. *Autism and the Myth of the Person Alone.* New York: New York University Press.

Billstedt, E., Gillberg, C. and Gillberg, C. 2005. Autism after adolescence: Population-based 13- to 22-year follow-up study of 120 individuals with autism diagnosed in childhood. *Journal of Autism and Developmental Disorders,* 35, 351-360.

Bimbrahw, J., Boger, J. and Mihailidis, A. 2012. Investigating the efficacy of a computerized prompting device to assist children with autism spectrum disorder with activities of daily living. *Assistive Technology,* 24(4), 286-298.

Birch, J. 2003. *Congratulations! It's Asperger's Syndrome.* London: Jessica-Kingsley Publishers.

Bishop-Fitzpartick, L., Minshew, N.J. and Eack, S. 2013. A systematic review of psychosocial interventions for adults with autism spectrum disorders. *Journal of Autism and Developmental Disorders,* 43, 687-694.

Bittles, A., Petterson, B., Sullivan, S., Hussain, R, Glasson E. and Montgomery, P., 2002. The influence of intellectual disability on life expectancy. *The Journals of Gerontology Series A: Biological Science and Medical Science,* 57, pp. 470-472

Blasco, R., Marco, A., Casas, R., Cirujano, D. and Picking, R. 2014. A smart kitchen for ambient assisted living. *Sensors,* 14, 1629-1653.

Bogdashina, O. 2003. *Sensory Perceptual Issues in Autism and Asperger Syndrome: Different Sensory Experiences – Different Perceptual Worlds.* London: Jessica Kingsley.

Boger, J., and Mihailidis, A. 2011. The future of intelligent assistive technologies for cognition: Devices under development to support independent living and aging-with-choice. *NeuroRehabilitation,* 28, 271-280.

Bolton, P., Macdonald, H., Pickles, A. et al. 1994. A case-control family history study of autism. *Journal of Child Psychology and Psychiatry,* 35, 877-900.

Bolton, P.F., Carcani-Rathwell, I., Hutton, J., Goode, S. et al. 2011. Epilepsy in autism: Features and correlates. *The British Journal of Psychiatry,* 198(4), 289-294.

Boucher, J., and Bowler, D.M. 2008. *Memory in Autism: Theory and Research.* Cambridge: Cambridge University Press.

Bower, L., 2000. *Creating a Healthy Household: The Ultimate Guide For Healthier, Safer, Less-Toxic Living.* Boise, ID: The Healthy House Institute.

Bowler, D.M., Gardiner, J.M. and Gaigg, S.B. 2007. Factors affecting conscious awareness in the recollective experience of adults with Asperger's syndrome. *Conscious Cognition,* 16, 124-143.

Braddock, D. 1999. Aging and developmental disabilities: Demographic and policy issues affecting American families. *Mental Retardation,* 37, 155-161.

Braddock, D. 2002. *The State of the States: Public Policy Toward Disability at the Dawn of the 21st Century.* Washington DC: American Association on Mental Retardation.

Braddock, D., and Mitchell, D. 1992. *Residential Services and Developmental Disabilities in the United States.* Washington DC: American Association on Mental Retardation.

Braddock, G. and Rowell, J. 2011. *Making Homes that Work: A Resource Guide for Families Living with Autism Spectrum Disorder and Co-Occurring Behaviors.* Eugene, OR: Creative Housing Solutions.

Brake, L.R., Schleien, S.J., Miller, K.D. and Walton, G. 2012. Photovoice: A tour through the camera lens of self-advocates. *Social Advocacy and Systems Change Journal,* 3(1), 44-53.

Brand, A. 2010. *Living in the Community: Housing Design for Adults with Autism.* London: Helen Hamlyn Centre, Royal College of Art.

Brand, A. and Gaudion, K. 2012. *Exploring Sensory Preferences: Living Environments for Adults with Autism.* London: Helen Hamlyn Centre for Design, Royal College of Art.

Brandt, R., Chong, G.H. and Martin, W.M. 2010. *Design Informed: Driving Innovation with Evidence-based Design.* New York: John Wiley & Sons.

Brereton, A. and Broadbent, K. 2007. *Act-Now Fact Sheet 35: Developing Gross Motor Skills.* Melbourne, Australia: Centre for Developmental Psychiatry and Psychology, Monash University. [online] Available at: <http://www.ibooksdaily.com/doc-detail/act-now-fact-sheet-35-faculty-of-medicine-nursing-and-558539/> [Accessed 16 April 2015].

Bruder, M.B., Kerins, G., Mazzarella, C., Sims, J., and Stein, N. 2012. Brief report: The medical care of adults with autism spectrum disorders: Identifying the needs. *Journal of Autism and Developmental Disorders,* 42, 2498-2504.

Brugha, T., McManus, S., Meltzer, H. et al. 2009. *Development and Testing of Methods for Identifying Cases of Autism Spectrum Disorder Among Adults in the Adult Psychiatric Morbidity Survey 2007.* Leeds, UK: The NHS Information Centre.

Brugha, T.S., Cooper, S.A., McManus, S. et al. 2012. Estimating the prevalence of autism spectrum condition in adults: Extending the 2007 adult psychiatric morbidity survey. *The Health and Social Care Information Centre (NHS).* [pdf] Available at <http://wenurses.info/MyNurChat/archive/LDdownloads/Est_Prev_Autism_Spec_Cond_in_Adults_Report.pdf> [Accessed 14 May 2014].

Brugha, T.S., McManus, S., Bankart, J., Scott, F., et al. 2011. Epidemiology of autism spectrum disorders in adults in the community in England. *Archives of General Psychiatry,* 68, 459-465.

Bryant, B., Soonwha, S. and Ok, M. 2012. Individuals with intellectual and/or developmental disabilities use of assistive technology devices in support provision. *Journal of Special Education Technology,* 27(2), 47-57.

Bryant, D., and Bryant, B. 2012. *Assistive Technology for People with Disabilities* (2nd ed.). Boston: Pearson.

Bryant, G., Seok, S. and Ok, M. 2012. Individuals with Intellectual and/or Developmental Disabilities Use of Assistive Technology Devices in Support Provision. *Journal of Special Education Technology,* 27(2), 41-57.

Buescher, A.V.S., Cidav, Z., Knapp, M. and Mandell, D.S. 2014. Costs of autism spectrum disorders in the United Kingdom and the United States. *JAMA Pediatrics,* 166(8), 721-728.

Bunn, S. 2001. *Self-Determination Resource Handbook.* Salem, OR: Oregon Department of Education.

Bureau of Labor Statistics, U.S. Department of Labor. 2015. *Persons with a Disability: Labor Force Characteristics – 2014.* [pdf] Available at: <http://www.bls.gov/news.release/pdf/disabl.pdf > [Accessed 30 June 2015].

Byers, E. S., Nichols, S. and Voyer, S.D. 2013. Challenging stereotypes: Sexual functioning of single adults with high functioning autism spectrum disorder. *Journal of Autism and Developmental Disorders,* 43, 2617-2627.

Cadenhead, J. 2014. Quietest Dishwasher by Decibel Rating. *Yale Appliance + Lighting Blog* [blog] 6 July. Available at: <http://blog.yaleappliance.com/bid/90427/Quietest-Dishwasher-By-Decibel-Rating-Reviews-Prices> [Accessed 20 June 2014].

Cambridge Cohousing. n.d. *Home.* [online] Available at: <http://www.cambridgecohousing.org> [Accessed 18 July 2015].

Careinfo. 2014. *Careinfo.* [online] Available at: <http://careinfo.org/> [Accessed 8 June 2014].

Carmien, S., Dawe, M., Fischer, G., Gorman, A. et al. 2005. Socio-technical environments supporting people with cognitive disabilities using public transportation. *ACM Transactions on Computer-Human Interaction (TOCHI),* 12(2), 233-262.

Carmien, S, Dawe, M., Fischer, G., Gorman, A., Kintsch, A. and Sullivan, J.F. 2005. Socio-technical environments supporting people with cognitive disabilities using public transportation. *ACM Transactions on Computer-Human Interaction,* 233-262.

Carr, E.G. and Owen-DeSchryve, J.S. 2007. Physical illness, pain and problem behavior in minimally verbal people with developmental disabilities. *Journal of Autism and Developmental Disorders,* 37, 413-424.

Cascio, C., McGlone, F., Folger, S., Tannan, V., Baranek, G., Pelphrey, K.A. and Essick, G. 2008. Tactile perception in adults with autism: a multidimensional psychophysical study. *Journal of Autism and Developmental Disorders,* 38(1), 127-137.

Cascio, C. J., Moana-Filho, E. J., Guest, S., Nebel, M. B., Weisner, J., Baranek, G. T. and Essick, G. K. 2012. Perceptual and neural response to affective tactile texture stimulation in adults with autism spectrum disorders. *Autism Research,* 5: 231–244.

Case-Smith, J. and Arbesman, M. 2008. Evidence-based review of interventions for autism used in or of relevance to occupational therapy. *The American Journal of Occupational Therapy,* 62(4), 416-429.

Cederlund, M., Hagberg, B., Billstedt, E., Gillberg, I.C. et al. 2008. Asperger syndrome and autism: A comparative longitudinal follow-up study more than 5 years after original diagnosis. *Journal of Autism and Developmental Disorders,* 38, 72-85.

Centers for Disease Control and Prevention (CDC). 2013. *Autism: Data and statistics.* [online] Available at: <http://www.dcd.gov/ncbddd/autism/data.html> [Accessed 10 July 2013].

Centers for Medicare and Medicaid Services. 2014. Medicaid Program; State Plan Home and Community-Based Services, 5-Year Period for Waivers, Provider Payment Reassignment, and Home and Community-Based Requirements for Community First Choice and Home and Community-Based Services (HCBS) Waivers. Final Rule. 42, CFR Part 430, 431 et al. 16 January 2014. *Federal Register,* 79(11) 2947-3038. [online] Available at: <http://www.gpo.gov/fdsys/pkg/FR-2014-01-16/pdf/2014-00487.pdf> [Accessed 18 April 2015].

Chalfont, G. E. 2011. Charnley Fold: A Practice Model of Environmental Design for Enhanced Dementia Day Care. *Social Care and Neurodisability,* 2(2), 71-79.

Chalfont, G. and Walker, A. 2013. *Dementia Green Care Handbook of Therapeutic Design and Practice.* Safehouse Books.

Chan, M., Estéve, D., Escriba, C. and Campo, E. 2008. A review of smart homes – Present state and future challenges. *Computer Methods and Programs in Biomedicine,* 91, 55-81.

Chen, S.C., Ryan-Henry, S., Heller, T., et al. 2001. Health status of mothers of adults with intellectual disability. *Journal of Intellectual Disability Research,* 45, 439-449.

Chen, W., Landau, S., Sham, P., et al. 2004. No evidence for a link between autism, MMR, and measles virus. *Psychological Medicine,* 34, 543-553.

Chenoweth, D., Estes, C. and Lee, C. 2009. The economic cost of environmental factors among North Carolina children living in substandard housing. *American Journal of Public Health,* 99(53), S666-S674.

Cidav, Z., Marcus, S.C., and Mandell, D.S. 2012. Implications of childhood autism for parental employment and earnings. *Pediatrics,* 129 (4), 617-623.

CityQuiet. 2014. *CityQuiet: serenity now!* [online] Available at: <http://www.citiquiet.com/> [Accessed 12 June 2014].

Clarke, J., and van Amerom, G. 2008. Asperger's syndrome: Differences between parents' understanding and those diagnosed. *Social Work in Health Care,* 46(3), 85-106.

Cohen, S. 1978. Environmental load and the allocation of attention. In Baum, A., Singer, J. and Valins, S., eds. *Advances in Environmental Psychology.* Volume 1. Hillsdale, NJ: Erlbaum.

CoHo Ecovillage. n.d. *Home.* [online] Available at: <https://www.cohoecovillage.org> [Accessed 18 July 2015].

Constantino, J.N., Lajonchere, C., Lutz, M., et al. 2006. Autistic social impairment in the siblings of children with pervasive developmental disorders. *American Journal of Psychiatry,* 163, 292-296.

Consumer Reports. 2014. *The best countertops for busy kitchens.* [online] Available at: <http://www.consumerreports.org/cro/news/2014/08/the-best-countertops-for-busy-kitchens/index.htm> [Accessed 10 July 2015].

Cooper Marcus, C. and Sachs, N. 2013. *Therapeutic Landscapes: An Evidence-Based Approach to Designing Healing Gardens and Restorative Outdoor Spaces.* New York: John Wiley & Sons.

Cooper, E., Knott, L., Schaak, G., Sloane, L. and Zovistoski, Z. June 2015. *Priced Out in 2014: The Housing Crisis for People with Disabilities.* Boston: Technical Assistance Collaborative, Inc.

Cornerstone Community Housing. n.d. *Willakenzie Crossing Apartments.* [online] Available at: < http://www.willakenziecrossing.com> [Accessed 18 July 2015].

Cornwell, E.Y. and Waite, L.J. 2009. Measuring social isolation among older adults using multiple indicators from the NSHAP study. *Journal of Gerontology,* 64, 138-146.

Countertop Guides. 2014. *CounterTop Guides: Consumer Buying Guides to Bathroom and Kitchen Countertops.* [online] Available at: <https://www.countertopguides.com/> [Accessed 12 June 2014].

Cowen, T. 2009. Autism as academic paradigm. *The Chronicle of Higher Education.* [online] Available at: <http://chronicle.com/article/Autism-as-Academic-Paradigm/47033> [Accessed 13 July 2009].

Crane, L., Goddard, L. and Pring, L. 2009. Sensory processing in adults with autism spectrum disorders. *Autism,* 13(3): 215-228.

Cummins, R.A. and Lau, A.L.D. 2004. Cluster housing and the freedom of choice: A response to Emerson (2004). *Journal of Intellectual & Developmental Disability,* 29(3), 198-201.

Cuvo, A,. May, M. and Post, T. 2001. Effects of living room, Snoezelen room, and outdoor activities on stereotypic behavior and engagement by adults with profound mental retardation. *Research in Developmental Disabilities,* 22, 183-204.

Czarnuch, S. and Mihailidis, A. 2011. The design of intelligent in-home assistive technologies: Assessing the needs of older adults with dementia and their caregivers. *Gerontechnology,* 10(3): 169-182.

Davidson, J. and Henderson, V.L. 2010. "Coming out" on the spectrum: Autism, identity and disclosure. *Social and Cultural Geography,* 11(2), 155-170.

Davis, J., Watson, N. and Cunningham-Burley, S. 2000. Disabled children, ethnography and unspoken understandings: The collaborative construction of diverse identities. In Christiansen, P. and James, A., eds. *Research with Children: Perspectives and Practices.* New York: Routledge. (220-259).

Department for Education and Skills. 2005. *Building Bulletin 77 Designing for People with Special Educational Needs and Disabilities in Schools.* [pdf] Available at: <www.torbay.gov.uk/bb77_designing_for_pupils_with_sen.pdf> [Accessed 14 March 2014].

Department of Family and Community Services. 2013. Design guidelines: Group accommodation. Sydney NSW: Department of Family and Community Services. [online] Available at: <http://www.adhc.nsw.gov.au/individuals/support/somewhere_to_live/group_accommodation> [Accessed 12 June 2013].

Dewsbury, G., and Ballard, D. 2012. Telecare: Supporting independence at home. *British Journal of Healthcare Assistants,* 6(2), 71-73.

Dicker, S. and Bennett, E. 2011. Engulfed by the spectrum: The impact of autism spectrum disorders on law and policy. *Valparaiso University Law Review,* 45(2), 415-455.

Dieffenbach, B. 2012. Developmental disabilities and independent living: A systematic literature review. *Master of Social Work Clinical Research Papers.* Paper 19. [pdf] Available at: <http://sophia.stkate.edu/msw_papers/19> [Accessed 25 May 2014].

Dohrmann Architects. n.d. *Multifamily Residential.* [online] Available at: <http://www.dohrmannarchitects.com/> [Accessed 8 June 2014].

Dong, L., Di, H., Tao, L., Xu, G. and Olivier, P. 2009. Visual focus of attention: Recognition in the Ambient Kitchen. In: *Computer Vision – ACCV 2009, 9th Asian Conference on Computer Vision.* Xi'an, China 23-27 September 2009. Berlin and Heidelberg: Springer.

Donvan, J. and Zucker, C. 2010. Autism's first child. *The Atlantic.* [online] Available at: <http://www.theatlantic.com/magazine/print/2010/10/autisms-first-child/308227/> [Accessed 13 July 2013].

Douglas, K.H., Wojcik, B.W. and Thompson, J.R. 2012. Is there an app for that? *Journal of Special Education Technology,* 27(2), 59-70.

Draheim, C.C., Williams, D.P. and McCubbin, J.A. 2002. Prevalence of physical activity and recommended physical activity in community-based adults with mental retardation. *Mental Retardation,* 40, 436-444.

Drake, R.E., Merrens, M.,R. and Lynde, D.W., eds. 2005. *Evidence-based Mental Health Practice: A Textbook.* New York: W.W. Norton.

Dudley, C., Emery, H. and Nicholas, D. 2012. *Mind the Gap: The Missing Discussion Around Transportation for Adolescents and Adults with Autism Spectrum Disorder.* Calgary: Autism Calgary, Autism Society of Edmonton Area, The Ability Hub. [online] Available at: <http://www.theabilityhub.org/resources/books-publications/mind-gap> [Accessed 3 November 2013].

Duffy, J. and Dorner, R. 2011. The pathos of "mindblindness": Autism, science and sadness in "theory of mind" narratives. *Journal of Literary and Cultural Disability Studies,* 5(2), 201-215.

Duggan, C. and Linehan, C. 2013. The role of 'natural supports' in promoting independent living for people with disabilities: A review of existing literature. *British Journal of Learning Disabilities,* 41, 199-207.

Easter Seals. 2012. *Neighborhood Wayfinding Assessment.* Easter Seals Project Action and CDC Healthy Aging Research Network. [online] Available at: <http://www.projectaction.org/> [Accessed 28 January 2014].

Eaves, L.C. and Ho, H.H. 2008. Young adult outcome of Autism Spectrum Disorders. *Journal of Autism and Developmental Disorders,* 13, 739-747.

Edwards, C.A., McDonnell, C. and Merl, H. 2012. An evaluation of a therapeutic garden's influence on the quality of life of aged care residents with dementia. *Dementia,* 12, 495-510.

Edwards, T.L., Watkins, E.E., Lotfizadeh, A.D. and Poling, A. 2012. Intervention research to benefit people with autism: How old are the participants? *Research in Autism Spectrum Disorders,* 6, 996-999.

Eiman, M. and Cuskelly, M. 2002. Paid employment of mothers and fathers of adults with multiple disabilities. *Journal of Intellectual Disability Research,* 46, 158-167.

Elasbbagh, M., Divan, G., Koh, Y.J., Kim, Y.S. et al. 2012. Global prevalence of autism and other pervasive developmental disorders. *Autism Research,* 5(3), 160-179.

Elliot, D. 2013. In autism, the importance of the gut. *The Atlantic.* [online] Available at: <http://www.theatlantic.com/health/archive/2013/06/in-autism-the-importance-of-the-gut/276648/> [Accessed 15 June 2013].

Ellison, N.B., Steinfield, C. and Lampe, C. 2007. The benefits of Facebook "friends:" Social capital and college students' use of online social network sites. *Journal of Computer-Mediated Communication,* 12 (4), 1143-1168.

Elwin, M., Ek, L., Schroder, A. and Kjellin, L. 2012. Autobiographical accounts of sensing in Asperger syndrome and high-functioning autism. *Archives of Psychiatric Nursing,* 26(5), 420-429.

Elysa, J.M., Hinkley, L.B.N., Hill, S.S. and Nagarajan, S.S. 2011. Sensory processing in autism: A review of neurophysiologic findings. *Pediatric Research,* 69 (5 Pt 2), 48R-54R.

Emerson, E. and McVilly, K. 2004. Friendship activities of adults with intellectual disabilities in supported accommodation in Northern England. *Journal of Applied Research in Intellectual Disabilities,* 17, 191-197.

Emerson, E., Robertson, J., Gregory, N., Hatton, C., Kessissoglou, S. Hallam, A., et al. 1999. *Quality and Costs of Residential Supports for People with Learning Disabilities: A Comparative Analysis of Quality of Costs in Village Communities, Residential Campuses and Dispersed Housing Schemes.* Hester Adrian Research Centre, University of Manchester, Manchester.

Emmerich, S.J., Gorfain, J.E., Huang, M. and Howard-Reed, C. 2003. *Air and Pollutant Transport from Attached Garages to Residential Living Spaces.* National Institute of Standards and Technology, Technology Administration, U.S. Department of Commerce, NISTIR 7072.

Engstrom, I., Ekstrom, L. and Emilsson, B., 2003. Psychosocial functioning in a group of Swedish adults with Asperger syndrome or higher functioning autism. *Autism,* 7(1), 99-110.

Enterprise Green Communities. 2015. *2015 Enterprise Green Communities Criteria.* [online] Available at: <http://www.enterprisecommunity.com/solutions-and-innovation/enterprise-green-communities/criteria> [Accessed 30 June 2015].

EPA(a). n.d. *United States Environmental Protection Agency Bisphenol A (BPA) Action Plan Summary.* [online] Available at: <http://www.epa.gov/oppt/existingchemicals/pubs/actionplans/bpa.html> [Accessed 10 July 2015].

EPA(b). n.d. *United States Environmental Protection Agency Consumer Safety Information sheet: Inorganic Arsenic Pressure-treated Wood.* [online] Available at: <http://www.epa.gov/oppad001/reregistration/cca/cca_consumer_safety.htm> [Accessed 10 July 2015].

EPA(c). n.d. *United States Environmental Protection Agency Greener Products.* [online] Available at: <http://www.epa.gov/greenerproducts/related/> [Accessed 10 July 2015].

Erickson, C.A., Stigler, K.A., Corkins, M.R. et al. 2005. Gastrointestinal factors in autistic disorder: A critical review. *Journal of Autism and Developmental Disorders,* 35, 713-727.

Erickson, W., Lee, C. and von Schrader, S. 2014. *2012 Disability Status Report: United States.* Ithaca, NY: Cornell University Employment and Disability Institute (EDI).

Esbensen, A.J., Seltzer, M.M., Lam, K.S.L. and Bodfish, J.W. 2009. Age-related differences in restricted repetitive beahviors in autism spectrum disorder. *Journal of Autism and Developmental Disorders,* 39, 57-66.

ESPA (Education and Services for People with Autism). n.d. *Residential.* [online] Available at: <http://www.espa.org.uk/residential/> [Accessed 18 July 2015].

European Commission. 2014. *Prevalence of Autism Spectrum Disorders (ASD) in the EU.* [online] Available at: <http://ec.europa.eu/health/major_chronic_diseases/ diseases/autistic/index_en.htm#fragment1> [Accessed 18 April 2015].

Evans, D.W., Canavera, K., Kleinpeter, F.L., Maccubbin, E. and Taga, K. 2005. The fears, phobias and anxieties of children with autism spectrum disorders and Down syndrome: Comparisons with developmentally and chronically age matched children. *Child Psychiatry and Human Development,* 36, 3-26.

Evans, G.W. 1982. *Environmental Stress.* New York: Cambridge University Press.

Evans, G.W. and Cohen, S. 1987. Environmental stress. In Stokols, D. and Altman, I., eds. *Handbook of Environmental Psychology.* Volume 1. New York: John Wiley and Sons. (571-610).

Evans, G.W. and McCoy, J. 1998. When buildings don't work: The role of architecture in human health. *Journal of Environmental Psychology,* 18(1), 85-94.

Farley, M.A., McMahon, W.M., Fombonne, E., Jenson, W.R., Miller, J., Gardner, M., Block, H., Pingree, B., Ritvo, E.R., Ritvo, R.A. and Coon, H. 2009. Twenty-year outcome for individuals with autism and average or near-average cognitive abilities. *Autism Research,* 2, 109-118.

Farmer-Dougan, V. 1994. Increasing requests by adults with developmental disabilities using incidental teaching by peers. *Journal of Applied Behavior Analysis,* 27, 533-544.

Farrell, S.J., Aubry, T. and Coulombe, D. 2004. Neighborhoods and neighbors: Do they contribute to personal well-being? *Journal of Community Psychology,* 32, 9-25.

Farrelly, C. 2012. Positive as a new paradigm for the medical sciences. *EMBO Reports (European Molecular Biology Organization),* 13(3), 186-187.

Fava, L. and Strauss, K. 2010. Multi-sensory rooms: Comparing effects of the Snoezelen and Stimulus Preference environment on the behavior of adults with profound mental retardation. *Research in Developmental Disabilities,* 31, 160-171.

Felce, D. and Perry, J. 2012. Diagnostic grouping among adults with intellectual disabilities and autistic spectrum disorders in staffed housing. *Journal of Intellectual Disability Research.* 56(12), 1187-1193.

Fennelly, L. and Crowe, T. 2013. *Crime Prevention Through Environmental Design.* Oxford, UK: Butterworth-Heinemann.

Fenton, A. and Krahn, T. 2007. Autism, neurodiversity and equality beyond the 'normal.' *Journal of Ethics in Mental Health,* 2(2), 1-6.

Fernell, E., Hedvall, A., Westerlund, J., Höglund, C. et al. 2011. Early intervention in 208 Swedish preschoolers with autism spectrum disorder: A prospective naturalistic study. *Research in Developmental Disabilities,* 32, 2092-2101.

Fisher, P. 2007. Experiential knowledge challenges 'noramlity' and individualized citizenship: Towards 'another way of being.' *Disability and Society,* 22, 283-298.

Fleming, R. and Purandare, N. 2010. Long-term care for people with dementia: Environmental design guidelines. *International Psychogeriatrics,* 22 (7), 1084-1096.

Fletcher, D. 2013. *Virginia's Plan to Increase Independent Living Options.* Commonwealth of Virginia, Department of Behavioral Health and Developmental Services. [pdf] Available at: <http://www.dbhds.virginia.gov/library/document-library/doj%20final_doj_housing_plan_3_6_13.pdf> [Accessed 15 July 2015].

Flopro SmartPlus. n.d. *SmartPlus hot water recirculation.* [online] Available at: < http://flopro.taco-hvac.com/products/systems/instant_hot_water/smartplus/index.html> [Accessed 10 July 2015].

Floyd, F.J. and Gallagher, E.M. 1997. Parental stress, care demands, and use of support services for school-age children with disabilities and behavior problems. *Family Relations,* 46, 359-371.

Fombonne, E. 2012. Autism in adult life. *The Canadian Journal of Psychiatry,* 57(5), 273-274.

Fombonne, E., Bolton, P., Prior, J. et al. 1997. A family study of autism: Cognitive patterns and levels in parents and siblings. *Journal of Child Psychology and Psychiatry,* 38, 667-683.

Forbo Flooring. 2014. *Safestep Grip by Forbo.* [online] Available at: <http://www.forbo-flooring.com/> [Accessed 15 July 2014].

Forrest, R. and Kearns, A. 2001. Social cohesion, social capital and the neighbourhood. *Urban Studies,* 38, 2125-2143.

Fournier, K.A., Hass, C.J., Naik, S.K., Ladha, N. and Cauraugh, J.H. 2010. Motor coordination in autism spectrum disorders: A synthesis and meta-analysis. *Journal of Autism and Developmental Disorders,* 40 (10), 1227-1240.

Freedman, R.I. and Boyer, N.C. 2000. The power to choose: Supports for families caring for individuals with developmental disabilities. *Health and Social Work,* 25, 59-68.

Freedman, R.I., Griffiths, D., Krauss, M.W. and Seltzer, M.M. 1999. Patterns of respite use by aging mothers of adults with mental retardation. *Mental Retardation,* 37, 93-103.

Freeley, C. 2010. *Evaluating the Transportation Needs and Accessibility Issues for Adults on the Spectrum in New Jersey.* In: Transportation Review Board, *89th Annual Meeting Compendium of Papers.* Washington D.C.: Transportation Research Board.

Fry, R. 2013. *A Rising Share of Young Adults Live in Their Parents' Home.* Pew Research Center. [pdf] Available at: <http://www.pewsocialtrends.org/files/2013/07/SDT-millennials-living-with-parents-07-2013.pdf> [Accessed 3 May 2014].

Fujiura, G.T. 1998. Demography of family households. *American Journal of Mental Retardation,* 103, 225-235.

Furstenberg, F.F., Raumbaut, R.G. and Settersten, R.A. 2005. On the frontier of adulthood: Emerging themes and new directions. In Settersten, R.A., Furstenberg, F.F. and Rumbaut, R.G., eds. *On the Frontier of Adulthood: Theory, Research, and Public Policy.* Chicago: University of Chicago Press. (3-29)

Gabler-Halle, D., Halle, J.W. and Chung, Y.B. 1993. The effects of aerobic exercise on psychological and behavioral variables of individuals with developmental disabilities: A critical review. *Research In Developmental Disabilities,* 14, 359-386.

Ganz, M.L. 2007. The lifetime distribution of the incremental societal costs of autism. *Archives of Pediatric and Adolescent Medicine,* 161, 343-349.

Gaudion, K. 2013. *Designing Everyday Activities - Living Environments for Adults with Autism.* London: Helen Hamlyn Centre for Design. [online] Available at: <http://www.kingwood.org.uk/printable-documents-research> [Accessed 3 March 2014].

Gaudion, K. 2014. *Picture-it: A Digital Tool to Support Living with Autism.* London: Helen Hamlyn Centre for Design, Royal College of Art. [online] Available at: <http://www.rca.ac.uk/research-innovation/helen-hamlyn-centre/research_lab/age_ability_research_lab/publications/> [Accessed 18 July 2015].

Gaudion, K. and McGinley, C. 2012. *Green Spaces: Outdoor Environments for Adults with Autism.* London: Helen Hamlyn Centre for Design.

Geboy, L., Diaz Moore, K. and Smith, E.K. 2012. Environmental gerontology for the future: Community-based living for the third age. *Journal of Housing for the Elderly,* 26, 44-61.

Geller, L. and Greenberg, M. 2010. Managing the transition process from high school to college and beyond: Challenges for individuals, families and society. *Social Work in Mental Health,* 8(1), 92-116.

Genworth. 2013. *Genworth Cost of Care Survey: Home Care Providers, Adults Day Health Care Facilities, Assisted Living Facilities and Nursing Homes.* [pdf] Available at: <https://www.genworth.com/dam/Americas/US/PDFs/Consumer/corporate/130568_032213_Cost%20of%20Care_Final_nonsecure.pdf> [Accessed 19 April 2015].

Gerhardt, P.F. and Lanier, I. 2011. Addressing the needs of adolescents and adults with autism: A crisis on the horizon. *Journal of Contemporary Psychotherapy,* 41(1), 37-45.

Geurts, H.M., Corbett, B. and Solomon, M. 2009. The paradox of cognitive flexibility in autism. *Trends in Cognitive Science,* 13(2), 74-82.

Geurts, H.M. and Jansen, M.D. 2012. A retrospective chart study: The pathway to a diagnosis for adults referred for ASD assessment. *Autism,* 16(3), 299-305.

Geurts, H.M. and Vissers, M.E. 2012. Elderly with autism: Executive functions and memory. *Journal of Autism and Developmental Disorders,* 42, 665-675.

Ghaziuddin, M. and Butler, E. 1998. Clumsiness in autism and Asperger syndrome: A further report. *Journal of Intellectual Disability,* 42, 43-48.

Ghaziuddin, M. and Zafar, S. 2008. Psychiatric comorbidity of adults with autism spectrum disorders. *Clinical Neuropsychiatry,* 5, 9-12.

Giarelli, E. and Gardner, M. 2012. *Nursing of Autism Spectrum Disorder: Evidence-Based Integrated Care Across the Lifespan.* New York: Springer.

Gibson, B.E., Secker, B., Rolfe, D., Wagner, F. et al. 2012. Disability and dignity-enabling home environments. *Social Science and Medicine,* 74, 211-219.

Gifford, R. 1997. *Environmental Psychology: Principles and Practice.* 2nd edition. Boston: Allyn and Bacon.

Gillberg, C. and Neville, B. 2010. Autism and epilepsy: Comorbidity, coexistence or coincidence? In Bax, M. and Gillberg, C., eds. *Comorbidities in Developmental Disorders.* London: MacKeith Press.

Gillberg, C., Bilstedt, E., Sundh, V. and Gillberg, I.C. 2009. Mortality in autism: A prospective longitudinal community-based study. *Journal of Autism and Developmental Disorders,* 40(3), 352-357.

Gillespie-Lynch, K., Sepeta, L., Wang, Y., Gomez, M.S. et al. 2011. Early childhood predictors of the social competence of adults with autism. *Journal of Autism and Developmental Disorders,* 42(2), 161-174.

Gillott, A. and Standen, P.J. 2007. Levels of anxiety and sources of stress in adults with autism. *Journal of Intellectual Disabilities,* 11, 359-370.

Gilmour, L., Schalomon, P.M. and Smith, V. 2012. Sexuality in a community-based sample of adults with autism spectrum disorder. *Research in Autism Spectrum Disorders,* 6(1), 313-318.

GiraffPlus. n.d. *The GiraffPlus Project.* [online] Available at: <http://www.giraffplus.eu/> [Accessed 10 July 2015].

Gitlin, L.N. 2003. Conducting research on home environments: Lessons learned and new directions. *The Geronotologist,* 43(5), 628-637.

Glannon, W. 2007. Neurodiversity. *Journal of Ethics in Mental Health,* 2(2), 1-5.

Glass Education Center. n.d. *Determining the right glass for the right acoustics.* [online] Available at: <http://educationcenter.ppg.com/glasstopics/determining_the_right_glass.aspx> [Accessed 10 July 2015].

Global Green. 2007. *Blueprint for Greening Affordable Housing.* Washington DC: Island Press.

Goin-Kochel, R.P., Mackintosh, V.H. and Myers, B.J. 2008. Parental reports on the efficacy of treatments and therapies for their children with autism spectrum disorders. *Research on Autism Spectrum Disorders,* 27, 70-84.

Golant, S. 2015. *Aging in the Right Place.* Baltimore: Health Professions Press.

Goldman, A. 2013. Temple Grandin on autism, death, celibacy and cows. *New York Times.* 12 April. [online] Available at: <http://www.nytimes.com/2013/04/14/magazine/temple-grandin-on-autism-death-celibacy-and-cows.html?_r=0> [Accessed 1 February 2014].

Goodwin, M.S., Groden, J., Velicer, W.F., Lipsitt, L.P., Baron, M.G., Hofmann, S.G. and Groden, G. 2006. Cardiovascular arousal in individuals with autism. *Focus on Autism and Other Developmental Disabilities,* 21(2), 100-123.

Graetz, J.E. 2010. Autism grows up: Opportunities for adults with autism. *Disability and Society,* 21(1), 33-47.

Graham, H.J. and Firth, J. 1992. Home accidents in older people: Role of primary health care team. *BMJ*, 305, 30-32.

Grandin, T. 2012. *Different... Not Less: Inspiring Stories of Achievement and Successful Employment from Adults with Autism, Asperger's and ADHD.* Arlington, TX: Future Horizons.

Grandjean, P. and Landrigan, P.J. 2006. Developmental neurotoxicity of industrial chemicals: A silent pandemic. *Lancet,* 368, 2167-2178.

Green, D., Charman, T., Pickles, A. Chandler, S. et al. 2008. Impairment in movement skills of children with autistic spectrum disorders. *Developmental Medicine and Child Neurology,* 51, 311-316.

Green Building Council. n.d. *United Kingdom Green Building Council Materials.* [online] Available at: <http://www.ukgbc.org/resources/key-topics/circular-economy/materials> [Accessed 10 July 2015].

Greenspan, S.I. and Wieder, S. 2006. *Engaging Autism: Using the Floortime Approach to Help Children Relate, Communicate, and Think.* Cambridge, MA: Da Capo/Perseus.

Grinde, B. and Grindal Patil, G. 2009. Biophilia: Does visual contact with nature impact on health and well-being? *International Journal of Environmental Research and Public Health,* 6(9), 2332-2343.

Groden, J., Goodwin, M.S., Baron, M.G., Groden, G. et al. 2005. Assessing cardiovascular responses to stressors in individuals with autism spectrum disorders. *Focus on Autism and Other Developmental Disabilities,* 20(4), 244-252.

Haigh Hygienic Solutions. 2014. *Bedpan & Incontinence Waste Disposal Systems for Care Homes.* [online] Available at: <http://www.haighprivatecare.com/> [Accessed 8 June 2014].

Hall, E.T. 1990. *The Hidden Dimension.* New York: Anchor Books.

Hamilton, D.K. 2003. The four levels of evidence-based practice. *Healthcare Design Magazine,* 3. [online] Available at: http://www.healthcaredesignmagazine.com/article/four-levels-evidence-based-practice [Accessed 16 April 2015].

Happé, F. and Charlton, R.A. 2012. Aging in autism spectrum disorders: A mini-review. *Gerontology,* 58(1), 70-78.

Happé, F. and Frith, U. 2006. The weak coherence account: Detail-focused cognitive style in autism spectrum disorders. *Journal of Autism and Developmental Disorders,* 36, 5-25.

Hare, D.J., Wood, C., Wastell, S. and Skirrow, P. 2015. Anxiety in Asperger's syndrome: Assessment in real time. *Autism,* 19(5), 542-552.

Harris, M. and Kinder, M., producers. 2013. *Interacting With Autism.* [online] Available at: <http://anim.usc.edu/videos/sensory-overload-interacting-with-autism-project-by-miguel-jiron/> [Accessed 29 June 2015]

Harker, M. and King, N. 2004. *Tomorrow's Big Problem: Housing Options for People with Autism. A Guide for Service Commissioners, Providers and Families.* London: National Autistic Society.

Harmon, A. 2014. *Asperger Love: Searching for Romance When You're Not Wired to Connect.* [e-book] New York Times and Byliner. Available at: <www.amazon.com> [Accessed 14 April 2015]

Hatton, C. Emerson, E., Robertson, J., Henderson, D. and Cooper, J. 1995. The quality and costs of residential services for adults with multiple disabilities: A comparative evaluation. *Research in Developmental Disabilities,* 16, 439-460.

Haugenhofer, M. D.K., Elings, M., Hassink, J. and Hine, R.E. 2010. The development of green care in western European countries. *Explore,* 6(2), 106-157.

Haveman, M., van Berkum, G., Reijinder, R. and Heller, T. 1997. Differences in service needs, time demands, and caregiving burden among parents of persons with mental retardation across the life cycle. *Family Relations,* 46, 417-425.

Hayes, G.R. and Hosaflook, S.W. 2013. HygieneHelper: Promoting awareness and teaching life skills to youth with autism spectrum disorder. In: *Proceedings of the 12th International Conference on Interaction Design and Children.* New York City, 24-27 June 2013.

Hayes, T.L., Cobbinah, K., Dishongh, T., Kaye, J.A., Kimel, J., Labhard, M., Leen, T., Lundell, J., Ozertem, U., Pavel, M., Philipose, M., Rhodes, K. and Vurgun, S. 2009. A study of medication-taking and unobtrusive, intelligent reminding. *Telemedicine and e-Health*, 15, 770-776.

Healthy House Institute. 2014. Healthy House Institute: for a Healthier Home. [online] Available at: <http://healthyhouseinstitute.com> [Accessed 18 May 2014].

Health Physics Society. n.d. *Environmental and background radiation – granite and stone countertops.* [online] Available at <https://hps.org/publicinformation/ate/q7834.html> [Accessed 10 July 2015].

Helfrich, D. and Adrian, M. 2008. Comfort, clarity and calm: Architecture for autism. *Autism Advocate,* 53(3), 1-6.

Heller, T. 2010. People with intellectual and developmental disabilities growing old: An overview. *Impact: Feature Issue on Aging and People with Intellectual and Developmental Disabilities,* 23(1), 2-3.

Heller, T., Caldwell, J. and Factor, A. 2007. Aging family caregivers: Policies and practices. *Mental Retardation and Developmental Disabilities Research Reviews,* 13, 136-142.

Heller, T., Miller, A.B. and Factor, A. 1998. Environmental characteristics of nursing homes and community based settings and the well-being of adults with developmental disabilities. *Journal of Intellectual Disability Research,* 42(5), 418-428.

Heller, T., Miller, A.B. and Hsieh, K. 2001. Eight year follow-up of the impact of environmental characteristics on well-being of adults with developmental disabilities. *Mental Retardation,* 40 (5), 366-378.

Heller, T., Stafford, P., Davis, L.A., Sedlezky, L. and Gaylord, V. eds., 2010. *Impact: Feature Issue on Aging and People with Intellectual and Developmental Disabilities, 23*(1). Minneapolis: University of Minnesota, Institute on Community Integration. [online] Available at: <http://ici.umn.edu/products/impat/231/2.html> [Accessed 25 September 2013].

Helt, M., Kelley, E., Kinsbourne, et al. 2008. Can children with autism recover? If so, how? *Neuropsychology Review,* 18(4), 339-366.

Hendricks, D.R. and Wehman, P. 2009. Transition from school to adulthood for youth with autism spectrum disorders. *Focus on Autism and Other Developmental Disabilities,* 24(2), 77-88.

Henninger, N.A. and Taylor, J.L. 2012. Outcomes in adults with autism spectrum disorders: A historical perspective. *Autism,* 17(1), 103-116.

Henry, C.N. 2011. Designing for autism: Lighting. *Arch Daily.* [online] Available at: <http://www.archdaily.com/177293/designing-for-autism-lighting/> [Accessed 14 April 2015].

Henry, C.N. 2013. Architecture for autism: Architects moving in the right direction. *Arch Daily.* [online] Available at: <http://www.archdaily.com/197788> [Accessed 11 July 2013].

Herbert, M.R. 2010. Contributions of the environment and environmentally vulnerable physiology to autism spectrum disorders. *Current Opinion in Neurology,* 23(2), 103-110.

Higashida, N. 2013. *The Reason I Jump: The Inner Voice of a Thirteen-Year-Old Boy with Autism.* (Yoshida, K.A and Mitchell, D., trans.) New York: Random House.

Hill, E.L. 2004. Evaluating the theory of executive dysfunction in autism. *Developmental Review,* 24, 189-233.

Hill, L., Trusler, K., Furniss, F. and Lancioni, G. 2012. Effects of multisensory environments on stereotyped behaviours asessed as maintained by automatic reinforcement. *Journal of Applied Research in Intellectual Disabilities,* 25, 509-521.

Hill-Smith, A.J. and Hollins, S.C. 2002. Mortality of parents of people with intellectual disabilities. *Journal of Applied Research in Intellectual Disability,* 15, 18-27.

Hilton, C.,L., Harper, J.D., Kueker, R.H., Lang, A.R., Abbacchi, A.M., Todorov, A., and LaVesser, P.D. 2010. Sensory responsiveness as a predictor of social severity in children wit high functioning autism spectrum disorders. *Journal of Autism and Developmental Disorders,* 40, 937-945.

Hintzen, A., Delespaul, P., van Os, J. and Myin-Germeys, I. 2010. Social needs in daily life in adults with pervasive developmental disorders. *Psychiatry Research,* 179(1), 75-80.

Hirshberg, J. 2011. IAQ and your health: A deeper look at VOCs and Formaldehyde Emissions. *Green Building Supply.* [online] Available at: <http://www.greenbuildingsupply.com/Learning-Center/Paints-Coatings-LC/IAQ-and-Your-Health-A-Deeper-Look-at-VOCs-and-Formaldehyde> [Accessed 3 March 2014].

Ho, A., Collins, S., Davis, K. et al. 2005. *A Look At Working-Age Caregivers' Roles, Health Concerns, And Need For Support.* New York: The Commonwealth Fund.

Holm, P., Holst, J. and Perlt, P. 1994. Co-write your own life: Quality of life as discussed in the Danish context. In Goode, D., ed., *Quality of Life for Persons with Disabilities: International Perspectives and Issues.* Cambridge, MA: Bookline Books.

Hong, H., Kim, J.G., Abowd, G.D. and Arriaga, R.I. 2012. Designing a social network to support the independence of young adults with autism. In: *CSCW '12: Proceedings of the ACM 2012 Conference on Computer Supported Cooperative Work,* 627-636.

Hooyman, N. and Gonyea, J. 1995. *Feminist Perspectives on Family Care: Policies for Gender Justice.* Thousand Oaks, CA: Sage.

Horn, S., Sharkey, S., Grabowski, D. and Barrett, R. 2012. Costs of care in Green House Home compared to traditional nursing home residents. Unpublished working paper. Cited in: The Green House Project. *Home Economics: The Business Case for the Green House Model.* [online] Available at: <http://thegreenhouseproject. org/doc/21/business-case-full-web.pdf> [Accessed 19 April 2015].

Housing and Support Alliance. n.d. *Shared ownership, homebuy and HOLD.* [online] Available at: <http://www.housingandsupport.org.uk/shared-ownership-homebuy-and-hold> [Accessed 30 June 2015].

Howard, B., Cohn, E. and Orsmond, G. 2006. Understanding and negotiating friendships: Perspectives from an adolescent with Asperger syndrome. *Autism,* 33(5), 489-507.

Howe, J., Horner, R.H. and Newton, J.S. 1998. Comparison of supported living and traditional residential services in the state of Oregon. *Mental Retardation,* 36, 1-11.

Howlin, P. 2000. Outcome in adult life for more able individuals with autism or Asperger syndrome. *Autism,* 4, 63-83.

Howlin, P. and Moss, P. 2012. In review: Adults with autism spectrum disorders. *Canadian Journal of Psychiatry,* 57(5), 275-283.

Howlin, P., Goode, S., Hutton, J. and Rutter, M. 2004. Adult outcomes for children with autism. *Journal of Child Psychology and Psychiatry,* 45, 212-229.

Howlin, P., Moss, P. Savage, S. et al. 2011. Outcomes and needs in mid-later adulthood. Presentation at the *International Meeting for Autism Research,* 13 May 2011. San Diego, CA. [cited in Howlin and Moss, 2012].

Hughes, V. 2 April 2011. Researchers track down autism rates across the globe. *Simons Foundation Autism Research Initiative.* [online] Available at: <http://sfari. org/news-and-opinion/news/2011/researchers-track-down-autism-rates-across-the-globe> [Accessed 2 August 2013].

Humphreys, S. 2005. Architecture and autism. *Autism London Bulletin.* [online] Available at: <http://www.autismlondon.org.uk/publications/bulletins.htm> [Accessed 18 September 2009].

Hundert, J., Walton-Allen, N., Vasdev, S., Cope, K. et al. 2003. A comparison of staff-resident interactions with adults with developmental disabilities moving from institutional to community living. *Journal on Developmental Disabilities,* 10, 93-112.

Hutton, J., Goode, S., Murphy, M. et al. 2008. New-onset pediatric disorders in individuals with autism. *Autism,* 12, 373-390.

HVAC Quick. 2014. *HVAC Quick.* [online] Available at: <http://www.hvacquick. com/> [Accessed 8 June 2014].

HVI. 2014. *Home Ventilating Institute.* [online] Available at: <http://hvi.org/> [Accessed 21 June 2014].

Hyde, T.M. and Weinberger, D.R. 1997. Seizures and schizophrenia. *Schizophrenia Bulletin,* 23(4), 611-622.

Illuminating Engineering Society (IES). 2014. *Light Logic for the 21ˢᵗ Century.* [online] Available at: <http://www.ieslightlogic.org/> [Accessed 12 June 2014].

Interagency Autism Coordinating Committee (IACC). 2011. *IACC 2010 Autism Spectrum Disorder Research Portfolio Analysis Report.* Washington, D.C.: U.S. Department of Health & Human Services.

Intille, S.S. 2002. Designing a home of the future. *Pervasive Computing,* 2, 80-86.

IOM (Institute of Medicine). 2008a. *Autism and the Environment: Challenges and Opportunities for Research. Workshop Proceedings.* Washington DC: National Academies Press.

IOM (Institute of Medicine). 2008b. *Retooling for an Aging America: Building the Health Care Workforce.* Washington DC: The National Academies Press.

IOM (Institute of Medicine). 2011. *Climate Change, the Indoor Environment, and Health.* Washington DC: The National Academies Press.

IOM (Institute of Medicine). 2013. *Fostering Independence, Participation, and Healthy Aging Through Technology: Workshop Summary.* Washington DC: The National Academies Press.

Isaac, V., Stewart, R., Artero, S., Ancelin, M.L. and Ritchie, K. 2009. Social activity and improvement in depressive symptoms in older people: A prospective community cohort study. *American Journal of Geriatric Psychiatry,* 17, 688-696.

ISO. 2014. *International Organization for Standardization.* [online] Available at: <http://www.iso.org/iso/home.html> [Accessed 8 July 2014].

ISO Store. 2014. *Sound Isolation Store.* [online] Available at: <http://isostore.com/products-by-use/floors/> [Accessed 23 June 2014].

Jackson, B. 1997. Community integration: Much more than "being there." Paper delivered at: *Annual Conference of the Australian Society for the Study of Intellectual Disability*, Brisbane. [online] Available at: <www.include.com.au/wp-content/uploads/2011/11/Integration.pdf> [Accessed 12 September 2013].

Jackson, L. 2008. *Current Practices and Programs: An Analysis of Current Programs, Guiding Principles, Challenges and Recommendations Regarding Housing for People with Developmental Disabilities.* Sacramento: Association of Regional Center Agencies.

Jackson Place Cohousing. n.d. *Home.* [online] Available at: <http://www.seattlecohousing.org> [Accessed 18 July 2015].

James, I.A., Mukaetova-Ladinska, E., Reichelt, F.K., Briel, R. et al. 2006. Diagnosing Aspergers syndrome in the elderly: A series of case presentations. *International Journal of Geriatric Psychiatry,* 21(10), 951-960.

Janicki, M.P., Dalton, A.J., Henderson, C. and Davidson, P., 1999. Mortality and morbidity among older adults with intellectual disability: Health services considerations. *Disability and Rehabilitations,* 21(5/6), pp. 284-294.

Jansiewics, E.M., Goldberg, M.C., Newshaffer, C.J., Denekia, M.B., Landa, R. and Mostoffsky, S.H. 2006. Motor signs distinguish children with high functioning autism and Asperger's syndrome from controls. *Journal of Autism and Developmental Disorders,* 63, 613-621.

Jenkens, R., Sult, T., Lessell, N., Hammer, D. and Ortigara, A. 2011. Financial implications of The Green House model. *Senior Housing and Care Journal,* 18(1), 3-21.

Jiron, M. 2013. Sensory overload. From Harris, M. and Kinder, M., producers. *Interacting with Autism.* [online] Available at: <http://anim.usc.edu/videos/sensory-overload-interacting-with-autism-project-by-miguel-jiron/> [Accessed 29 June 2015].

Jolous-Jarnshidi, B., Cromwell,H.C., McFarland, A.M. and Meserve, L.A. 2010. Perinatal exposure to polychlorinated biphenyls alters social behaviors in rats. *Toxicology Letters,* 199, 136-143.

Jones, C.R.G., Happé, F., Baird, G., Simonoff, E., Simonoff, E., Marsden, A.J.S., Tregay, J., Phillips, R.J., Goswami, U., Thomson, J.J. and Charman, T. 2009. Auditory discrimination and auditory sensory behaviours in autism spectrum disorders. *Neuropsychologia,* 47: 2850-2858.

Jones, R.S.P., Zahl, A. and Huws, J.C. 2001. First-hand accounts of emotional experiences in autism: A qualitative analysis. *Disability & Society,* 16(3), 393-401.

Jones, R.T., Pettus, W. and Pyatok, M. 1995. *Good Neighbors: Affordable Family Housing.* New York: McGraw Hill.

Jordan, C.J. and Caldwell-Harris, C.L. 2012. Understanding differences in neurotypical and autism spectrum special interests through Internet forums. *Intellectual and Developmental Disabilities,* 50(5), 391-402.

JTM. 2014. *JTM: Commercial Laundry and Dishwashing Specialists.* [online] Available at: <http://www.jtmservice.co.uk/> [Accessed 4 June 2014].

Kamio, Y., Inada, N. and Koyama, T. 2012. A nationwide survey on quality of life and associated factors of adults with high-functioning autism spectrum disorders. *Autism.* doi: 10.1177/1362361312436848.

Kampert, A.L. and Goreczny, A.J. 2007. Community involvement and socialization among individuals with mental retardation. *Research in Developmental Disabilities,* 28, 278-286.

Kaplan, R. 2001. The nature of the view from home: Psychological benefits. *Environment and Behavior,* 33, 507–542.

Kaplan, R. and Kaplan, S. 1989. *The Experience of Nature. A Psychological Perspective.* Cambridge: Cambridge University Press.

Kaplan, S. 1995. The restorative benefits of nature: Toward an integrative framework. *Journal of Environmental Psychology,* 15, 169-182.

Kapp, S.K., Gantman, A. and Laugeson, E.A. 2011. Transition to adulthood for high-functioning individuals with autism spectrum disorders. In Mohammadi, M-R., ed. *A Comprehensive Book on Autism Spectrum Disorders.* Rijeka, Croatia: InTech. (451-478)

Kargas, N., Lopez, B., Reddy, V. and Morris, P. 2015. The relationship between auditory processing and restricted, repetitive behaviors in adults with autism spectrum disorders. *Journal of Autism and Developmental Disorders,* 45: 658-668.

Karst, J. and Hecke, A. 2012. Parent and family impact of autism spectrum disorders: A review and proposed model for intervention evaluation. *Clinical Child and Family Psychology Review,* 15(3), 247-277.

Kassirer, J.P. and Campion, E.W. 1994. Peer review: Crude and understudied, but indispensable. *Journal of the American Medical Association,* 272, 96-97.

Katz, N. 2013. Frigidaire, American Range and Gaggenau side-swing wall ovens (ADA). *Yale Appliance + Lighting Blog* [blog] 2 August. Available at: <http://blog.yaleappliance.com/bid/91046/Frigidaire-American-Range-and-Gaggenau-Side-Swing-Wall-Ovens-ADA> [Accessed 20 June 2014].

Kawasaki, Y., Yokota, K., Shinomiya, M., Shimizu, Y. et al. 1997. Brief report: Electroencephalographic paroxysmal activities in the frontal area emerged in middle childhood and during adolescence in a follow-up study of autism. *Journal of Autism and Developmental Disorders,* 27, 605-620.

Kern, J.K., Trivedi, M., Garver, C.R., Grannemann, B.D. et al. 2006. The pattern of sensory processing abnormalities in autism. *Autism,* 10, 480-494.

Kern, J.K., Trivedi, M.H., Grannemann, B.D., Garver, C.R., Johnson, D.G., Andrews, A.A., Schroeder, J.L. 2007. Sensory correlations in autism. *Autism,* 11, 123-134.

Kientz, J.A., Goodwin, M.S. and Hayes, G.R. 2013. *Interactive Technologies for Autism: Synthesis Lectures on Assistive, Rehabilitative, and Health-preserving Technologies.* San Rafael, CA: Morgan & Claypool Publishers.

Kim, Y.S., Leventhal, B.L., Koh, Y.J. et al. 2011. Prevalence of autism spectrum disorders in a total population sample. *American Journal of Psychiatry,* 168(9), 904-912.

Kinnaer, M., Baumers, S. and Heylighen, A. 2014. How do people with autism (like to) live? In Langdon, P.M., Lazar, J., Heylighen, A. and Dong, H., eds., *Inclusive Designing: Joining Usability, Accessibility and Inclusion.* London: Springer-Verlag.

Kinnaer, M., Baumers, S. and Heylighen, A. 2015. Autism-friendly architecture from the outside in and the inside out: An explorative study based on autobiographies of autistic people. *Journal of Housing and the Built Environment.* [online] Available from: <http://link.springer.com/article/10.1007%2Fs10901-015-9451-8>. [10 July 2015].

Kirigin, K.A. 2001. The teaching-family model: A replicable system of care. *Residential Treatment for Children & Youth,* 18(3), 99-110.

Kloos, B. and Shah, S. 2009. A social ecological approach to investigating relationships between housing and adaptive functioning for persons with serious mental illness. *American Journal of Community Psychology,* 44, 316-326.

Knapp, M., Romeo, R. and Beecham, J. 2009. Economic cost of autism in the U.K. *Autism,* 13(3), 317-336.

Kobayashi, R., Muraia, T. and Yoshinaga, K. 1992. A follow-up study of 201 children with autism in Kyushu and Yamaguchi areas, Japan. *Journal of Autism and Developmental Disorders,* 22, 395-411.

Koritsas, S. and Iacono, T. 2009. Limitations to life participation and independence due to secondary conditions. *American Association on Intellectual and Developmental Disabilities,* 114(6), 437-448.

Kozma, A., Mansell, J. and Beadle-Brown, J. 2009. Outcomes in different residential settings for people with intellectual disability: A systematic review. *American Journal on Intellectual and Developmental Disabilities,* 114(3), 193-222.

Krauss, M.W., Seltzer, M.M. and Jacobson, H.T. 2005. Adults with autism living at home or in non-family settings: Positive and negative aspects of residential status. *Journal of Intellectual Disability Research,* 49, 111-124.

Kuhlthau, K., Orlich, F., Hall, T.A. et al. 2010. Health-related quality of life in children with autism spectrum disorders: Results from the autism treatment network. *Journal of Autism and Developmental Disorders,* 40, 721-729.

Kurtz, Z. Tookey, P. and Ross, E. 2009. Epilepsy in young people: 23 year follow up of the British national child development study. *British Medical Journal,* 7128, 339-342.

Laberg, T., Aspelund, H. and Thygesen, H. 2005. *Smart Home Technology: Planning and Management in Municipal Services.* Directorate for Social and Health Affairs, the Delta Centre. [online] Available at: <www.shdir.no/deltasenteret> [Accessed 2 June 2014].

Lainhart, J.E. 1999. Psychiatric problems in individuals with autism, the parents and sibling. *International Review of Psychiatry,* 11, 278-298.

Lakin, K.C., Doljanac, R., Byun, S., Stancliffe, R.J. et al. 2008. Choice making among Medicaid Home and Community-Based Services (HCBS) and ICF/MR recipients in six states. *American Journal of Mental Retardation,* 113, 325-342.

Lancioni, E., Dijkstra, A., O'Reilly, M., Groenweg, J. and Van den Hof, E. 2000. Frequent versus nonfrequent verbal prompts delivered unobtrusively: Their impact on the task performance of adults with intellectual disability. *Education and Training in Mental Retardation and Developmental Disabilities,* 35(4), 428-433.

Landesman, S. 1986. Quality of life and personal life satisfaction: Definition and measurement issues. *Mental Retardation,* 24, 141-143.

Landrigan, P.J. 2010. What causes autism? Exploring the environmental contribution. *Current Opinion in Pediatrics,* 22, 219-225.

Landrigan, P.J. and Goldman, L.R. 2011. Children's vulnerability to toxic chemicals: A challenge and opportunity to strengthen health and environmental policy. *Health Affairs,* 30(5), 1-9.

Lang, R., Koegel, L.K., Ashbaugh, K. Regester, A. et al. 2010. Physical exercise and individuals with autism spectrum disorders: A systematic review. *Research in Autism Spectrum Disorders,* 4, 565-576.

Larkin, M. 1997. Approaches to amelioration of autism in adulthood. *The Lancet,* 349, 186.

Larsson, M., Weiss, B., Janson, S., Sundell, J. and Bornehag, C-G. 2008. Associations between indoor environmental factors and parental-reported autistic spectrum disorders in children 6-8 years of age. *NeuroToxiology,* 30, 822-831.

Laufenberg, T. 2004. *Stabilized Engineered Wood Fiber for Accessible Trails.* U.S. Department of Agriculture, Forest Service, FPL-GTR-155. [online] Available at: <http://www.access-board.gov/research/completed-research/stabilized-engineered-wood-fiber-for-accessible-trails> [Accessed 12 June 2014].

Lawton, M.P. 1980. *Environment and Aging.* Monterey, CA: Brooks/Cole.

Lawton, M.P. and Nahemow, L. 1973. Ecology and the aging process. In Eisdorfer, C. and Lawton, M.P. eds. *The Psychology of Adult Development and Aging.* Washington DC: American Psychological Association. (619-674)

Lazarus, R.S. 1966. *Psychological Stress and the Coping Process.* New York: McGraw-Hill.

Lazarus, R.S. and Cohen, J.B. 1977. Environmental stress. In Altman, I. and Wohlwill, J.F., eds. *Human Behavior and Environment: Advances in Theory and Research.* Volume 2. New York: Springer. (89-127)

Lee, Y., Ahn, C. and Jang, M. 2011. Health promoting spatial design characteristics of Korean apartment house in user benefit perspective. In: *SHB2011, 5th International Symposium on Sustainable Healthy Buildings.* Seoul, Korea 10 February 2011.

Lee, Y., Hwang, J., Lim, S., Lee, H. and Kim, J.T. 2012. Identifying space planning guidelines for elderly care environments from the holistic health perspective. In: *SHB2012, 6th International Symposium on Sustainable Healthy Buildings.* Seoul, Korea 27 February 2012.

Leekam, S.R., Nieto, C., Libby, S.J., Wing, L. and Gould, J. 2007. Describing the sensory abnormalities of children and adults with autism. *Journal of Autism and Developmental Disorders,* 37, 894-910.

Lifshitz, H., Merrick, J. and Morad, M. 2008. Health status and ADL functioning of older persons with intellectual disability: Community residence versus residential care centers. *Research in Developmental Disabilities,* 29, 301-315.

Lin, L-Y., Orsmond, G.I., Coster, W.J. and Cohn, E.S. 2011. Families of adolescents and adults with autism spectrum disorders in Taiwan: The role of social support and coping in family adaptation and maternal well-being. *Research in Autism Spectrum Disorders,* 5(1), 144-156.

Ling-Yi, L., Shu-Hing, Y. and Ya-Tsu, Y. 2012. A study of activities of daily living and employment in adults with autism spectrum disorders in Taiwan. *International Journal of Rehabilitation Research,* 35(2), 109-115.

Liptak, G.S., Kennedy, J.A. and Dosa, N.P. 2011. Social participation in a nationally representative sample of older youth and young adults with autism. *Journal of Developmental and Behavioral Pediatrics,* 32(4), 277-283.

Liss, M., Saulnier, C., Fein, D. and Kinsbourne, M. 2006. Sensory and attention abnormalities in autistic spectrum disorders. *Autism,* 10(2): 155-172.

Livable Housing Australia. 2012. *Livable Housing Design Guidelines.* Department of Social Services, Australian Government. [online] Available at: <http://livablehousingaustralia.org.au/> [Accessed 12 June 2013].

Losh, M., Childress, D., Lam, K. et al. 2008. Defining key features of the broad autism phenotype: A comparison across parents of multiple- and single-incidence autism families. *American Journal of Medical Genetics, Part b: Neuropsychiatric Genetics,* 147(B), 424-433.

Lotan, M., Gold, C. and Yalon-Chamovitz S. 2009. Reducing challenging behavior through structured therapeutic intervention in the controlled multi-sensory environment (Snoezelen): Ten case studies. *International Journal on Disability and Human Development,* 8(4), 377-392.

Lowry, S. 1990. Accidents at home. *British Medical Journal,* 300, 104-106.

Luckasson, R. and Schalock, R. 2012. Human functioning, supports, assistive technology, and evidence-based practices in the field of intellectual disability. *Journal of Special Education Technology,* 27(2), 3-10.

Lund, R., Nilsson, C.J. and Avlund, K. 2010. Can the higher risk of disability onset among older people who live alone be alleviated by strong social relations? A longitudinal study of non-disabled men and women. *Age and Ageing,* 39, 319-326.

Madsen, T., Kucher, Y. and Olle, T. 2004. *Growing Up Toxic: Chemical Exposures and Increases in Developmental Disease.* Los Angeles: Environmental California Research and Policy Center.

Mahan, S. and Kozlowski, A.M. 2011. Adults with autism spectrum disorders. In Matson, J.L. and Sturmey, P., eds. *International Handbook of Autism and Pervasive Developmental Disorders.* New York: Springer Science and Business Media. (521-538)

Mahmood, A., Chaudhury, H., Michael, Y., Campo, M., Hay, K. and Sarte, A. 2012. A photovoice documentation of the role of neighborhood physical and social environments in older adults' physical activity in two metropolitan areas in North America. *Social Science & Medicine,* 74, 1180-1192.

Manjoivioina, J. and Prior, M. 1995. Comparison of Asperger's syndrome and high-functioning autistic children on a test of motor impairment. *Journal of Autism and Developmental Disorder,* 25, 23-29.

Mankowski, E. and Rappoport, J. 1995. Stories, identity, and the psychological sense of community. In Wyer, R.S. ed. *Knowledge and Memory: The Real Story. Advances in Social Cognition (No. 8).* Hillsdale, NJ: Erlbaum.

Mansell, J. 2006. Deinstituionalisation and community living: Progress, problems and priorities. *Journal of Intellectual and Developmental Disability,* 31(2), 65-76.

Mansell, J., Beadler-Brown, J., Macdonald, S. and Ashman, B. 2003. Functional grouping in residential homes for people with intellectual disabilities. *Research in Developmental Disabilities,* 24, 170-182.

Marco, E.J., Hinkley, L.B.N., Hill, S.S. and Nagarajan, S.S. 2011. Sensory processing in autism: A review of neurophysiological findings. *Pediatric Research,* 69(5Pt 2), 48R-54R.

Marriage, S., Wolverton, A. and Marriage, K. 2009. Autism spectrum disorder grown up: A chart review of adult functioning. *Journal of Canadian Academy of Child and Adolescence Psychiatry,* 18(4), 322-328.

Massey, M. 2012. *The Dopamine diaries.* [blog] Available at: <https://margaretmassey.wordpress.com> [Accessed 18 July 2015].

Matson, J.L. and Boisjoli, J.A. 2009. An overview of developments in research on persons with intellectual disabilities. *Research in Developmental Disabilities,* 30, 587-591.

Matson, J.L. and Rivet, T.T. 2008. Characteristics of challenging behaviours in adults with autistic disorder, PDD-NOS, and intellectual disability. *Journal of Intellectual and Developmental Disability,* 33(4), 323-329.

Matson, J.L. and Wilkins, J. 2008. Nosology and diagnosis of Asperger's syndrome. *Research in Autism Spectrum Disorders,* 2(2), 288-300.

Mayo Clinic. 2014. *Allergy-proof your home.* [online] Available at: <http://www.mayoclinic.org/diseases-conditions/allergies/in-depth/allergy/art-20049365> [Accessed 4 May 2014].

Maytum, M. 2013. *Sweetwater Spectrum: Life with Purpose.* San Francisco, CA: Leddy Maytum Stacy Architects Brochure.

McArdle J. 1998. *Resource Manual for Facilitators in Community Development.* Volumes I and II. Melbourne: Vista Publications.

McGlaughlin, A., Gorfin, L. and Saul, C. 2004. Enabling adults with learning disabilities to articulate their housing needs. *British Journal of Social Work,* 34, 709-726.

McIlwain, L. 2013. The day my son went missing. *New York Times.* 12 Nov [online] Available at: <http://www.nytimes.com/2013/11/13/opinion/wandering-is-a-major-concern-for-parents-of-children-with-autism.html> [Accessed 7 August 2015]

Medical Architecture. n.d. [online] Available at: <http://www.medicalarchitecture.com/> [Accessed 8 June 2014].

Memon, M., Wagner, S.R., Pedersen, C.F., Beevi, F.H.A. and Hansen, F.O. 2014. Ambient assisted living healthcare frameworks, platforms, standards, and quality attributes. *Sensors,* 14, 4312-4341.

Mesibov, G.B. and Shea, V. 2011. Evidence-based practices and autism. *Autism,* 15(1), 114-133.

Mesibov, G.B., Schopler, E. and Sloan, J.L. 1983. Service development for adolescents and adults in North Carolina's TEACCH program. In Schopler, E. and Mesibov, G.B. eds. *Autism in Adolescents and Adults.* New York: Plenum Press. (411-432)

Messbauer, L. 2008. *Multi-Sensory Environment - A protocol for individuals with autism.* [online] Available at: <http://www.lmessbauer.com/content/multi-sensory-environment-%E2%80%93-protocol-individuals-autism> [Accessed 8 August 2013].

Messbauer, L. 2009. *Why should a Multi-Sensory Environment be White in Color?* [online] Available at: <http://www.lmessbauer.com/content/why-should-multi-sensory-environment-be-white-color> [Accessed 8 August 2013].

Messbauer, L. 2012. *Designing Your Own MSE Room for Treatment.* [online] Available at: <http://www.lmessbauer.com/content/designing-your-own-mse-room-treatment> [Accessed 8 August 2013].

Michael Singer Studio. 2014. *Individuals with Autism Spectrum Conditions: A Population Positively Affected by Sustainable Practices, A New Model of Shared Housing,* report. Michael Singer Studio, Vermont and Florida.

Mihailidis, A., Boger, J.N., Craig, T. and Hoey, J. 2008. The COACH prompting system to assist older adults with dementia through handwashing: An efficacy study. *BMC Geriatrics,* 8: 28-46.

Mikiten, E. 2008. Housing Consortium of the East Bay: Lincoln Oaks Apartments. [video online] Available at: <http://www.youtube.com/watch?v=3rB4Gm5CZMA> [Accessed 12 October 2009].

Milner, P. and Kelly, B. 2014. Community participation and inclusion: People with disabilities defining their place. *Disability and Society,* 24(1), 47-62.

Millan, A. 2010. *Autism: Believe in the Future. From Infancy to Independence.* New York: iUniverse, Inc.

Minnesota Technical College Task Force. 1993. *Educational Opportunities for Developmental Disabilities Service Providers.* St. Paul, MN: Governor's Planning Council on Developmental Disabilities.

Minshew, N.J. and Hobson, J.A. 2008. Sensory sensitivities and performance on sensory perceptual tasks in high-functioning individuals with autism. *Journal of Autism and Developmental Disorders,* 38, 1485-1498.

Minshew, N.J., Sung, K., Jones, B.L. and Furman, J.M. 2004. Underdevelopment of the postural control system in autism. *Neurology,* 63, 2056-2061.

Missouri Autism Guidelines Initiative. 2012. *Autism Spectrum Disorders: Guide to Evidence-Based Interventions. A 2012 Consensus Publication.* [pdf] Available at: <http://autismguidelines.dmh.mo.gov/documents/Interventions.pdf> [Accessed 16 April 2015].

Montes, G. and Halterman, J.S. 2006. Characteristics of school-age children with autism. *Journal of Developmental and Behavioral Pediatrics,* 27(5), 379-385.

Montes, G. and Halterman, J.S. 2008. Child care problems and employment among families with preschool-aged children with autism in the United States. *Pediatrics,* 122(1).

Mostafa, M. 2008. An architecture for autism: Concepts of design intervention for the autistic user. *Archnet-IJAR, International Journal of Architectural Research,* 2(1), 189-211.

Mostafa, M. 2010. Housing adaptation for adults with autism spectrum disorder. *Open House International,* 35, 37-48.

Mostofsky, S.H., Powell, S.K., Simmonds, D.J., Goldberg, M.C. et al. 2009. Decreased connectivity and cerebellar activity in autism during motor task performance. *Brain,* 132(9), 13-25.

Mottron, L. et al. 2006. Enhanced perceptual functioning in autism: An update and eight principles of autistic perception. *Journal of Autism and Developmental Disorders,* 36 (1), 27-43.

Mouridsen, S.E., Bronnum-Hansen, H., Rich, B. et al. 2008. Mortality and causes of death in autism spectrum disorders: An update. *Autism,* 12, 403-414.

Muller, E., Schuler, A. and Yates, G.B. 2008. Social challenges and supports from the perspective of individuals with Asperger syndrome and other autism spectrum disabilities. *Autism,* 12(2), 173-190.

Murphy, G.H., Beadle-Brown, J., Wing, L., Gould, J. et al. 2005. Chronicity of challenging behaviours in people with severe intellectual disabilities and/or autism: A total population sample. *Journal of Autism and Developmental Disorders,* 35(4), 405-418.

Murray, W. 1996. Planning residential environments with persons with mental retardation. *Journal of Planning Literature,* 11(2), 155-166.

Muselman, D.M., Woodruff, E. and Kellar-Guenther, Y. 2010. *Changes in Quality of Life for Group Home Residents of the Bob and Judy Charles SmartHome: An Exploratory Analysis.* Denver: University of Colorado Denver, Colorado WIN Partners. [pdf] Available at: <http://www.ucdenver.edu/academics/colleges/medicalschool/departments/pediatrics/research/programs/psi/Resources/Documents/Smarthome%20Research.pdf> [Accessed 15 April 2015].

National Autistic Society. n.d. *Environment and surroundings.* [online] Available at: <http://www.autism.org.uk/living-with-autism/at-home/environment.aspx> [Accessed July 15, 2015].

National Center on Birth Defects and Developmental Disabilities, Centers for Disease Control and Prevention. 2012. *Key Findings: Trends in the Prevalence of Developmental Disabilities in U.S. Children, 1997-2008.* [online] Available at: <http://www.cdc.gov/ncbddd/features/birthdefects-dd-keyfindings.html> [Accessed 1 August 2013].

National Complete Streets Coalitions. n.d. *Smart Growth America.* [online] Available at: <http://www.smartgrowthamerica.org/complete-streets> [Accessed 18 June 2014].

National Core Indicators. 2011. *NCI Data Brief.* Issue 3. April [online] Available at: <http://www.nationalcoreindicators.org/upload/core-indicators/DATA_BRIEF_-_Autism_-_April_4_2011_-_No_3_1.pdf> [Accessed 27 September 2013].

National Council on Disability. 2010. *The State of Housing in America in the 21st Century: A Disability Perspective.* Washington DC: National Council on Disability.

National Gateway to Self Determination. n.d. *What is self-determiniation and why is it important?* [online] Available at: <http://www.ngsd.org > [Accessed 30 June 2015]

National Health Service. n.d. *Telecare and Telehealth Services in the UK.* [online] Available at: <http://www.nhs.uk/Planners/Yourhealth/Pages/Telecare.aspx> [Accessed 10 July 2015].

National Research Council (of National Academies). 2011. *Health Care Comes Home: The Human Factors.* Washington DC: National Academies Press.

NCAC. 2014. *National Council of Acoustical Consultants.* [online] Available at: <http://ncac.com/> [Accessed 16 June 2014].

Neighborhood Wayfinding Assessment. 2012. *Easter Seals Project Action and CDC Healthy Aging Research Network.* [online] Available at: <http://www.projectaction.org/> [Accessed 28 January 2014].

Neßelrath, R., Haupert, J., Frey, J. and Brandherm, B. 2011. Supporting persons with special needs in their daily life in a smart home. In: *7th International Conference on Intelligent Environments Proceedings.* Nottingham, UK 25-28 July 2011.

Newman, L., Wagner, M., Knockey, A.-M. et al. 2011. *The Post-High School Outcomes of Young Adults with Disabilities up to 8 Years after High School: A Report from the National Longitudinal Transition Study-2 (NLTS2)* (NCSER 2011-3005). Menlo Park, CA: SRI International. [online] Available at: <http://www.nlts2.org/reports/2009_04/index.html> [Accessed 16 April 2015].

Newschaffer, C.J., Croen, L.A., Daniles, J. et al. 2007. The epidemiology of autism spectrum disorders. *Annual Review of Public Health, 28,* 235-258.

NKBA. 2014. *National Kitchen and Bath Association.* [online] Available at: <http://www.nkba.org/> [Accessed 8 July 2014].

Nordin, V. and Gilberg, C. 1998. The long term course of autistic disorder: Update on follow-up studies. *Acta Pscyhiatric Scandinavia, 97,* 99-108.

NREL. 2014. *National Renewable Energy Laboratory.* [online] Available at: <http://www.nrel.gov/> [Accessed 12 July 2014].

O'Connor, K. and Kirk, I. 2008. Brief report. Atypical social cognition and social behaviours in autism spectrum disorder: A different way of processing rather than an impairment. *Journal of Autism and Developmental Disorders, 38,* 1989-1997.

Odom, S.L., Collet-Klingenberg, L., Rogers, S.J. and Hatton, D.D. 2010. Evidence-based practices in interventions for children and youth with autism spectrum disorders. *Preventing School Failure,* 54(4), 275-282.

Olivier, P., Xu, G., Monk, A. and Hoey, J. 2009. Ambient kitchen: Designing situated services using a high fidelity prototyping environment. In: *2nd International Conference on Pervasive Technologies Related Assistive Environments.* Corfu, Greece 9-13 June 2009. New York: ACM.

Olsson, I., Steffenburg, S. and Gillberg, C. 1988. Epilepsy in autism and autisticlike conditions: A population-based study. *Archives of Neurology, 45,* 666-668.

O'Neill, M. and Jones, R.S. 1997. Sensory-perceptual abnormalities in autism: A case for more research? *Journal of Autism and Developmental Disorders, 33,* 631-642.

Orsmond, G., Shattuck, P.T., Cooper, B.P., Sterzing, P.R. and Anderson, K.A. 2013. Social participation among young adults with an autism spectrum disorder. *Journal of Autism and Developmental Disorders,* 43(11), 2710-9.

Orsmond, G.I., Krauss, M.W. and Seltzer, M.M. 2004. Peer relationships and social and recreational activities among adolescents and adults with autism. *Journal of Autism and Developmental Disorders,* 34(3), 245-256.

O'Shaughnessy, C.V. 2013. *National Spending for Long-Term Services and Supports, 2011.* Washington, DC: National Health Policy Forum.

Ousley, O. and Mesibov, G. 1991. Sexual attitudes and knowledge of high-funcitoning adolescents and adults with autism. *Journal of Autism and Developmental Disabilities,* 21, 471-481.

Oyane, N.M.F. and Bjorvatn, B. 2005. Sleep disturbances in adolescents and young adults with autism and Asperger syndrome. *Autism,* 9(1), 83-94.

Ozonoff, S., Lisif, A-M., Baguio, F. et al. 2010. A prospective study of the early behavioral signs of autism spectrum disorder. *Journal of American Academy of Child and Adolescent Psychiatry,* 49(3), 248-268.

Ozonoff, S., Pennington, B.F. and Rogers, S.J. 1991. Executive function deficits in high-functioning autistic individuals: Relationship to theory of mind. *Journal of Child Psychology and Psychiatry,* 32 (7), 1081-1105.

Page, J. and Boucher, J. 1998. Motor impairments in children with autistic disorder. *Child Language and Teaching Therapy,* 14, 233-259.

Palmen, A., Didden, R. and Lang, R. 2011. A systematic review of behavioral intervention research on adaptive skill building in high-functioning young adults with autism spectrum disorder. *Research in Autism Spectrum Disorders,* 6(2), 602-617.

Pandya, S.M., Wolkwitz, K. and Feinberg, L.F. 2006. *Support For Working Family Caregivers: Paid Leave Policies In California And Beyond.* San Francisco: CA: Family Caregiver Alliance.

Paperstone. n.d. *Paperstone Products.* [online] Available at <http://www.paperstoneproducts.com/> [Accessed 24 May 2014].

Parish, S., Seltzer, M.M., Greenberg, J.S. et al. 2004. Economic implications of caregiving at midlife: Comparing parents with and without children who have developmental disabilities. *Mental Retardation,* 42, 413-426.

Parish, S.L. and Cloud, J.M. 2006. Financial well-being of young children with disabilities and their families. *Social Work,* 47(4), 415-424.

Parish, S.L. and Lutwick, Z.E. 2005. A critical analysis of the emerging crisis in long-term care for people with developmental disabilities. *Social Work,* 50, 345-354.

Parish, S.L. and Whisnant, A.K. 2005. Policies and programs for children and youth with disabilities. In Jenson, J.M. and Fraser, M.W., eds. *Social Policies for Children and Families: A Risk and Resilience Perspective.* Thousand Oaks, CA: Sage. (167-194).

Partnership for People with Disabilities. n.d. *Person-Centered Planning: Centers for Medicare and Medicaid Services' Definition.* [online] Available at: <http://www.medicaid.gov/mltss/docs/PCP-CMSdefinition04-04.pdf> [Accessed 13 May 2014].

Pelphrey, K., Shultz, S., Hudac, C. and Vander Wyk, B. 2011. Constraining heterogeneity: The social brain and its development in autism spectrum disorder. *Journal of Child Psychology and Psychiatry,* 52(6), 631-644.

Pennington, B.F. and Ozonoff, S. 1996. Executive functions and developmental psychopathology. *Journal of Child Psychology and Psychiatry,* 37, 51-87.

Perera, F.P., Rauh, V.,Whyatt, R.M.,Tsai, W.Y., Tang, D., Diaz, D., Hoepner, L., Barr, D., Tu, Y.H., Camano, D., Kenney, P. 2006. Effect of prenatal exposure to airborne policyclic aromatic hydrocarbons on neurodevelopment in the first 3 years of life among inner-city children. *Environmental Health Perspective,* 114, 1287-1292.

Perkins, D., Florin, P., Rich, R. Wandersman, A. and Chavis, D. 1990. Participation and the social and physical environmental of residential blocks: Crime and community context. *American Journal of Community Psychology,* 32(6), 691-705.

Perkins, D.D. and Long, D.A. 2002. Neighborhood sense of community and social capital: A multi-level analysis. In Fisher, A.T., Sonn, C.C. and Bishop, B.J. eds. *Psychological Sense of Community: Research, Applications, and Implications.* New York: Kluwer Academic/Plenum Publishers. (291-316).

Perkins, E.A. and Moran, J.A. 2010. Aging adults with intellectual disabilities. *Journal of the American Medical Association,* 304(1), 91-92.

Perkins, E.Z. and Berkman, K.A. 2012. Into the unknown: Aging with autism spectrum disorders. *American Journal on Intellectual and Developmental Disabilities,* 117(6), 478-496.

Perry, N. 2009. *Adults on the Autism Spectrum Leave the Nest: Achieving Supported Independence.* London: Jessica Kingsley Publishers.

Peterson, C.B., Prasad, N.R. and Prasad, R. 2012. The future of assistive technologies for dementia. *Gerontechnology,* 11(2), 195-202.

Phakos, C. 2013. *What is the best option for sound barrier flooring for multi-family housing?* US Green Building Council's Green Home Guide. [online] Available at: <http://greenhomeguide.com/askapro/question/what-is-the-best-option-for-sound-barrier-flooring-for-multi-family-housing-that-requires-sound-control> [Accessed 28 September 2013].

Pham, C., Jackson, D., Schoning, J., Bartindale, T., Plotz, T. and Olivier, P. 2013. FoodBoard: Surface contact imaging for food recognition. In: *UbiComp '13.* Zurich, Switzerland 8-12 September 2013. New York: ACM.

Pickett, J., Xiu, E, Tuchman, R., Dawson, G. et al. 2011. Mortality in individuals with autism, with and without epilepsy. *Journal of Child Neurology,* 26, 932-939.

Piven, J. and Rabins, P. 2011. Autism spectrum disorders in older adults: Toward defining a research agenda. *Journal of the American Geriatrics Society,* 59, 2151-2155.

Plimley, L.A. 2007. A review of quality of life issues and people with autism spectrum disorders. *British Journal of Learning Disabilities,* 35, 205-213.

Pollack, D. 2009. *Neurodiversity in Higher Education: Positive Reponses to Specific Learning Differences.* Malden, MA: John Wiley and Sons.

Portes, A. 1998. Social capital: Its origins and applications in modern sociology. *Annual Review of Sociology,* 24, 1-24.

Posada, M., Garcia Primo, P., Ferrari, M.J. and Martin-Arribas, M.C. 2007. *European Autism Information System (EAIS) Report on the 'Autism Spectrum Disorders Prevalence Data and Accessibiity to Services' Questionnaire (Q-EAIS)*. Madrid: Research Institute for Rare Diseases, Instituto de Salud Carlos III. [online] Available at: <http://ec.europa.eu/health/ph_information/dissemination/diseases/docs/autism1.pdf> [Accessed on 15 April 2015].

Program Design, Inc. 2005. *A Guide to Supported Living in Florida*. Florida Developmental Disabilities Council, Inc. [online] Available at: <http://apd.myflorida.com/customers/supported-living/living-guide/docs/introduction.pdf> [Accessed 10 May 2014].

Prouty, R.W., Smith, G. and Lakin, K.C. 2003. *Residential Services for Persons with Developmental Disabilities*. Minneapolis, MN: Research and Training Center on Community Living, University of Minnesota.

Putnam, R.D. 1993. *Making Democracy Work*. Princeton, NJ: Princeton University Press.

Putnam, R.D. 1995. Bowling alone. *Journal of Democracy*, 6, 65-78.

Pynoos, J., Steinman, B.A., Nguyen, A.Q.D. and Bressette, M. 2012. Assessing and adapting the home environment to reduce falls and meet the changing capacity of older adults. *Journal of Housing for the Elderly*, 26, 137-155.

QuietRock. n.d. *QuietRock Sheetrock*. [online] Available at <http://www.quietrock.com/> [Accessed 20 May 2014].

Randell, M. and Cumella, S. 2009. People with an intellectual disability living in an intentional community. *Journal of Intellectual Disability Research*, 53(8), 716-726.

Rapoport, A. 1990. *The Meaning of the Built Environment: A Nonverbal Communication Approach*. Tuscon: University of Arizona Press.

Rayens, N. 1980. The less you've got, the less you get: Functioning grouping, a cause for concern. *Mental Retardation*, 18, 217-220.

Reichow, B. and Volkmar, F.R. 2011. Evidence-based practices in autism: Where we started. In Reichow, B., Doehring, P., Cicchetti, D.V., and Volkmar, F.R., eds. *Evidence-based Practices and Treatments for Children with Autism*. New York: Springer. (3-24).

Reichow, B., Volkmar, F.R. and Cicchetti, D.V. 2008. Development of the evaluative method for evaluating and determining evidence-based practices in autism. *Journal of Autism and Developmental Disorders*, 38(7), 1311-1319.

Renty, J. and Roeyers, H. 2006. Satisfaction with formal support and education for children with autism spectrum disorder: The voices of the parents. *Child: Care, Health and Development*, 32(3), 371-385.

Resnik, D.D. and Blackbourn, J. 2009. *Opening Doors: A Discussion of Residential Options for Adults Living with Autism and Related Disorders*. Phoenix, AZ: Urban Land Institute, Southwest Autism Research and Resource Center, and Arizona Board of Regents. [pdf] Available at: <http://www.autismcenter.org/sites/default/files/files/openingdoors_print_042610_001.pdf> [Accessed 15 April 2015].

Rhoades, C. and Browning, P. 1977. Normalization at what price? *Mental Retardation,* 15, 24.

Rice, C.E., Rosanoff, M., Dawson, G., Durkin, M.S. et al. 2010. Evaluating changes in the prevalence of the autism spectrum disorders (ASDs). *Public Health Reviews,* 34(2). [online] Available at: <http://www.publichealthreviews.eu/upload/pdf_files/12/00_Rice.pdf> [Accessed on 15 April 2015].

Richdale, A.L. and Schreck, K.A. 2009. Sleep problems in autism spectrum disorders: Prevalence, nature and possible biopsychosocial aetiologies. *Sleep Medicine Reviews,* 13, 403-411.

Richlite, 2014. *Richlite: Eco-friendly paper-based fiber composites.* [online] Available at: <http://www.richlite.com/> [Accessed 12 July 2014].

Risk and Policy Analysts, Ltd. 2011. *Assessing the Health and Environmental Impacts in the Context of Socio-Economic Analysis Under Research. Final Report. Part 1: Literature Review and Recommendations.* Prepared for European Commission Directorate − General Environment. [pdf] Available at: <http://ec.europa.eu/environment/chemicals/reach/pdf/publications/reach_sea_part%201_final_publ.pdf> [Accessed 19 April 2015].

Robertson, J. and Emerson, E. 2006. *A Systematic Review of the Comparative Benefits and Costs of Models of Providing Residential and Vocational Supports to Adults with Autism Spectrum Disorder.* Report for the National Autistic Society, Institute for Health Research, Lancaster University.

Robertson, J., Emerson, E., Pinkney, L., Caesar, E., Felce, D., Meek, A., Carr, D., Lowe, K., Knapp, M. and Hallam, A. 2005. Community-based residential supports for people with intellectual disabilities and challenging behaviour: The views of the neighbours. *Journal of Applied Research in Intellectual Disabilities,* 18 (1), 85-92.

Robertson, S.M. 2010. Neurodiversity, quality of life, and autistic adults: Shifting research and professional focuses onto real-life challenges. *Disability Studies Quarterly,* 30(1). [online] Available at: <http://dsq-sds.org/article/view/1069/1234> [Accessed 16 November 2010].

Robertson, S.M. and Ne'eman, A.D. 2008. Autistic acceptance, the college campus, and technology: Growth of neurodiversity in society and academia. *Disability Studies Quarterly,* 28(4). [online] Available at: <http://dsq-sds.org/article/view/146/146> [Accessed 16 April 2015].

Robinette, J., Charles, S., Mogle, J. and Almeida, D. 2013. Neighborhood cohesion and daily well-being: Results from a diary study. *Social Science & Medicine,* 96, 174-182.

Robison, J.E. 2007. *Look Me in the Eye: My Life with Asperger's.* New York: Crown.

Rockwool. 2014. *Rockwool: Firesafe insulation.* [online] Available at: <http://www.rockwool.com/> [Accessed 12 July 2014].

Rodaway, P. 1994. *Sensuous Geographies: Body, Sense and Place.* London: Routledge.

Rodin, J. and Langer, E. 1977. Long-term effects of a control-relevant intervention with the institutional aged. *Journal of Personality and Social Psychology,* 35(2), 897-902.

Roizen, N.J. and Patterson, D. 2003. Down's syndrome. *The Lancet,* 361, 1281–1289.

Rowe, J.W. and Kahn, R.L. 1997. Successful aging. *The Gerontologist,* 37, 433–440.

Roy, M., Dillo, W., Emrich, H.M. and Ohlmeier, M.D. 2011. Asperger's syndrome in adulthood. *The Neurotypical Site.* [online] Available at: <http://www.theneurotypical.com/aspergers_in_adulthood.html> [Accessed 19 April 2015].

Rydzewska, E. 2012. Destination unknown? Transition to adulthood for people with autism spectrum disorders. *British Journal of Special Education,* 39(2), 87–93.

Sackett, D., Staus, S., Richardson, W., Rosenberg, W. et al. eds. 2000. *Evidence-Based Medicine: How to Practice and Teach EBM.* Edinburgh: Churchill Livingstone.

Sackett, D.L., Rosenberg, W.M.C., Gray, J.A.M., Haynes, R.B. et al. 1996. Evidence based medicine: What it is and what it isn't. *BMJ,* 312, 71.

Safestep. n.d. *Safestep Grip by Forbo.* [online] Available at <http://www.forbo-flooring.com/> [Accessed 20 May 2014].

Salamon, M. 2014. Adults with autism at risk for many health problems: Study. *HealthDay.* [online] Available at: <http://consumer.healthday.com/cognitive-health-information-26/autism-news-51/adults-with-autism-at-higher-odds-for-other-ailments-687631.html> [Accessed 17 April 2015].

Saldaña, D., Álvarez, R.M., Lobatón, S., Lopez, A.M., Moreno, M. and Rojano, M. 2009. Objective and subjective quality of life in adults with autism spectrum disorders in southern Spain. *Autism,* 13(3), 303–316.

Sampson, R.J., Morenoff, J.D. and Gannon-Rowley, T. 2002. Assessing "neighborhood effects": Social processes and new directions in research. *Annual Review of Sociology,* 28, 443–478.

Sanchez, P., Vazquez, F. and Serrano, L. 2011. Autism and the built environment. In Williams, T. ed. *Autism Spectrum Disorders - From Genes to Environment.* [online] Available at: <http://www.intechopen.com/books/autism-spectrum-disordersfrom-genes-to-environment/autism-and-the-built-environment> [Accessed 21 August 2013].

Sansal, K.E., Edes, B.Z. and Binatli, A.O. 2012. Effects of indoor lighting on depression probability and academic performance in a population of Turkish adolescents. In: *The Fifth Conference Balkan Light 2012 Proceedings,* Belgrade, Serbia. [online] Available at: <http://2012.experiencinglight.nl/doc/20.pdf> [Accessed 17 April 2015].

Sanoff, H. 1991. *Visual Research Methods in Design.* New York: Van Nostrand Reinhold.

Sanoff, H. 2000. *Community Participatory Methods in Design and Planning.* New York: Wiley.

Sarason, S.B. 1977. *The Psychological Sense of Community: Prospects for a Community Psychology.* London: Jossey-Bass.

Saxby, H., Thomas, M., Felce, D. and de Kock, U. 1986. The use of shops, cafes and public houses by severely and profoundly mentally handicapped adults. *British Journal of Mental Subnormality,* 32, 69–81.

Saxon, S.V., Etten, M.J. and Perkins, E.A. 2010. *Physical Change and Aging: A Guide for the Helping Professions.* 5th edition. New York: Springer.

SCGH. 2014. *Sierra Club Green Home.* [online] Available at: <http://www.scgh.com/> [Accessed 7 August 2015]

Schalock, R.L., Luckasson, R.A. and Shogren, K.A. 2007. The renaming of *mental retardation:* Understanding the change to the term *intellectual disability. Intellectual and Developmental Disabilities,* 45(2), 116-124.

Schleien, S.J., Brake, L., Miller, K.D. and Walton, G. 2013. Using Photovoice to listen to adults with intellectual disabilities on being part of the community. *Annals of Leisure Research,* 16(3), 212-229.

Schleien, S., Green, F. and Stone, C. 1999. Making friends within inclusive community recreation programs. *Journal of Leisurability,* 26(3). [online] Available at: <http://lin.ca/sites/default/files/attachments/V26N3A4.htm> [Accessed 25 April 2014].

Schön, D.A. 1983. *Reflective Practitioner: How Professionals Think in Action.* New York: Basic Books.

Schreibman, L. 2005. *The Science and Fiction of Autism.* Cambridge, MA: Harvard University Press.

Schuhow, D.A. and Zurakowski, T.L. 2012. Evidence-based care of the older client with autism. In Giarelli, E., and Gardner, M., eds. *Nursing of Autism Spectrum Disorder: Evidence-Based Integrated Care Across the Lifespan.* New York: Springer. (353-385)

Scott, I. 2009. Designing learning spaces for children on the autism spectrum. *Good Autism Practice,* 10(1), 36-51.

Seligman, M. 2011. *Flourish: A Visionary New Understanding of Happiness and Well-Being.* New York: Free Press.

Sellin, B. 1993. *Ik wil geen inmiij meer zijn: Berichten uit een autistische kerker.* Rotterdam: Thoth. Translation of: "Ich will kein Inmich mehr sein: Botschaften aus einem autistischen Kerker." Köln: Kiepenheuer & Witsch [quoted in Baumers and Heylighen, 2010].

Seltzer, M.M. and Krauss, M.W. 2001. Quality of life of adults with mental retardation/developmental disabilities who live with family. *Mental Retardation and Developmental Disabilities Research Review,* 7, 105-114.

Seltzer, M.M., Krauss, M.W. Shattuck, P.T., Orsmond, G., Swe, A., and Lord, C. 2003. The symptoms of autism spectrum disorders in adolescence and adulthood. *Journal of Autism and Developmental Disorders,* 33, 565-581.

Seltzer, M.M., Shattuck, P. Abbeduto, L. and Greenberg, J.S. 2004. Trajectory of development in adolescents and adults with autism. *Mental Retardation and Developmental Disabilities Research Reviews,* 10, 234-247.

Selye, H. 1956. *The Stress of Life.* New York: McGraw-Hill.

Selye, H. 1974. *Stress Without Distress.* Philadelphia: Lippincott.

Sensorium. n.d. *Sensorium – Caring with Technology.* [online] Available at: <http://www.sensorium.co.uk/Home.aspx> [Accessed 10 July 2015].

Sergeant, L., Dewsbury, G. and Johnstone, S. 2007. Supporting people with complex behavioural difficulties and autistic spectrum disorder in a community setting: An inclusive approach. *Housing, Care and Support,* 10(1), 23–30.

Sharpe, D.L. and Baker, D.L. 2011. The financial side of autism: Private and public costs. In Mohammadi, M–R., ed. *A Comprehensive Book on Autism Spectrum Disorders.* Rijeka, Croatia: InTech. (275–296).

Shattuck, P.T., Narendorf, S.C., Cooper, B., Sterzing, P.R. et al. 2012. Postsecondary education and employment among youth with an autism spectrum disorder. *Pediatrics,* 129(6), 1042–1049.

Shattuck, P.T., Seltzer, M.M., Greenberg, J.S., Orsmond, G.I., Bolt, D., Kring, S. et al. 2007. Change in autism symptoms and maladaptive behaviors in adolescents and adults with an autism spectrum disorder. *Journal of Autism and Developmental Disorders,* 13, 129–135.

Shavelle, R.M. and Strauss, D. 1998. Comparative mortality of persons with autism in California, 1980–1996. *Journal of Insurance Medicine,* 30, 220–225.

Shavelle, R.M., Strauss, D. and Pickett, J. 2001. Causes of death in autism. *Journal of Autism and Other Developmental Disabilities,* 31, 569–576.

Shea, V. and Mesibov, G.B. 2005. Adolescents and adults with autism. In Volkmar, F.R., Paul, R., Klin, A., and Cohen, D., eds. *Handbook of Autism and Pervasive Developmental Disorder: Volume 1: Diagnosis, Development, Neurobiology and Behavior.* 3rd edition. New York: John Wiley and Sons. (288–311).

Sheppard-Jones, K., Prout, H.T. and Kleinert, H. 2005. Quality of life dimensions for adults with developmental disabilities: A comparative study. *Mental Retardation,* 43, 281–291.

Sherwin, S. 1998. A relational approach to autonomy in health care. In Feminist Health Care Ethics Research Network and Sherwin, S., eds. *The Politics of Women's Health.* Philadelphia: Temple University Press. (19–47).

Shiovitz-Ezra, S. and Ayalon, L. 2010. Situational versus chronic loneliness as risk factors for all-cause mortality. *International Psychogeriatrics,* 22, 455–462.

Shtayermann, O. 2007. Peer victimization in adolescents and young adults diagnosed with Asperger's syndrome: A link to depressive symptomatology, anxiety symptomatology and suicidal ideation. *Issues in Comprehensive Pediatric Nursing,* 30(3), 87–107.

Siebelink, E.M. 2006. Sexuality and people with intellectual disabilities: Assessment of knowledge, attitudes, experiences and needs. *Mental Retardation,* 44(4), 283–294.

Sigman, M., Spence, S.J. and Wang, A.T. 2006. Autism from developmental and neuropsychological perspectives. *Annual Review of Clinical Psychology,* 2, 327–355.

Silverman, C. 2008. Fieldwork on another planet: Social science perspectives on the autism spectrum. *BioSocieties,* 3(3), 325–341.

Simonoff, E., Pickles, A., Charman, T., Chandler S., Louscas, T. and Baird, G. 2008. Psychiatric disorders in children with autism spectrum disorders: Prevalence, comorbidity, and associated factors in a population-derived sample. *Journal of the American Academy of Child and Adolescent Psychiatry,* 47, 921–929.

Sinclair, J. 1999. *Why I dislike "person first" language.* [online] Available at: <http://autismmythbusters.com/general-public/autistic-vs-people-with-autism/jim-sinclair-why-i-dislike-person-first-language/> [Accessed 16 April 2015].

Sinclair, J. 2005. *Autism Network International: The development of a community and its culture.* [online] Available at: <http://www.autreat.com/History_of_ANI.html> [Accessed 16 April 2015].

Sinclair, J. 2010. Cultural commentary: Being autistic together. *Disability Studies Quarterly,* 30 (1). [online] Available at: <http://dsq-sds.org/article/view/1075/1248> [Accessed 1 December 2010].

Singer, E. 2013. Matthew Goodwin: Bridging disciplines for autism care. *Simons Foundation Autism Research Initiative.* 8 April. [online] Available at: <http://sfari.org/news-and-opinion/investigator-profiles/2013/matthew-goodwin-bridging-disciplines-for-autism-care> [Accessed 25 January 2014].

Skeels, M.M., Unruh, K.T., Powell, C. and Pratt, W. 2010. Catalyzing social support for breast cancer patients. *Proceedings of the ACM CHI 2010,* 173-1822.

Skjaeveland, O. and Garling, T. 1997. Effects on interactional space on neighboring. *Journal of Environmental Psychology,* 17, 181-198.

Smart Home Design Centers. 2014. *SCGH: Greenhome.* [online] Available at: <http://www.scgh.com/> [Accessed 8 June 2014].

Smith, C.L. 1991. Measures and meaning in comparisons of wealth equality. *Social Indicators Research,* 24, 367-392.

Smith, L.E., Greenberg, J.S. and Mailick, M.R. 2012. Adults with autism: Outcomes, family effects, and the multi-family group psychoeducation model. *Current Psychiatry Report,* 14, 732-738.

Smith, L.E., Maenner, M.J. and Seltzer, M.M. 2012. Developmental trajectories in adolescents and adults with autism: The case of daily living skills. *Journal of American Academy of Child and Adolescent Psychiatry,* 51(6), 622-631.

Smith, P.A. 2012. Aging in autism. *Perspectives on Gerontology,* 17(2), 69-75.

Smith, R.S. and Sharp, J. 2013. Fascination and isolation: A grounded theory exploration of unusual sensory experiences in adults with Asperger Syndrome. *Journal of Autism and Developmental Disabilities*, 43(4), 891-910.

Smolders, K.C.H.J. and de Kort Y.A.W. 2012. Bright light effects on mental fatigue. In: *Proceedings of Experiencing Light.* Eindhoven, the Netherlands 12-13 November 2012.

Smolders, K.C.H.J. and de Kort, Y.A.W. 2014. Bright light and mental fatigue: Effects on alertness, vitality, performance and physiological arousal. *Journal of Environmental Psychology,* 12, 1-15.

Smull, M. and Sanderson, H. 2005. *Essential Lifestyle Planning for Everyone.* United Kingdom: The Learning Community.

Social Care, Local Government and Care Partnership Directorate, Department of Health. 2014. *Think Autism: Fulfilling Lives, the Strategies for Adults with Autism in England – An Update.* London: Department of Health. [pdf] Available at: <https://www.gov.uk/government/publications/think-autism-an-update-to-the-government-adult-autism-strategy> [Accessed 15 July 2014].

Solomon, A. 2008. The autism rights movement. *New York Magazine.* [online] Available at: <http://nymag.com/print/?/news/features/47225/> [Accessed 23 March 2012].

Solomon, A. 2012. *Far from the Tree: Parents, Children and the Search for Identity.* New York: Schribner.

Solomon, O. 2010. Sense and the senses: Anthropology and the study of autism. *Annual Review of Anthropology,* 39, 241-259.

Spreat, S. and Conroy, J.W. 2002. The impact of deinstitutionalization on family contact. *Research in Developmental Disabilities,* 23, 202-210.

Spreat, S., Conroy, J.W. and Rice, D.M. 1998. Improve quality in nursing homes or institute community placement? Implementation of OBRA for individuals with mental retardation. *Research in Developmental Disabilities,* 19, 507-518.

Stancliffe, R.J., Abery, B.H. and Smith, J. 2000. Personal control and the ecology of community living settings: Beyond living-unit size and type. *American Journal on Mental Retardation,* 105, 431-454.

Stancliffe, R.J., Lakin, K.C., Larson, S., Engler, J. et al. 2010. Choice of living arrangements. *Journal of Intellectual Disability Research,* 55(8), 746-762.

Standifer, S. 2011. Fact sheet on autism employment. *Autism Works: National Conference on Autism and Employment.* [pdf] Available at: <www.autismhandbook. org/images/5/5d/AutismFactSheet2011.pdf> [Accessed 8 August 2015].

Steingard, R.J., Zimnitzky, B., DeMaso, D.R., Bauman, M.L. and Bucci, J.P. 1997. Sertraline treatment of transition-associated anxiety and agitation in children with autistic disorder. *Journal of Child and Adolescent Psychopharmacology,* 7, 9-15.

Sterling, L., Dawson, G., Estes, A. and Greenson, J. 2008. Characteristics associated with presence of depressive symptoms in adults with autism spectrum disorder. *Journal of Autism and Developmental Disorders,* 38, 1011-1018.

Stevenson, R.A., Siemann, J.K., Schneider, B.C., Eberly, H.E. et al. 2014. Multisensory temporal integration in autism spectrum disorders. *The Journal of Neuroscience,* 34(3), 691-697.

Stewart, M.E., Bargard, L., Pearson, J. et al. 2006. Presentation of depression in autism and Asperger syndrome: A review. *Autism,* 10, 103-116.

Stokes, M. and Kaur, A. 2005. High-functioning autism and sexuality: A parental perspective. *Autism,* 9(3), 266-289.

Stokes, M., Newton, N. and Kaur, A. 2007. Stalking, and social and romantic functioning among adolescents and adults with autism spectrum disorder. *Journal of Autism and Developmental Disorders,* 37(1), 1969-1986.

Strouse, M.C., Carroll-Hernandez, T.A., Sherman, J.A. and Sheldon, J.B. 2003. Turning over turnover: The evaluation of a staff scheduling system in a community-based program for adults with developmental disabilities. *Journal of Organizational Behavior Management,* 23(2/3), 45-63.

Strouse, M.C., Sherman, J.A. and Sheldon, J.B. 2013. Do good, take data, get a life, and make a meaningful difference in providing residential services! In: Reed, D.D., DiGennaro Reed, F.D. and Luiselli, J.K., eds. *Handbook of Crisis Intervention and Developmental Disabilities.* New York: Springer. (441-465).

Stuart-Hamilton, I., Griffith, G., Totsika, V., Nash, S., Hastings, R.P., Felce, D. and Kerr, M. 2009. *The Circumstances and Support Needs of Older People with Autism.* Report for the Welsh Assembly Government. Cardiff: Welsh Assembly. [pdf] Available at: <http://www.ssiacymru.org.uk/resource/p_o_Older_people_with_ASD_-_Research_Report_-_September_2009.pdf> [Accessed 26 April 2014].

Stuart-Hamilton, I. and Morgan, H. 2011. What happens to people with ASD in middle age and beyond? Report of a preliminary on-line study. *Advances in Mental Health and Intellectual Disabilities,* 5, 22-28.

Surie, D., Baydam, B. and Lindgren, H. 2013. Proxemics awareness in Kitchen As-A-Pal: Tracking objects and human in perspective. In: *9th International Conference on Intelligent Environments.* Athens, Greece 18-19 July 2013.

Sweetwater Spectrum. n.d. *Life With Purpose.* [online] Available at: <http://www.sweetwaterspectrum.org/home0.aspx> [Accessed 18 July 2015].

Szatman, P., Bartolucci, G. Bremner, R., Bond, S. and Rich, S. 1989. A follow-up study of high-functioning autistic children. *Journal of Autism and Developmental Disabilities,* 19, 213-225.

Tammet, D. 2007. *Born on a Blue Day: Inside the Extraordinary Minds of an Autistic Savant.* New York: Free Press.

Tantam, D. 1991. Asperger's syndrome in adulthood. In Frith, J., ed. *Autism and Asperger Syndrome.* Cambridge, U.K.: Cambridge University Press. (147-183).

Tarkett/Johnsonite. 2014. *Tarkett Flooring Solutions.* [online] Available at: <http://www.tarkett.com/> [Accessed 2 June 2014].

Taylor, J.L. 2009. The transition out of high school and into adulthood for individuals with autism and for their families. *International Review of Research in Mental Retardation,* 38, 1-32.

Taylor, J.L. and Seltzer, M.M. 2010. Changes in the autism behavioral phenotype during the transition to adulthood. *Journal of Autism and Developmental Disorders,* 40, 1431-1446.

Temple, V.A., Anderson, C. and Walkley, J.W. 2000. Physical activity levels of individuals living in a group home. *Journal of Intellectual and Developmental Disability,* 25(4), 327-341.

Terman, M. and McMahan, I. 2012. *Chronotherapy: Resetting Your Inner Clock to Boost Mood, Alertness, and Quality Sleep.* New York: Avery.

The Arc. 2014. *The 2014 Federal Home and Community-Based Services Regulation: What You Need to Know.* [online] Available at: <http://www.thearc.org/document.doc?id=4596> [Accessed 19 April 2015].

The Arc Jacksonville. n.d. *The Arc Jacksonville Village.* [online] Available at: <http://www.arcjacksonville.org/thearcvillage/> [Accessed 18 July 2015].

The Arc North Carolina. 2008. *A Closer Look at Housing Choices: A Housing Resource Guide for People with Developmental Disabilities.* [online] Available at: <http://www.arcnc.org/housing-resources> [Accessed 21 November 2013].

The Green House Project. 2012. *Home Economics: The Business Case for the Green House Model.* [online] Available at: <http://thegreenhouseproject.org/doc/21/business-case-full-web.pdf> [Accessed 19 April 2015].

Theoharides, T.C. and Zhang, B. 2011. Neuro-inflammation, blood-brain barrier, seizures and autism. *Journal of Neuroinflammation,* 8, 168.

Think College. n.d. *College options for people with intellectual disabilities.* [online] Available at: <http://www.thinkcollege.net/> [Accessed 10 July 2015].

Thomaz, E., Bettadapura, V., Reyes, G., Sandesh, M., Schindler, G., Plotz, T., Abowd, G.D. and Essa, I. 2012. Recognizing water-based activities in the home through infrastructure-mediated sensing. In: *UbiComp 2012.* Pittsburgh, PA, USA 5-8 September 2012. New York: ACM.

Thompson, J., Bradley, V., Buntinx, W., Schalock, R., Shogren, K. et al. 2009. Conceptualizing supports and the support needs of people with intellectual disability. *Intellectual and Developmental Disabilities,* 47(2),135-146.

Thompson, T., Robinson, J. and Dietrich, M.S. 1996. Architectural features and perceptions of community residences for people with mental retardation. *American Journal on Mental Retardation,* 101, 292-314.

Thorn, S.H., Pittman, A., Myers, R.E. and Slaughter, C. 2009. Increasing community integration and inclusion for people with intellectual disabilities. *Research in Developmental Disabilities,* 30, 891-901.

Throne, J.M. 1979. Deinstitutionalisation: Too wide a swath. *Mental Retardation,* 17, 171-175.

Tomchek, S.D.,and Dunn, W. 2007. Sensory processing in children with and without autism: A comparative study using the short sensory profile. *American Journal of Occupational Therapy,* 61, 190-200.

Tordman, S., Anderson, G.M., Botbol, M., Brailly-Tabard, S. et al. 2009. Pain reactivity and plasma ß-endorphin in children and adolescents with autistic disorder. *Plos One,* 4(8): e5289.

Totsika, V., Felce, D., Kerr, M. and Hastings, R.P. 2010. Behavior problems, psychiatric symptoms and the quality of life for older adults with intellectual disability with and without autism. *Journal of Autism and Developmental Disorders,* 40, 1171-1178.

Townley, G. and Kloos, B. 2009. Development of a measure of sense of community for individuals with serious mental illness residing in community settings. *Journal of Community Psychology,* 37(3), 362-380.

Travers, J. and Tincani, M. 2010. Sexuality education for individuals with autism spectrum disorders: Critical issues and decision making guidelines. *Education and Training in Autism and Developmental Disabilities,* 45(2), 284-293.

Trembath, D., Germano, C., Johanson, G. and Dissanayake, C. 2012. The experience of anxiety in young adults with autism spectrum disorders. *Focus on Autism and Other Developmental Disabilities,* 27(4): 213-224.

Tuchman, R. and Rapin, I. 2002. Epilepsy in autism. *Lancet Neurology,* 1, 352-358.

Tuchman, R., Moshe, S.L. and Rapin, I. 2009. Convulsing toward the pathophysiology of autism. *Brain Development,* 31, 95-103.

Tunstall Solutions. 2014. *Tunstall Solutions.* [online] Available at: <http://uk.tunstall.com/solutions> [Accessed 7 August 2015].

Turner-Brown, L.M., Perry, T.D., Dichter, G.S., Bodrish, J.W. et al. 2008. Brief report: Feasibility of social cognition and interaction training for adults with high functioning autism. *Journal of Autism and Developmental Disorders,* 38, 1777-1784.

Tyler, C.V., Schramm, S.C., Karafa, M., Tang, A.S. and Jain, A.K. 2011. Chronic disease risks in young adults with autism spectrum disorder: Forewarned is forearmed. *American Journal of Intellectual and Developmental Disabilities,* 116 (5), 371-80.

Tyler, C.V., White-Scott, S., Ekvall, S.M. and Abulafia, L. 2008. Environmental health and developmental disabilities: A life span approach. *Community Health,* 31(4), 287-304.

Ulrich, R. 1999. Effects of gardens on health outcomes: theory and research. In Barnes, M. and Cooper Marcus, C., eds. *Healing Gardens: Therapeutic Benefits and Design Recommendations.* New York: John Wiley & Sons.

Ulrich, R.S., Zimring, C., Zhu, X., DuBose, J.R. et al. 2008. A review of the research literature on evidence-based healthcare design. *Health Environments Research and Design,* 1(3), 61-125.

Underwood, L., McCarthy, J. and Tsakanikos, E. 2010. Mental health of adults with autism spectrum disorders and intellectual disability. *Current Opinions in Psychiatry,* 23, 421-426.

Unger, D.G. and Wandersman, A. 1982. Neighboring in an urban environment. *American Journal of Community Psychology,* 10, 493-509.

United Nations. 2006. *Convention on the Rights of Persons with Disabilities.* [online] Available at: <http://www.un.org/disabilities/convention/conventionfull.shtml> [Accessed on 15 April 2015].

Urbano, M.R., Hartmann, K., Deutsch, S.I., Polychronopoulos, G.M.B. et al. 2013. Relationships, sexuality, and intimacy in autism spectrum disorders. In Fitzgerald, M., ed. *Recent Advances in Autism Spectrum Disorders. Volume 1.* Intech. [online] Available at: <http://www.intechopen.com/books/recent-advances-in-autism-spectrum-disorders-volume-i/relationships-sexuality-and-intimacy-in-autism-spectrum-disorders> [Accessed 17 April 2015].

U.S. Department of Health and Human Services. 2002. Notice. *Federal Register,* 67, 69223-69225.

U.S. Department of Health and Human Services. 2006. *The Supply of Direct Support Professionals Serving Individuals with Intellectual Disabilities and Other Developmental Disabilities: Report to Congress.* Washington DC. [pdf] Available at: <http://aspe. hhs.gov/daltcp/reports/2006/DSPsupply.pdf> [Accessed 17 April 2015].

Vallee, J., Cadot, E., Roustit, D., Parizot I. and Chauvin, P. 2011. The role of daily mobility in mental health inequalitites: The interactive influence of activity space and neighbourhood of residence on depression. *Social Science & Medicine*, 73, 1133-1144.

Van Alphen, L.M., Dijker, A.J.M., van den Borne, H.H.W. and Curfs, L.M.G. 2009. The significance of neighbours: Views and experiences of people with intellectual disability on neighbouring. *Journal of Intellectual Disability Research,*53(8), 745-757.

Van Alphen, L.M., Duker, A.J.M., van den Borne, B.H.W. and Curfs, L.M.G. 2010. People with intellectual disability as neighbours: Towards understanding the mundane aspects of social integration. *Journal of Community & Applied Social Psychology,* 20, 347-362.

Van Bougondien, M.E., Reichle, N.C. and Schopler, E. 2003. Effects of a model treatment approach on adults with autism. *Journal of Autism and Developmental Disorders,* 33, 131-140.

Van Bourgondien, M. and Schopler, E. 1996. Intervention for adults with autism. *Journal of Rehabilitation*, 62, 65-71.

van den Berg, A., Hartig, T. and Staats, H. 2007. Preference for nature in urbanized societies: Stress, restoration, and the pursuit of sustainability. *Journal of Social Issues*, 63(1), 79-96.

van den Berg, A., Maas, J., Verheij, R. and Groenewegen, P. 2010. Green space as a buffer between stressful life events and health. *Social Science & Medicine*, 70, 1203-1210.

van Hoof, J., Kort, H.S.M.,Duijnstee, M.S.H., Rutten, P.G.S. and Hensen, J.L.M. 2010. The indoor environment and the integrated design of homes for older people with dementia. *Building and Environment,* 45, 1244-1261.

Vanderbilt Sleep Disorders Center. 2013. *Suggestions for better sleep.* Vanderbilt Department of Neurology. [online] Available at: <http://www.mc.vanderbilt.edu/ root/vumc.php?site=neurology&doc=44094> [Accessed 18 June 2014].

Vardouli, T., Chondros, C., Voulipiro, E. and Antonopoulou, E. 2012. CommonSENSE: A participatory design toolkit for shaping physical space through real-time data. In: *2012 Eight International Conference on Intelligent Environments.* Washington DC: ICEE Computer Society. (64-71) [online] Available at: <http:// dl.acm.org/citation.cfm?id=2358083> [Accessed 18 July 2015].

Venter, A., Lord, C. and Shopler, E. 1992. A follow-up study of high-functioning autistic children. *Journal of Child Psychology and Psychiatry,* 33(3), 489-507.

Viets, E. 2009. Lessons from evidence-based medicine: What healthcare designers can learn from the medical field. *HERD,* 2(2), 73-87.

Volkmar, F.R. and Cohen, D.J. 1991. Comorbid association of autism and schizophrenia. *American Journal of Psychiatry,* 148, 1705-1707.

Wahl, H-W. and Weisman, G.D. 2003. Environmental gerontology at the beginning of the new millennium: Reflections on its historical, empirical and theoretical development. *The Gerontologist,* 43 (5), 616-627.

Walker, R.B. and Hiller, J.E. 2007. Places and health: A qualitative study to explore how older women living alone perceive the social and physical dimensions of their neighborhoods. *Social Science and Medicine,* 65, 1154-1165.

Walsh, P.N., Emerson, E., Lobb, C., Hatton, C., Bradley, V., Schalock, R.L. and Moseley, C. 2007. *Supported Accommodation Services for People with Intellectual Disabilities: A Review of Models and Instruments Used to Measure Quality of Life in Various Settings.* Dublin, Ireland: National Disability Authority.

Ward, M.J. and Meyer, R.N. 1999. Self-determination for people with developmental disabilities and autism: Two advocates' perspectives. *Focus on Autism and Other Developmental Disabilities,* 14(3), 133-139.

Ward Thompson, C., Roe, J., Aspinall, P., Mitchell, R. et al. 2012. More green space is linked to less stress in deprived communities: Evidence from salivary cortisol patterns. *Landscape and Urban Planning,* 105, 221-229.

Watling, R.L, Deitz, J. and White, O. 2001. Comparison of sensory profile scores of young children with and without autism spectrum disorders. *American Journal of Occupational Therapy,* 55, 416-412.

Weden, M.M., Carpiano, R.M. and Robert, S.A. 2008. Subjective and objective neighborhood characteristics and adult health. *Social Science and Medicine,* 66, 1256-1270.

Wedmore, H.V. 2011. *Autism Spectrum Disorders and Romantic Intimacy.* Graduate Theses and Dissertations, Digital Repository at Iowa State University. [online] Available at: <http://lib.dr.iastate.edu/cgi/viewcontent.cgi?article=1112&context=etd> [Accessed 1 July 2015].

Wehmeyer, J., Buntinx, W., Lachapelle, Y., Luckasson, R., Schalock, R., Verdugo, M. et al. 2008. The intellectual disability construct and its relation to human functioning. *Intellectual and Developmental Disabilities*, 46(4), 311-318.

Wehmeyer, M.L., Tasse, M.J., Davies, D.K. and Stock, S. 2012. Support needs of adults with intellectual disability across domains: The role of technology. *Journal of Special Education Technology*, 27(2), 11-21.

Weller, A.C. 2001. *Editorial Peer Review: Its Strengths and Weaknesses.* Medford, NJ: Information Today, Inc.

Wendt, D.C. and Slife, B.D., 2007. Is evidence-based practice diverse enough? Philosophy of science considerations. *American Psychologist,* 62(6), 613-614.

Westen, D. and Bradley, R. 2005. Empirically supported complexity: Rethinking evidence-based practice in psychotherapy. *Current Directions in Psychological Science,* 14(5), 266-271.

Westin, A.F. 1967. *Privacy and Freedom.* New York: Athenaum.

White, G.W., Simpson, J.L. Gonda, C., Ravesloot, C. and Coble, Z. 2010. Moving from independence to interdependence: A conceptual model for better understanding community participation of centers for independent living consumers. *Journal of Disability Policy Studies,* 20(4), 233-240.

Whitehurst, T. 2006. The impact of building design on children with autistic spectrum disorders. *Good Autism Practice,* 7(1), 31-38.

Whitehurst, T. 2007. *Evaluation of Features Specific to an ASD Designed Living Accommodation.* Clent, West Midlands, UK: Sunfield Research Institute.

Wickelgren, I. 2012. The importance of being social. *Scientific American.* [online] Available at: <http://blogs.scientificamerican.com/streams-of-consciousness/2012/04/24/the-importance-of-being-social/?print=true> [Accessed 17 April 2015].

Williams, D. 1991. *Nobody Nowhere: The Extraordinary Autobiography of An Autistic.* New York: Crown.

Williams, J.G., Higgins, J.P. and Brayne, C.E. 2006. Systematic review of prevalence studies of autism spectrum disorders. *Archives of Disease in Childhood,* 91(1), 8-15.

Williams, S. and Boult, M. 2009. *Post Action Reviews – Property A, South Oxfordshire and Poprerty B, West Oxfordshire. Report 1: The Main Report.* London: Det Norske Veritas Ltd.

Wilson, J.C. 2008. *Weather Reports form the Autism Front: A Father's Memoir of His Autistic Son.* Jefferson, NC: McFarland and Company.

Wilson-Kovacs, D., Ryan, M.K., Haslam, S.A. and Rabinovich, A. 2008. Just because you can get a wheelchair in the building doesn't necessarily mean that you can still participate: Barriers to the career advancement of disabled professionals. *Disability & Society,* 23, 705-717.

Wilson, P.G., Reid, D.H. and Green, C.W. 2006. Evaluating and increasing in-home leisure activity among adults with severe disabilities in supported independent living. *Research in Developmental Disabilities,* 27, 93-107.

Windham, G.C., Zhang, L.,Runier, R., Croen, L.A. and Grether, J.K. 2006. Autism spectrum disorders in relation to distribution of hazardous air pollutants in the San Francisco Bay area. *Environmental Health Perspective,* 114, 1438-1444.

Wing, L. 1981. Asperger's syndrome: A clinical account. *Psychological Medicine,* 11, 115-129.

Wobbrock, J.O., Kane, S.K., Gajos, K.Z., Harada, S. and Froehlich, J. 2011. Ability-based design: Concept, principles and examples. *ACM Transactions on Accessible Computing,* 3(3), 1-36.

Wolbring, G. and Leopatra, V. 2013. Sensors: Views of staff of a disability service organization. *Journal of Personalized Medicine,* 3, 23-39.

Wolf, M.M., Kirigin, K.A., Fixsen, D.L, Blasé, K.A. and Braukmann, C.J. 1995. The teaching-family model: A case study in data-based program development and refinement. *Journal of Organizational Behavior Management,* 15(1-2), 11-68.

Wolfensberg, W. 1972. *The Principle of Normalization in Human Services.* Toronto: National Institute on Mental Retardation.

Wolff, S. and McGuire, R.J. 1995. Schizoid personality in girls: A follow-up study: What are the links with Asperger's syndrome? *Journal of Child Psychology and Psychiatry,* 36, 793-817.

Woo, C.C. and Leon, M. 2013. Environmental enrichment as an effective treatment for autism: A randomized controlled trial. *Behavioral Neuroscience,* 127(4), 487-497.

World Health Organization (WHO). 1993. *International Statistical Classification of Disease and Related Health Problems. 10ᵗʰ Revision. ICD-10. Volumes 1-3.* Geneva: World Health Organization.

World Health Organization (WHO). 2002. *Towards A Common Language for Functioning, Disability and Health.* ICF. Geneva, Switzerland: World Health Organization. [pdf] Available at: <http://www.who.int/classifications/icf/training/icfbeginnersguide.pdf> [Accessed 7 August 2015]

World Health Organization Quality of Life Group (WHOQOL), 1995. The World Health Organization Quality of Life Assessment (WHOQOL): Position paper from the World Health Organization. *Social Science and Medicine,* 41(10), 1403-1409.

Wright, S.D., Brooks, D.E., D'Astous, V. and Grandin, T. 2013. The challenge and promise of autism spectrum disorders in adulthood and aging: A systematic review of the literature (1990-2013). *Autism Insights,* 5, 21-73.

Wu, M., Birnholtz, J., Richards, B., Baecker, R. and Massimi, M. 2008. Collaborating to remember: A distributed cognition account of families coping with memory impairments. *Proceedings of ACM CHI,* 825-834.

Wurlitzer, C. 2014. The Best Induction Cooktops 2014. *Yale Appliance + Lighting Blog* [blog] 5 May. Available at: <http://blog.yaleappliance.com/best-induction-cooktops-2014> [Accessed 20 June 2014].

Young, J., Corea, C., Kimani, J. and Mandell, D. 2010. *Autism Spectrum Disorders (ASDs) Services: Final Report on Environmental Scan.* Columbia, MD: IMPAQ International, LLC.

Young, N. 2014. Elder tech. *CBC Radio, Spark blog.* [blog] 22 June. Available at: <http://www.cbc.ca/spark/blog/2014/06/22/elder-tech/> [Accessed 12 July 2014].

Yudell, M., Tabor, H., Dawson, G., Rossi, J. et al. 2013. Priorities for autism spectrum disorder risk communication and ethics. *Autism,* 17(6), 701-722.

Zamprelli, J. 2009. *Housing persons with an intellectual disability in intentional communities: Identifying relevant physical and governance structures.* Canada Mortgage and Housing Corporation. [online] Available at: <http://www.cmhc.ca/en/inpr/rehi/rehi_011.cfm> [Accessed 27 May 2014].

Zeisel, J. 2013. Improving person-centered care through effective design. *Generations, Journal of the American Society on Aging.* 37(3),45-52.

Zeisel, J., Silverstein, N.M., Hyde, J., Levkoff, S., Lawton, M.P. and Holmes, W. 2003. Environmental correlates to behavioral health outcomes in Alzheimer's special care units. *The Gerontologist,* 43 (5), 697-711.

Zeisel, J. and Tyson, M. 1999. Alzheimer's treatment gardens. In Cooper Marcus, C. and Barnes, M., eds., *Healing Gardens: Therapeutic Benefits and Design Recommendations.* New York: John Wiley & Sons.

Zimring, C. 1982. The built environment as a source of psychological stress: Impacts of buildings and cities on satisfaction and behavior. In Evans, G.W., ed. *Environmental Stress.* New York: Cambridge University Press. (151-178)

Zlotnik, J.L. and Galambos, C. 2004. Evidence-based practices in health care: Social work possibilities. Editorial. *Health and Social Work.* [online] Available at: <http://staging.knowledgeplex.org/news/46698.html>. [Accessed 13 April 2006].

RESEARCH AND INFORMATION SOURCES USED IN DEVELOPING GOALS AND GUIDELINES

KEY

Population

AC:	Autistic children and/or teens
AA:	Autistic adults (also includes mixed sample, e.g. those with autism and other developmental disabilities)
R:	Non-ASC but similar behaviors/symptoms (e.g. elopement among seniors with dementia)
G:	Standards/practices for general population
V:	Manufacturer or vendor literature

Basis for

✓:	Quality of life goals
+:	Design guidelineS

Sources of Empirical Studies (Including Literature Reviews of Empirical Research, Evidence-Based or Research-Informed Guidelines, and Demographic/Statistical Profiles)

Source	Population	Safety-Security	Clarity-Familiarity	Sensory Balance	Privacy-Social	Choice-Independence	Health-Wellness	Dignity	Durability	Affordable	Neighborhood Access
		For Goals (✓) and Guidelines (+)									
Abbott and McConkey, 2006	AA					+	+	+			+
Ahrentzen, 2002	G		✓+								
Ahrentzen and Steele, 2009	AA/AC	+	+	+	+	+	+		+		
Algase et al, 2009	R	✓									
Altman and Chermers, 1980	G				✓						
Amado et al, 2013	AA						+				
Anderson et al, 2012	AA	✓									
Archea, 1977	G				+						
Armitage, 2013	G	+									
Bagatell, 2010	AA				✓						
Baker et al, 2008	AA/AC	+		+							
Barnes and Cooper Marcus, 1999	G						+				
Barnes and Design in Caring Environments Study Group, 2002	R				+			+			
Baron-Cohen and Wheelwright, 2004	AA/AC				✓						
Baron-Cohen et al, 2009	AA/AC		✓								
Baum et al, 1982	G						✓				
Baumers and Heylighen, 2010	AA	✓	✓+								
Baumers and Heylighen, 2014	AA	✓	+		✓						
Bauminger et al, 2004	AC				✓						
Ben-Sasson et al, 2009	AA/AC			✓							
Berman et al, 2008	G						+				
Bhat et al, 2011	AA/AC								✓		
Bogdashina, 2003	AA/AC			✓							
Bolton et al, 2011	AA	✓					✓				
Brand and Gaudion, 2012	AA			✓+							
Brand, 2010	AA	+	+	+	+	✓+	+	+	+	+	+
Brereton and Broadbent, 2007	AC								✓		
Bryant and Bryant, 2012	R	+									
Carmien et al, 2005	R					+					
Cascio et al, 2008	AA/AC	+		+	+					+	
Chalfont and Walker, 2013	AA/R						+				

Source	Population	Safety-Security	Clarity-Familiarity	Sensory Balance	Privacy-Social	Choice-Independence	Health-Wellness	Dignity	Durability	Affordable	Neighborhood Access
						For Goals (✓) and Guidelines (+)					
Chan et al, 2008	R					✓					
Cohen, 1978	G		✓								
Cuvo et al, 2001	R			+			+				
Davidson and Henderson, 2010	AA				✓						
Draheim et al, 2002	R						✓				
Dudley et al, 2012	AC					+					+
Duggan and Linehan, 2013	R					✓					
Edwards et al, 2012	R	+									
Elwin et al, 2012	AA		+	+							
Emerson et al, 1999	R										✓
Emmerich et al, 2003	G						+				
Evans and Cohen, 1987	G		✓								
Evans and McCoy, 1998	G		+								
Evans, 1982	G		✓				✓				
Farley et al, 2009	AA		+			+		✓ +			✓ +
Farrell et al, 2004	G	✓						✓			✓
Fennelly and Crowe, 2013	G	+									
Fleming and Purandare, 2010	R	+		+	+		+				
Forrest and Kearns, 2001	G										✓
Fournier et al, 2010	AA/AC	+		+			+				
Freeley, 2009	AA					+					
Frith, 2003	AA/AC		✓								
Gabbler-Hall et al, 1993	AA/AC						✓				
Gaudion and McGinley, 2012	AA	+		+	+	+	+		+		
Geboy et al, 2012	R							+			
Geurts and Vissers, 2012	AA		✓								
Geurts et al, 2009	AA		✓								
Ghaziuddin and Butler, 1998	AC	✓									
Gibson et al, 2012	AA							✓			
Golant, 2015	R							+			
Goodwin et al, 2006	AC						✓				
Green et al, 2008	AC	✓									
Greenhouse, 2012	R	+									
Groden et al, 2005	AC						✓				
Hall, 1990	G				✓						
Happé and Charlton, 2010	AA			✓			✓				
Happé and Frith, 2006	AA/AC		✓								

Source	Population	For Goals (✓) and Guidelines (+)									
		Safety-Security	Clarity-Familiarity	Sensory Balance	Privacy-Social	Choice-Independence	Health-Wellness	Dignity	Durability	Affordable	Neighborhood Access
Heller et al, 2007	AA/R		+	+			+				+
Hill, 2004	AA		✓								
Hilton et al, 2010	AA/AC			✓							
Jackson, 1997	AA/R			+	+	+	+				+
Jackson, 2008	AA					✓					
Jansiewics et al, 2006	AC	✓									
Jones et al, 2001	AA		+	+			+				
Kaplan, 2001	G			+			+				
Kaplan, 1995	G			+			+				
Kaplan and Kaplan, 1989	G						+				+
Kapp et al, 2011	AA			✓							
Kern et al, 2006	AA/AC			✓			✓				
Kern et al, 2007	AA/AC			✓							
Kinnaer et al, 2014	AA		✓	+	✓+						
Kloos and Shah, 2009	R						✓				
Kozma, et al, 2009	R					+	+				+
Lang et al, 2010	G						✓				
Lawton and Nahemow, 1973	R							✓+			
Lawton, 1980	R						✓+	✓+			
Lazarus, 1966	G						✓				
Lazarus and Cohen, 1977	G						✓				
Lee et al, 2011	R	+		+	+	+					
Lee et al, 2012	R	+	+	+	+	+	+	+	+		
Leekham et al, 2007	AA/AC			✓							
Liptak et al, 2011	AA				✓						
Manjoiviona and Prior, 1995	AC	✓									
Marco et al, 2011	AC			✓							
Matson and Rivet, 2008	AA	✓									
Messbauer, 2009	AA/R/G			+							
Michael Singer Studio, 2014	AA/AC	+	+	+	+	+	+	+	+	+	
Milner and Kelly, 2009	R										✓
Minshew et al, 2004	AC	✓									
Mostafa, 2010	AC		+			+	+				
Mostafa, 2008	AC		✓	+							
Mottron et al, 2006	AA/AC		✓								
Muller et al, 2008	AA				✓						
Murphy et al, 2005	AA	✓									
Muselman and Woodruff, 2010	R							✓			

Source	Population	For Goals (✓) and Guidelines (+)									
		Safety-Security	Clarity-Familiarity	Sensory Balance	Privacy-Social	Choice-Independence	Health-Wellness	Dignity	Durability	Affordable	Neighborhood Access
National Autism Society, 2014	AA		+	+			+				
National Council on Disability, 2010	R									✓	
National Research Council, 2011	R	+									
O'Connor and Kirk, 2008	AA		✓								
O'Neill and Jones, 1997	AA/AC			✓							
Orsmond et al, 2004	AA				✓						
Osborn, 2009	AA							✓ +			+
Ousley and Mesilov, 1991	AA							✓			
Page and Boucher, 1998	AC	✓									
Pennington and Ozonoff, 1996	AA		✓								
Perkins and Berkman, 2012	AA			✓							
Pynoos et al, 2012	R	+									
Rapoport, 1990	G		✓ +		✓						
Rhoades and Browning, 1977	G										✓
Rodin and Langer, 1977	G					✓	✓				
Sampson et al, 2002	G	✓						✓			✓
Saxon, Etten and Perkins, 2010	AA			✓							
Schuhow and Zurakowski, 2012	AA						✓				
Selye, 1956, 1974	G						✓				
Sergeant et al, 2007	AA/AC		✓ +	+		+	+		✓ +		
Shattuck et al, 2012	AA				✓						
Siebelink, 2009	AA		+					✓ +			
Singer, 2013	AC		✓								
Skjaeveland and Garling, 1997	G										✓
Smith and Sharp, 2013	AA/AC			+	+						
Smolders and de Kort, 2014	G			+			✓	+			
Stancliffe et al, 2011	AA					✓					✓
Standifer, 2011	AA								✓		
Stevenson et al, 2014	AA/AC		✓								
Stokes et al, 2007	AA							✓			
Strouse et al, 2013	R	+		+			+				
Temple et al, 2000	R						✓				
Terman and McMahon, 2012	G						✓				
Thompson et al, 1996	R							✓ +			+
Tomchek and Dunn, 2007	AA/AC		✓								
Tyler et al, 2011	AA						+				+
Tyler et al, 2008	R						✓				

Source	Population	Safety-Security	Clarity-Familiarity	Sensory Balance	Privacy-Social	Choice-Independence	Health-Wellness	Dignity	Durability	Affordable	Neighborhood Access
		For Goals (✓) and Guidelines (+)									
Ulrich, 1999	R			+			+				
Unger and Wandersman, 1982	G										✓
Urbano, 2013	AA							✓			
Van Alphen et al, 2009	AA				+		+				
Van Bourgondien & Schloper, 1996	AA						+				
Van den Berg et al, 2007	G						+				
Van den Berg et al, 2010	G						+				+
Van Hoof et al, 2010	R	+		+							
Wahl and Weisman, 2003	R							+			
Walker and Hiller, 2007	G	✓						✓			✓
Ward Thompson et al, 2012	G						✓				
Watling et al, 2001	AA/AC			✓							
Weden et al, 2008	G	✓						✓			✓
Wedmore, 2011	AA		+					✓+			
Westin, 1967	G				✓						
Wickelgren, 2012	G				✓						
Williams and Boult, 2009	AA	+	+	+	+	+	+	+	+		✓ +
Woo and Leon, 2013	AA/AC			✓							
Wu et al, 2008	R					+					
www.designadvisor.org	G								+		
Zamprelli, 2009	R	+	+			+	+				
Zeisel and Tyson, 1999	R	+									
Zeisel et al, 2003	R	✓ +					+				
Zeisel, 2013	R	+	+		+	+		+			

Reflective Practice: Residential Visits by Authors (all in US)

Source	Population	For Goals (✓) and Guidelines (+)									
		Safety-Security	Clarity-Familiarity	Sensory Balance	Privacy-Social	Choice-Indpependence	Health-Wellness	Dignity	Durability	Affordable	Neighborhood Access
29 Palms (AZ), 2014: Interviews, site visit	AA/R		+		+						
Center for Discovery (NY), 2012: Interviews, site visit	AC	✓		✓			✓	✓	✓		
Community Living Options (KS), 2009: Interviews, two sites visits	AA/R	✓			✓	✓			✓	✓	
First Place (AZ), 2014: Interviews, site visit	AA						+				+
Hello Housing (CA), 2009: Interviews, three sites visits	AA/R	✓+					+		✓+	✓	✓
Lincoln Oaks (CA), 2009: Interviews, site visit	AA/R		+		+	+				+	
Milagros Independent Housing (CA), 2009: Interviews, site visit	AA/R	+			+	+				+	
Mission Bay Senior Housing (CA), 2009: Interviews, site visit	R				+						
Mt. Bethel Village (NJ), 2013: Interviews, site visit	AA	✓	✓						✓		
Stoney Pine (CA), 2009: Interviews, site visit	AA/R	+			+	+				+	
Sweetwater Spectrum (CA), 2012, 2013: Interviews, site visits	AA	✓	✓	✓	✓	✓	✓	✓	✓		✓

Reflective Practice: Sources of Experts' Experiences, Assessments

Source	Population	Safety-Security	Clarity-Familiarity	Sensory Balance	Privacy-Social	Choice-Independence	Health-Wellness	Dignity	Durability	Affordable	Neighborhood Access
		For Goals (✓) and Guidelines (+)									
American Association of People with Disabilities, 2012	AA	+									+
AIA, 2012	G					+					+
Autism Society of Delaware, 2006	AA							✓ +			
Beaver, 2006, 2010	AC	+	+	+			+		+		
Birch, 2003	AA		✓								
Brereton and Broadbent, 2007	AA								✓		
Department of Family and Community Services, 2013	AA/R/G	+	+	+		+	+		+	+	
Dorhmann, 2014	AA			+							
Donvan and Zucker, 2010	AA		✓			✓					✓
Easter Seals Project Action, 2012	AA	+				+	+				+
Enterprise Green Communities, 2015	G/M	+					+				
Fleishmann, 2012	AC		✓								
Grandin, 1995	AA		✓	✓							
Grandin, 2012	AA		✓								
Harris and Kinder, 2013	AA/AC			✓							
Harker and King, 2004	AA				+		+	✓ +			+
Harmon, 2013	AA							✓			
Health Physics Society, n.d	G								+		
Healthy House Institute, 2014	G						+		+		
Higashida, 2013	AC	✓	✓								
Humphreys, 2005	AA/AC			+							
Katz, 2013	G					+					
Laufenberg, 2004	G					+					
Livable Housing Australia, 2012	G	+									
Maytum, 2013	AA	+		+			+		+	+	+
McGlaughin et al, 2004	R					+		+			
Medical Architecture, 2014	AA		+				+				
Mikiten, 2008	AA/R/G		+								

Source	Population	For Goals (✓) and Guidelines (+)									
		Safety-Security	Clarity-Familiarity	Sensory Balance	Privacy-Social	Choice-Indpendence	Health-Wellness	Dignity	Durability	Affordable	Neighborhood Access
National Complete Streets, n.d.	G	+									+
Perry, 2009	AA									✓	✓
Robison, 2007	AA				✓	✓					
Scott, 2009	A					+	+				
Sinclair, 2010	AA				✓+						
Tammet, 2007	AA		✓								
The Arc, North Carolina, 2008	AA					+					+
Whitehurst, 2007	AC	+	+								
Williams, 1991	AA			✓							
Wilson, 2008	AA			✓							

Manufacturer Literature (includes Manufacturer Societies)

Source	Population	Safety-Security	Clarity-Familiarity	Sensory Balance	Privacy-Social	Choice-Indpendence	Health-Wellness	Dignity	Durability	Affordable	Neighborhood Access
		Goals (√) and Guidelines (+)									
Acoustikblok, 2014	V			+							
Careinfo.org, 2014	V						+				
CityQuiet.com, 2014	V			+							
Countertop Guides, 2014	V								+		
Haigh Hygiene Solutions, 2014	V						+				
Hirshberg, 2011	V						+				
Home Ventilation Institute, 2014	V						+				
HVAC Quick, 2014	V			+							
Illuminating Engineering Society, 2014	V		+	+							
International Organization for Standardization, 2014	V			+							
JTM, 2014	V		+				+				
National Council of Acoustical Consultants, 2014	V			+							
National Kitchen and Bath Association, 2014	V						+				
National Renewable Energy Lab, 2014	V									+	
Paperstone, nd	V								+		
Phakos, 2013	V			+							
QuietRock, nd	V			+							
Richlite, 2014	V								+		
Rockwell Firesafe Insulations, 2014	V			+							
Safestep Grip by Forbo, nd	V	+							+		
Smart Home Design Centers, 2014	V									+	
Tarkett/Johnsonite, 2014	V	+							+		
Wurlitzer, 2014	V	+									

CHAPTER FOUR IMAGE SOURCES

4.1   Dan Burden: www.pedbikeimages.org

4.2   Dan Burden: www.pedbikeimages.org

4.4   PNWRA: https://www.flickr.com/photos/pnwra/456613376/in/photolist

4.5   Dan Burden: www.pedbikeimages.org

4.6   Laura Sandt: www.pedbikeimages.org

4.7   La Citta Vita: https://www.flickr.com/photos/la-citta-vita/5963839865/in/album-72157627253745768/

4.8   Dan Burden: www.pedbikeimages.org

4.9   Julia Diana: www.pedbikeimages.org

4.10   Saxbald Photography: https://www.flickr.com/photos/saxbaldphotography/15861416154/

4.11   Dan Burden: www.pedbikeimages.org

4.12   Tonu Mauring: https://www.flickr.com/photos/mauring/4693617948/in/dateposted/

4.15   Bill Young: https://www.flickr.com/photos/by_photo/8611668563

4.16   Tulane Public Relations: CC BY 2.0 (http://creativecommons.org/licenses/by/2.0)], via Wikimedia Commons

4.18   Chris and Karen Highland: https://www.flickr.com/photos/frederickhomesforsale/15349971806/in/photostream/

4.19   La Citta Vita: https://www.flickr.com/photos/la-citta-vita/7802551914/in/album-72157631113816934/

4.20   Steve Cadman: https://www.flickr.com/photos/stevecadman/771343750

4.24   Jeremy Levine: https://www.flickr.com/photos/jeremylevinedesign/14677931596/in/dateposted/

4.25   CTJ71081: https://www.flickr.com/photos/55267995@N04/15441945530/in/photolist

4.26   Arya Ganesh G: https://www.flickr.com/photos/32297395@N06/8727491369/in/dateposted/

4.27   JJ and Chris: https://www.flickr.com/photos/26834393@N04/16360602849/

4.28   Karen Roe: https://www.flickr.com/photos/karen_roe/7278319748/in/album-72157629914684502/

4.29   Sonja Lovas: https://www.flickr.com/photos/sonjalovas/4038233322/

4.30   Arya Ganesh G: https://www.flickr.com/photos/32297395@N06/8727993501/in/dateposted/

4.31   Ms. Phoenix: https://www.flickr.com/photos/32020964@N08/5088256083/

4.33   Mikhail Golub: https://www.flickr.com/photos/golub/11534713823/in/dateposted/

4.34   Ceylon Tea Trails: https://www.flickr.com/photos/teatrails/6901830565/

4.35   Emily May: https://www.flickr.com/photos/emilysnuffer/15786351717/in/dateposted/

4.36   Fairfax County Fate House: https://www.flickr.com/photos/fairfaxcounty/5572652258/in/album-72157626257883699/

4.37   David Rothamel: https://www.flickr.com/photos/realestatezebra/3208848276/

4.38   Ines Hegedus-Garcia: https://www.flickr.com/photos/miamism/16232696048/in/album-72157650183126928/

4.40   Nic McPhee: https://www.flickr.com/photos/nics_events/2238345539/

4.41   Simon Mason: https://www.flickr.com/photos/simoncmason/3076460913/in/dateposted/

4.44   Seier+Seier: https://www.flickr.com/photos/seier/8544665520/

4.45   Mikhail Golub: https://www.flickr.com/photos/golub/11534671434/in/dateposted/

4.46   John M: https://www.flickr.com/photos/jsmjr/1400270486/

4.49   Tim Collins: https://commons.wikimedia.org/wiki/File:Templestowe_Kitchen.jpg

4.50   Nancy Hugo: https://www.flickr.com/photos/nancyhugo/421729935/in/album-72157604941769227/

4.51   Jordanhill School D&T Dept: https://www.flickr.com/photos/designandtechnologydepartment/4013738194/in/photostream

4.52   Bill Wilson: https://www.flickr.com/photos/okchomeseller/14776687637/

4.53   Atlanta Scott: https://www.flickr.com/photos/atlantascott/3388086143/in/dateposted/

4.56   Nancy Hugo: https://www.flickr.com/photos/nancyhugo/444867414/in/dateposted/

4.57   Jason Flakes, US DOE Solar Decathlon: https://www.flickr.com/photos/solar_decathlon/10179876934/in/album-72157636058705006/

4.58   Leelooshka: https://www.flickr.com/photos/leelooshka/8418198896/

4.59   Nancy Hugo: https://www.flickr.com/photos/nancyhugo/418234930/

4.60   Bay Dragon: https://www.flickr.com/photos/thiesson/3785337/

4.61   Brian and Rita Burke: https://www.flickr.com/photos/kennarealestate/3583306682/in/photolist

4.63   Homestilo: https://www.flickr.com/photos/homestilo/14302084244/in/photostream/

4.64   Nicolas Will: https://www.flickr.com/photos/numb3r/5998610525/

4.66   Emily May: https://www.flickr.com/photos/emilysnuffer/11919505985/in/dateposted/

4.67   Rubbermaid Products: https://www.flickr.com/photos/rubbermaid/5093015443/in/photostream/

4.69   Tim Collins: https://commons.wikimedia.org/wiki/File:Bedroom_Mitcham.jpg

4.70   Russell Street: https://www.flickr.com/photos/russellstreet/6919591439/

4.71   Jeremy Levine: https://www.flickr.com/photos/jeremylevinedesign/2818734013/in/dateposted/

4.72   Holland & Green Architecture: https://www.flickr.com/photos/84063900@N02/7697116148/

4.74   Design Milk: https://www.flickr.com/photos/designmilk/14205693493

4.75   Geoffrey Fairchild: https://www.flickr.com/photos/gcfairch/4367100484/

4.76   Memphis CVB: https://www.flickr.com/photos/ilovememphis/17370796535/

4.78   Heritage: https://www.flickr.com/photos/hhandr/13837280834/

4.79   Sean MacEntee: https://www.flickr.com/photos/smemon/5441137613/in/photolist-9hPfDt-9hSs5U

4.83   Ciell: https://commons.wikimedia.org/wiki/File:Snoezelruimte.JPG#/media/File:Snoezelruimte.JPG

4.84   Maegan Tintari: https://www.flickr.com/photos/lovemaegan/4665584710/in/photostream/

4.85   Bill Wilson: https://www.flickr.com/photos/okchomeseller/16043983551/

4.86   Jesus Rodriguez: https://www.flickr.com/photos/jmrodri/8050934318/

4.88   PJM: https://commons.wikimedia.org/wiki/File:6%22x6%22_porcelain_floor_tiles.jpg#/media/File:6%22x6%22_porcelain_floor_tiles.jpg

4.89   Maegan Tintari: https://www.flickr.com/photos/lovemaegan/4665584678/in/photostream/

4.90   Stephen Harris: https://www.flickr.com/photos/96227967@N05/15119157216/

4.91   Rubbermaid Products: https://www.flickr.com/photos/rubbermaid/6979511593/in/
album-72157629577493969/

4.92   FD Richard: https://www.flickr.com/photos/50697352@N00/979556610/

4.93   FE Group Bangkok: https://commons.wikimedia.org/wiki/File:Home_Office_FeStep_of_Fe_Group_Bangkok_
Thailand.jpg

4.94   University of Exeter: https://www.flickr.com/photos/26126239@N02/8496950061/

4.96   Blinds Online: https://www.flickr.com/photos/blindsonline/15634122958/in/dateposted/

4.97   Jeremy Levine: https://www.flickr.com/photos/jeremylevinedesign/2815613330

4.99   Dave Dugdale: https://www.flickr.com/photos/davedugdale/3955153414/

4.100   Jeremy Levine: https://www.flickr.com/photos/jeremylevinedesign/3134290901/in/dateposted/

4.101   Team EarthLED: https://www.flickr.com/photos/62324368@N06/5927232012/in/photostream/

4.102   Steve Larkin: https://www.flickr.com/photos/124705972@N06/14431885421/

4.103   Aurimas: https://www.flickr.com/photos/needoptic/5185370545/

4.104   Lightyears.dk: https://www.flickr.com/photos/lightyearsdk/5761042716

4.105   Fairfax County Fate House: https://www.flickr.com/photos/fairfaxcounty/5572060459/in/
album-72157626257883699/

4.106   Susan Serra: https://www.flickr.com/photos/kitchendesigner/7625804886/in/dateposted/

4.107   Scott Lewis: https://www.flickr.com/photos/99781513@N04/16247413828/in/dateposted/

4.108   Joffre Essley: https://www.flickr.com/photos/homesower/8393039807/

4.109   Architecture, Food & One: https://www.flickr.com/photos/7542656@N02/523818915/

4.110   D-Kuru: [CC BY-SA 3.0 at (http://creativecommons.org/licenses/by-sa/3.0/at/deed.en)], via Wikimedia Commons

4.112   Alex Kehr: https://www.flickr.com/photos/alexkehr/103727672/

4.113   Raysonho: https://commons.wikimedia.org/wiki/File:NestProtect.JPG#/media/File:NestProtect.JPG

4.114   Scott Lewis: https://www.flickr.com/photos/99781513@N04/16988997702/in/photolist

4.116   Scott Lewis: https://www.flickr.com/photos/99781513@N04/16601145734/in/photostream/

4.117   Tunstall: http://www.flickr.com/photos/tunstalltelehealthcare/6841243861/in/set-72157629244864767

4.118   Maschinenjunge: https://commons.wikimedia.org/wiki/File:RFID_Chip_003.JPG

4.119   Scott Lewis: https://www.flickr.com/photos/99781513@N04/17098717782/in/dateposted/

4.120   Jiuguang Wang: https://www.flickr.com/photos/jiuguangw/4982410844

4.122   Conan: https://www.flickr.com/photos/conanil/7047934677/in/photolist

4.123   Scott Lewis: https://www.flickr.com/photos/99781513@N04/16360064819/

4.124   Ted Eytan: https://www.flickr.com/photos/taedc/13138979395/

4.125   Carlisle HVAC: https://www.flickr.com/photos/carlislehvac/12822663943/in/photolist

4.127   Anubis100: https://en.wikipedia.org/wiki/File:Thermoholz_vergleich.JPG

4.128   Blinds Online: https://www.flickr.com/photos/blindsonline/15795870946/in/photostream/

4.129   Mauroguanandi: https://www.flickr.com/photos/mauroguanandi/14797295908

4.130   Rosenfeld Media: https://www.flickr.com/photos/rosenfeldmedia/3265589106/

4.132   Detlef Schobert: https://www.flickr.com/photos/detlefschobert/2553492137/in/photolist

INDEX

29 Palms 179–80

A

AASPIRE (Academic Autistic Spectrum
    Partnership in Research and Education) 194
ability-based design 190
access, visual 58, 100, 105, 109–10, 113, 121
accessibility 76–80
accessibility guidelines 92
accessible recreation 87
accident prevention 44–5, 72, 117, 139, 152, 165
accumulated effects 53
acoustics
    design guidelines 155–7
    acoustical consultants 155
    acoustical insulation, buffers 144
    and assistive technologies 161
    bathrooms 129
    bedrooms 126
    dining areas 114
    flooring 168
    heating 146–7
    high-pitched sounds 157
    laundry rooms 139
    living rooms 112
    multi-sensory environments 135
    overall home 93
    staff office 142
    and storage solutions 141
    ventilation 144
Acoustikblok 155–6
activists 7–8
activities of daily living (ADLs) 61
activity, gross motor 44–5, 71–2, 104, 107, 110,
    123, 134
activity, physical 66, 67, 87, 96
activity rooms 106
adaptive behaviors 16–17, 48, 49, 65
adults with ASD 9–11, 63–4
Advancing full spectrum housing (Ahrentzen and
    Steele, 2009) 34, 181, 184

advocacy 25–7, 193–7
affordability 72–6
affordable housing 61, 73, 75, 177, 178, 183–4
aging population 23, 63
air conditioning 146–7
air purifiers 136
air quality 66
Airmount Woods 182–3
alarms 158, 159
Allendale Housing, Inc. 177
allergen reduction 145, 167
Altman, I. 58
Alzheimer's 19, 46
Ambient Intelligent environments 190
Ambient Kitchen 191
amenities, neighborhood and community 41,
    83–4
American Academy of Pediatrics 30
American Institute of Architects 32
American Psychological Society 6, 9
anxiety 64
    see also stress
apartment-based living arrangements 176–80
appliances 152–4
Arc Village 184
Archea, John 58
architecture 32–3
Asperger's syndrome 5, 6–7, 55, 70
aspirations 3, 11–12, 16, 17, 27, 82, 171
    see also preferences, residential
assessment methods 29, 33, 36, 82, 193–5
assistive technologies 158–63, 190–3
attached homes 13, 14–15
auditory integration training 51
Augusto, J.C. 190
autism, definitions and labeling xi, 6–7
Autism Act 2009 6
Autism and Development Disabilities Monitoring
    Network 3
autism interventions and evidence-based practice
    30–1
Autism Network International (ANI) 26, 56, 57

Autism Society of Delaware 60, 69
Autism Speaks 1, 8, 15, 18, 27
Autism Spectrum Condition (ASC) 2
Autism Spectrum Disorder (ASD) 2, 6–7
Autistic Self Advocacy Network (ASAN) 26, 38
autobiographies, as research tools 46, 48
auto-ethnographic profiles 36
Autreat 57, 59

B

Bagatell, Nancy 56–7
Baio, J. 3, 5
Baron-Cohen, Simon 26, 48
Basas, C.G. 188
bathrooms
  design guidelines 128–33
  accident prevention 45
  close to communal living areas 113
  and daily living tasks 62
  en-suite bathrooms 17, 19, 23
  lighting 149, 150
  as personal space 69
bathtubs 128, 130–1
Baumers, Stijn 46, 49, 58–9
bed occupancy sensors 162
bedrooms
  design guidelines 124–7
  as personal space 53, 69
Beechwood 177
behavioral issues, in adulthood 10–11
behaviors, challenging 45
behaviors, disruptive 45
behaviors, maladaptive 65
BEING 67
belonging, sense of 78–9
benefits of autism 25–6
Bergen County's United Way 177, 184
Berkman, K.A. 74
Billstedt, E. 14, 16
biographical profiles 36
Bisphenol A (BPA) 166
blackout shades 126, 168
Blasco, R. 191
blind corners 121
blinds 145, 148, 165, 168, 169
Bluetooth 161
Bogdashina, O. 51
boundaries, personal 57–8
Brand, A, 53, 62, 195
building codes 43
built-in furniture 127
Bureau of Autism Services of the State of
  Pennsylvania 172–3

C

cabinetry 115–17, 139, 166
Cambridge Cohousing 186–8
carbon monoxide detectors 158, 159
care and support
  costs 3, 22–5, 72–6
  definitions 13
  facilitated by good design 42
  preferences for 17–22
  statistics 14–15
care workers
  and good design 42, 131, 138
  low pay 23
  and personal space 60, 142–3
  separate office 60, 106, 142–3
carpets 123, 167, 169
catatonia 64
ceilings 93, 107, 121, 123, 156
Center for Discovery, The (TCFD) 53–4, 174
Center for Health Design 33
Centers for Disease Control and Prevention 5
Centers for Medicare and Medicaid Services
  (CMS) 18
challenges, providing 62–3, 71
challenging behaviors 45
Charles House (Boulder) 69
chemicals 66, 116, 119–20, 131, 164–70
childhood disintegrative disorder 6–7
choice 3, 19, 26, 61–3, 91, 193–7
circulation 105, 113
clarity (quality of life goal) 47–50
cleaning products 167
closets 125, 150
cluster homes 13
clutter, avoiding 103, 112, 116, 140–1
COACH (Cognitive Orthosis for Assisting
  aCtivities in the Home) 192
Cochrane Collaboration 29
co-design workshops 82, 195
Cohen, Sheldon 49
CoHo Ecovillage 185–6
cohousing 184–7
color
  appropriate use of 93, 107, 114
  choice of 164
  of lighting 68, 148, 150
  sensory rooms 134
  used to highlight features 125, 137, 165
Combating Autism Act (2006) 1
common rooms/ communal areas
  bathrooms 128, 129
  dining areas 114
  gathering areas 90, 97, 99, 187
  living rooms 111–13
  multiple functionality of spaces 103
  sensory considerations 53
  and sociability 106
  storage 140
  visual access/ overview 105

commonSENSE 196–7
communication 6–10, 36, 49–50, 65, 193–4
community development financial institutions
    (CDFIs) 75
community inclusion 77–9, 83–90
community land trusts 75
community living
    design guidelines 83–90
    community inclusion 77–9, 83–90
    intentional communities 79, 173, 184–5
    new visions 172–89
    separate communities 78–9
    trend towards 3, 24
Community Living Options 25, 174
Community Participation Project (CPP) 78–9
community-based participatory research (CBPR)
    194–5
comorbidity 10, 63–4
Complete Streets 88
compost 116
computer simulated environments 196
condensation 162
"conditions" vs. "disorders" 26
contingency funds 92
continuity, importance of 48
control, need for 57–8
cooking 16, 66, 114–20, 191
cool pavement 98
cooling systems 146–7
Cornerstone Community Housing 178
corridors and hallways 103, 104–5, 109, 121–3
costs of care 3, 22–5, 72–6
countertops 115, 117, 119–20, 139
courtyards 98–9
Crime Prevention Through Environmental
    Design (CPTED) 43–4
crowding 60
cues, visual 88, 103
Cummins, R.A. 78
Cure Autism Now 1
curtains and blinds 104, 126, 145, 165, 168

D

"daily hassles" 65
daily living skills 16
damage (to building/ fittings) 72
Dawson, Michelle 48
decks 90, 168
decor
    calming 93
    indicating private/public area distinction 125
    varied ambience 95
    see also color
deficit-based definitions of disability 25–6, 36,
    47–8
definitions of autism 6–7
deinstitutionalization 171–2
dementia 46, 50

depression 48, 64, 67
design guidelines 81–170
detectors 99, 130, 139, 151, 158, 159
    see also sensors
developmental disabilities 42, 61, 65
diagnosis criteria 6–7, 9–10
Diagnostic and Statistical Manual of Mental
    Disorders (DSM) 6, 50
dignity 68–71
dimmer switches 148
dining areas 114
disability benefits 17–18
Disability Opportunity Fund 75
disability rights 25, 51–3, 184, 185, 196
Disability Studies Quarterly 36
disruptive behaviors 45
"do no harm" principle 46
Dohrmann Architects 179–80
Donvan, John 77–8
doormats 110
doors and doorways
    door sensors 147, 158
    doorways 107, 121–3
    inward opening 128
    lock systems 159
    materials 169
    preview windows/ sidelights 104–5
    and privacy 107
Dorner, R. 36
"down time," need for 56
drain 131, 139
drains 118
drawers 117, 154
drugs and medication 64
dryers 136, 138, 153
Duffy, J. 36
duplex models of housing 174–6
durability 71–2
dust 145

E

eating areas see dining areas
Eaves, L. 15
education 11, 30–1, 179, 188–9
electrical outlets 94, 151, 165
elevators 121
elopement 45–6, 113, 158, 165
emergency call systems 162
employment 73–4
enhanced perceptual functioning (EPF) 48
en-suite bathrooms 17, 19, 23
Enterprise Green Communities 67
entry areas 109–10
entry/ exit systems 159–60
environmental design 31–4
environmental stress 48–9, 65
environmental toxins 166
    see also toxic chemicals

epilepsy 44, 64
  see also seizure disorders
epoxy-based paints 165–6
e-Servant 191
ESPA 177
ethnographic research 51, 53, 56
European Autism Interventions 1–2
evidence-based design (EBD) 31–4
evidence-based medicine 29–30
evidence-based practices (EBP) 29–39
  in autism intervention 30–1
executive functioning (EF) 47
exercise 66, 67, 87, 96

F

fall prevention 44–5, 72, 110, 118, 131
familiarity 47–50
family care
  costs of care 22
  in the future 173
  greatest source of care 24
  location of home near to family 86
  natural supports 62
  support for family carers 24
family co-residence 16, 172
  see also parental home
family home 14, 17, 21
Family-Teaching Home model 25, 174–6
fans 126, 129, 138–9, 144, 162
farmstead communities 184
faucets 118
fencing 101
fiberboard 116, 129
financial constraints 17–18
finishes 62, 116, 164, 166–7, 169–70
First Place 179–80
First Place Academy 179–80, 188–9
first-person accounts, incorporating 36
Fleishmann, Carly 48
flexible design 92, 103, 106, 111, 175–6
flood detectors 130, 139, 159
flooring
  bathrooms 128, 131–2
  durability 169
  hallways and corridors 123
  kitchens 118
  laundry rooms 139
  odor-prevention 167
  soundproofing 168
floorplan 102–8
fluorescent bulbs 148
food 7, 52, 73
  see also cooking; dining areas
FoodBoard 191
formaldehyde 116, 120, 165–6
Foundation for Senior Living (FSL) 179, 180
friendships, fostering 54–60

functionality of spaces 49–50, 102–3, 111, 114, 121
funding, of care and support 22–5
furnishings 102, 107
furniture
  bedrooms 125–7
  built-in furniture 127
  furniture placement 112–13
  materials 170
  movability of 164

G

garages 145
garbage 116, 118
gardens 67, 96–101
gastrointestinal problems 11
gathering areas 90, 97, 99, 187
Gaudion, K. 53, 82, 195
GiraffPlus 192
glare, avoiding 168
glass 105, 129, 165, 168
Goodwin, Matthew 53–4, 65
Grandin, Temple 49, 74
Grant, Xenia 57
Green Cabinet Source 116
green care 67
green design features 75
Green House Project 19, 25
green spaces 87, 95
Groden, J. 65
group homes
  definitions 13
  detail of sharing arrangements 17
  images of 18–19
  vs. institutions 17
  new visions 172–89
  number of residents 59–60
  statistics 14–15

H

hallways and corridors 103, 104–5, 109, 121–3
Hamlyn Centre for Design 67
handles, knobs and levers 154
handrails 43, 123, 130, 131
hardscape 98, 101
Harmon, Amy 70
healing gardens 97
health (quality design goals) 63–8
health, mental 64, 65, 67–8
health conditions, related 7–8
healthcare facility design 32–3
heating systems 126, 135, 146–7
Helen Hamlyn Centre for Design of the Royal
  College of Art 53, 195
Henry, C.N. 33
HEPA air filtration 145
Herbert, M. 7

Hester, Randy 195
Heylighen, Ann 46, 49, 58–9
Higashida, Naoki 45, 48
high ceilings 93, 107, 121, 123
"high-functioning" autism spectrum disorder 7
high-pitched sounds 157
Ho, H. 15
hob see stove
Home and Community-Based Services (HCBS) 18, 26–7
home monitoring system 162
Home of the Future Consortium 62
Home Ownership for People with Long-Term Disabilities (HOLD) 75
home-like environment
    bathrooms 128
    floorplan strategies 103
    kitchens 116–17
    materials 164
    overall home 95
    and safety 46
    short hallways 121
homestead communities 184
hospital design 32
hospital living 12, 14, 16
housemates 92, 106
    see also social interaction
housing crisis/ global recession 3
housing preference surveys 18–19
    see also preferences, residential
housing types 12–22, 172–89
Howlin, P. 12, 14, 16
humidity 66, 162
HVAC 145, 147
Hydrostream 191–2
hypersensitivity 50–1, 98, 155
hypoallergenic materials 167
hyposensitivity 50–1, 98

I

identity-first language xi–xii, 9
"impairment"-based models 42–3
"imprisonment," avoiding 46
income 72–6
incontinence 128, 136, 137
independent living
    and choice goals 61–2
    goals of 16, 69
    quality of life design goals 59, 61–3
    statistics 12–15, 16
individualized living spaces 19
indoor air quality 66–7
information overload 48–9
informed choice 193–7
injury to others 44
insecticides 167
Institute of Medicine 66
institutionalized living

avoiding an institutional feel 30, 93, 101, 103, 116–17, 121, 125, 128, 132, 164, 167, 170
declining trend 3, 16, 170, 171–2
deinstitutionalization 171–2
integrated-continuum settings 188–9
intellectual disabilities 7–8, 61, 64, 78
Intelligent Assistive Technology Systems Lab (IATSL) 192
intelligent environments 190, 196–7
intentional communities 79, 173, 184–5
Interacting with Autism 51–2
intercom/ camera systems 160
interdependency 185
intermediate care program 172
International Classification of Diseases 6
International Classification of Functioning, Disability and Health 25
internet 57–8
intimacy 69–70, 124
ironing boards 139
islands, kitchen 115
isolation, overcoming 54–60, 62

J

Jackson Place Cohousing 185
Jiron, Miguel 51, 52
"just-in-time-teaching" 63

K

Kapp, S.K. 55–6
keyless locks 159
Kingwood Trust 53, 67, 69
Kinnaer, M. 49, 53, 58
Kitchen As-A-Pal 191
kitchenettes 124
kitchens
    design guidelines 115–20
    accident prevention 45
    and daily living tasks 62
    lighting 150
    meanings of spaces 49
    separate laundry area from 108, 136
    smart kitchens 191
Kloos, B. 65
Krauss, M.W. 14

L

lamps 150
    see also lighting
Lau, A.L.D. 78
laundry rooms 108, 136–9
layout of accommodation 102–8
Leadership Institute 188–9
LED bulbs 148, 150
Leddy Maytum Stacy 181
LEED certification 66–7, 175

legibility 102
Leopatra, V. 158
life expectancy 9, 23
lighting
  design guidelines 148–51
  bathrooms 129, 130
  in closets 125
  floorplan strategies 107
  hallways and corridors 122
  and health 67–8
  kitchens 118
  light bulbs 148, 149
  living rooms 112
  outdoor spaces 96
  outside 99
  overall home 93
  recessed LED lighting 150
  in storage areas 140, 150
lived experience, in research 35–6
Living Building Challenge 67
living rooms 111–13
location of home 68, 76–80, 83–90
lock systems (doors) 159
lockable cabinets 115
lockable fuse boxes 159
loneliness 59
long-term care 22–5
long-term medication 64
low-income living 17–18

M

macerators 137
Madeline Corporation 177
maladaptive behaviors 65
Marmoleum 167, 169
Massey, Margaret 188
materials 164–70
McGinley, C. 82, 195
McIlwain, Lori 45
MDF 116, 166
meaningful activity 61–2
meanings of spaces 49–50
Medex fibreboard 116
media centers 126
Medicaid 18
medical model of disability 25, 42, 56, 158
medication 64
mental health 64, 65, 67–8
Mesibov, G.B. 31
Messbauer, Linda 134–5
Michael Singer Studio 175
Miller, Diane 196
Missouri Autism Guidelines Initiative 31
moisture 129, 136, 145
mortality rates 9
Moss, P. 12–15
motion detectors (avoiding) 99, 151

motor coordination 44–5, 71–2, 104, 107, 110, 123, 134
Mottron, L. 48
multiple functionality of spaces 49–50, 102–3, 111, 114, 121
multiple residents 59, 104, 106, 109, 111, 114, 116, 128, 142, 146, 161
multi-sensory environments 134–5
multi-story residence 89, 121, 122, 129, 175
Murray, W. 27

N

nameplates, avoiding 116
National Autistic Society 69
National Professional Development Center on Autism Spectrum Disorders (NPDC) 31
natural environment, importance of 87, 95, 96–101, 122, 125
natural light
  design guidelines 148–51
  bathrooms 129
  floorplan strategies 103, 107
  hallways and corridors 122
  kitchens 118
  living rooms 112
  outdoor spaces 96
  overall home 93
natural supports 62
neighbors
  acceptance of autistic neighbors 77, 85
  accessibility and support 76–80, 83, 89, 100
  neighborhood design guidelines 83–90
  and security from crime 44
  similarity to neighboring houses 69, 85
neurocognitive conditions xii, 10, 35
neurodevelopmental conditions xii, 3–4, 6, 9, 16, 35
neurodiversity 8, 25–6, 37
neurotoxins 66
neurotypical (NT) xii, 41, 56, 64
New Horizons in Autism 184
New Jersey Community Development Corporation 177
nightlighting 150
NIMBY (Not in My Backyard) 77, 85
noise
  and assistive technologies 161
  bathrooms 129
  bedrooms 126
  communal areas 112
  and flooring 168
  heating 146–7
  kitchens 119
  laundry rooms 139
  local area 86
  sensory rooms 135
  soundproofing 155–7
  staff rooms/ offices 142

ventilation 144
and windows 168
non-toxic materials, finishes 115–16, 119, 120,
131, 166–7, 169
non-verbal communication 49–50
normalization (vs. choice) 26
nursing homes 19, 25

O

obesity 64, 66, 87
obsessive compulsive disorders (OCD) 64
Odom, S.L. 31
odors
bathrooms 129
dining areas 114
kitchens 119
laundry rooms 138
sealing flooring 167
sensory sensitivities 52
ventilation 144–5
office (support workers') 60, 106, 108, 142–3
older adults 10, 19, 51
older people's housing 19, 25, 45, 61–2, 189–90
Olmstead 188
options, viable 61–2, 194
Orchard Commons 177
order, creating a sense of 47–50
outcome goals 11–12, 17
outdoor spaces
design guidelines 96–101
and health goals 67
for laundry 137
living room transition to 113
materials 168
ovens 117, 153
overcrowding 60, 112
overload of stress/ information 48–9

P

paints 165–6
panic alarms 162
parental home 14–15, 16, 73–4, 79
parental support 22–3, 55–6
parking 89, 94
Parkview Services 185
participatory action research (PAR) 194–5
participatory decision-making 197
participatory design 195–7
participatory process 185
participatory strategies 194
particleboard 116, 120, 166
paths 97, 99, 100
pavement 98
pedestrian-friendly neighborhoods 86, 88, 94
peer review, importance of 33
perceptual functioning 47–8
periphery seating 111, 112

Perkins, E.Z. 74
Perry, N. 79
personal space, need for 58–9, 92
personalization 92
person-centered planning 11–12, 193, 194
person-environment perspective 11
person-first language xi–xii, 9
person-in-environment (PIE) 42
pervasive developmental disorder 6–7
pesticides 167
pets 92
Photovoice 82
physical elements "offering a grip" 46
physical health 7–8, 64, 87
pipework, concealed 133
pollution 86, 164
porches/ covered entryways 100, 109, 110, 150
positive biology 42–3
practitioners, as experts 39
predictability 47–50
preferences, residential
finding out about 17, 18–22, 84, 91
means to assess 193–4
and research 35–6, 39
pressed wood 116
prevalence rates 5–9, 10
preview windows/ sidelights 104–5, 124
primary functions of rooms 50
privacy
and assistive technologies 161, 191, 193
bathrooms 128–33
bedrooms 124–7
floorplan strategies 106
and laundry 136
and neighborhood design 89
outside 99
private spaces 53, 69
quality of life design goals 57–60, 69
property exit sensors 158
proprioception 71–2, 98, 134
psychiatric disorders 10
public transport 76, 83, 84

Q

quality of life design goals 41–80
QuietRock 156

R

ramps 121–3
randomized controlled trials 29–30, 31, 35
recycling 116
reflective experience 35–6
repetitive behaviors 6–8, 11, 64, 72
Research Design Connections 33
research funding for autism 1–2
research integrity 35
research-informed approach (RIA) 35–7

residential alternatives 12–22, 172–89
residential home program 172
Resnik, D. 74, 75, 189
restoration 42, 49, 50
RFID (radio frequency identification) 161, 190, 191
risk
  dignity of 70–1
  gardens shouldn't be risk-free 96
  providing a degree of challenge 62–3, 71
Robert Woods Johnson Foundation 19, 25
Robertson, Scott 9, 26, 37
Robinson, Ricki 52
Robison, John 51
robots 163, 192
Rockwool 155
roommates 92, 106
  see also social interaction
routines 49
rubbish disposal 116, 118
rural communities 2, 21, 79, 184

S

Sackett, D. 29
safety and security goal 43–7
SAIL Housing 178–9
Sanoff, Henry 195
Sarason, S.B. 78
Schön, D. 35
school, transition from 11
seating
  entryways 109
  floorplan strategies 102–3, 106
  kitchens 115
  living rooms 111–13
  outdoor spaces 96–7, 100
  overall home 93
  and storage solutions 140
second skin system 175
security goal 43–7
sedentary lifestyles 66
seizure disorders 9, 44, 64, 162
self-advocacy 26–7, 39, 82, 193–7
self-care assistance 45
self-determination 58, 61, 69–71, 193
self-injury 44–5, 51, 72
self-sufficiency 77
sensors 158–63, 197
sensors, motion 99, 151
sensory issues
  accumulated effects 53
  and aging 11, 64
  enhanced perceptual functioning (EPF) 48
  environmental design 93
  flexibility in design 107–8
  and food 114
  gardens 98
  multi-sensory environments 134–5

sensory balance (quality of life goal) 50–4
sensory neutral spaces 93, 112
sensory profiling tool 53
sensory recalibration spaces 107
sensory rooms 108, 134
sensory stimulation 7
sensory wristbands 54
sensory zones 98
sensory-neutral residences 53
Sergeant, L. 48, 72
service animals 92
sexual intimacy 69–70, 124
Shah, S. 65
shared equity home ownership 75
shared home model 19
  see also group homes
shared living arrangements 59–60
Shea, V. 31
shelving 81, 116–17, 118, 125, 127
showers 128, 130, 132
sightlines 58, 105, 109, 110, 143
signs 43, 88, 94
Silverstein, Daniel 34
Sinclair, James 9, 56, 57, 59
single-story residences 93, 104, 121
sinks 118, 131, 137, 139, 154
size of group homes 93
size of rooms/ areas 107, 128
Sketch-Up 196
sleep 66, 67, 126
slip-resistant flooring 118, 132
sluice washing machines 137
small houses 93
smaller spaces 49, 93–4
smart devices 28
smart home technology 19, 24, 158–63, 189–93
Smart Kitchen 191
smoke alarms 158, 159
Snoezelen Rooms 135
social interaction
  assistive technologies 191–2
  and hallways 122
  and layout 106
  living rooms 111–13
  overall home 83
  quality of life design goals 41–2, 54–60
  togetherness (sharing social spaces) 54–60
Social Mirror 191–2
social networks 55, 89
Social Security Income (SSI) 17–18, 73–4
sociality 59
solar heating 146
solarium 146, 175
Solomon, A. 1, 7
Solomon, O. 35
soundproofing 155–7
Southwest Autism Research and Resource Center (SARRC) 179, 189
spectrum condition, autism as xi, 2–3, 42

stability 47–50
staff rooms/ offices 60, 106, 108, 142–3
stairs 45, 121–3
statistics on autism 3, 5–9
step-free homes 104, 109
stigma 69, 163
stims 51, 56
storage
   design guidelines 140–1
   bedrooms 124, 126
   kitchen 116, 118
   laundry rooms 138
   open or closed 81, 125, 141
stove 117, 118, 153
strengths-based viewpoints 36
stress
   and green spaces 87
   as health issue 64–5
   and layout 105
   stress overload 48–9
support workers
   and good design 42, 131, 138
   low pay 23
   personal space 60, 142–3
   separate office 60, 106, 108, 142–3
supported independent living (SIL) 68
supported living model 174
supportive housing 188
supportive living arrangements 177
surveys
   alternatives to 27, 36, 82, 193–5
   conventional types 18–19, 27
Sweetwater Spectrum 180–2
switches 144, 148, 151, 165
systematic reviews 29, 31
systematizing behavior 26

T

Taft Community College Transition to
   Independent Living Program 189
Tammet, Daniel 49
taps 118
TCFD Duplex Model 175–6
technology
   design guidelines 158–63
   bathrooms 130–1
   door/ window sensors 147
   and independence 362–3
   "just-in-time-teaching" 63
   kitchens 118
   laundry rooms 139
   local transportation 76
   mobile technology 62
   safety features on appliances 152–4
   wristband sensors 54
   see also smart home technology
telehealth packages 158, 160–1
televisions 126

temperature controls 126, 135, 146–7
terminology xi–xii, 9
territoriality 58–9
texture 51, 52, 93, 97–8, 107, 119
The Arc Village 184
The Center for Discovery (TCFD) 53–4, 174
Thermablok 156
thermal controls 126, 135, 146–7
thermostat 147
Thompson, C. Ward 67
thresholds 97, 100, 104, 109–10, 121, 130, 145
timers vs. motion sensors 99, 151
togetherness (sharing social spaces) 54–60
toilets 132
toxic chemicals 66, 116, 119–20, 131, 165–7
transition to adulthood 11
Transitional Academy 188
transitional spaces 107, 122
transportation, public 76, 83, 84
Triplett, Donald 74, 77–8

U

Ubiquitous Computing Group 191
Ulrich, R. 32, 33
unemployment 73–4
United Nations Convention on the Rights of
   Persons with Disabilities 61
United Way, Bergen County 177, 184
universal design 92, 181

V

Van Hoof, J. 66
Vardouli, T. 196
variety 59, 87, 95, 97, 111, 113
ventilation
   design guidelines 144–5
   bathrooms 129
   bedrooms 125
   dining areas 114
   hallways and corridors 122
   kitchens 119
   laundry rooms 136, 138
   living rooms 112
   overall home 93
vestibular input 98
Viets, E. 32, 33
views 95, 101, 122, 126
village communities 79, 184
Virgona + Virgona Architects 184
virtual world 57–8
visitors 89, 94, 106, 109, 128
visual access/ overview 58, 100, 105, 109, 110,
   113, 121
visual cues 88, 103
visual elements 94, 103
VOCs (volatile organic compounds) 164, 165–6

W

wall cavities 176
wall decals 107
walls
 bathrooms 130–2
 curving 121
 paints 166
 and privacy 90, 105
 reinforcement 130, 154
 soundproofing 126, 156–7
wandering 45–6, 113, 158, 165
wants and needs 17–22
Ward Thompson, C. 67
washing machines 137, 138, 153
waste disposal systems 118, 133
water 118, 130, 149, 153, 159, 192
wayfinding 88, 102
Wedmore, H.V. 70
Welcome HOME 196
welfare benefits 17–18, 73–4
WELL Building Standard 67
wellness 63–8
Wessex experiment 171
wet-area fittings 149
wheelchair users
 bathrooms 128
 circulation around the home 113
 laundry rooms 138
 and lighting glare 149
 ramps 121–3
 and storage solutions 140
 thresholds 104, 121
wifi 126, 190
Willakenzie Crossing 177–8
Williams, Donna 49, 57
Wilson, James C 53
window coverings 104, 126, 145, 165, 168
window seats 103, 112, 122
windows
 bathrooms 129
 and dignity 68
 flooring 104
 laminated glass 165
 laundry rooms 138
 lighting 149
 materials 170
 noise levels 168
 overall home 95
 preview windows/ sidelights 104–5, 124
 ventilation 144
 window sensors 147, 158
 see also natural light

Wobbrock, J.O. 190
Wolbring, G. 158
wood, pressed 116
work and employment 73–4
World Health Organization 2, 5, 6, 25
Wright, S.D. 36, 37
wristband sensors 54

Y

yards *see* gardens; outdoor spaces

Z

zero-step threshold or entry 100, 104, 109
Zero-VOC (volatile organic compounds) 164,
 165–6
zoning 85
Zucker, Caren 77–8

Printed and bound by CPI Group (UK) Ltd, Croydon, CR0 4YY

16/04/2025

14658342-0002